T0075279

Contemporary Interventional Ultrasonography in Urology

Contemporary Interventional Ultrasonography in Urology

Edited by

Osamu Ukimura, MD, PhD
Department of Urology, Kyoto Prefectural University of Medicine, Kyoto, Japan

Inderbir S. Gill, MD, MCh
Section of Laparoscopic & Robotic Surgery, Glickman Urological Institute, Cleveland Clinic Foundation, Cleveland, OH, USA

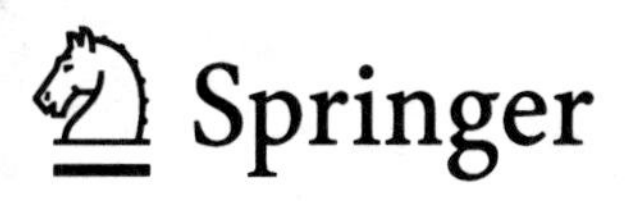

Editors
Osamu Ukimura, MD, PhD
Department of Urology
Kyoto Prefectural University of Medicine
Kyoto
Japan

Inderbir S. Gill, MD, MCh
Section of Laparoscopic & Robotic Surgery
Glickman Urological Institute
Cleveland Clinic Foundation
Cleveland, OH, USA

ISBN 978-1-84800-216-6 ISBN 978-1-84800-217-3 (eBook)
DOI 10.1007/978-1-84800-217-3

British Library Cataloguing in Publication Data

Library of Congress Control Number: 2008939890

Printed on acid-free paper

Springer Science + Business Media
springer.com

Foreword

Ultrasonography has evolved from a branch of acoustics that deals with the study and use of sound waves to an important clinical modality in assessing varied structures and organ systems throughout the body. Much of the work began in the 1940s after World War II by examining intracranial abnormalities, and later intrathoracic and intra-abdominal structures. The quality of images gradually improved with the development of gray-scale and real-time imaging, and more recently color and power Doppler studies. Further advancement in minimally ablative technology has utilized ultrasonography to monitor interventional procedures such as renal prostate biopsy and ablative therapy of varied malignancies, in addition to the development of increasing diagnostic appreciations.

Intraoperative ultrasonography has been used by general surgeons in biliary, pancreatic, and vascular surgery and its role in urology is primarily related to the identification of renal calculi at the time of pyelolithotomy or nephrolithotomy. With the development of lithotripsy and percutaneous renal surgery, ultrasound is used in addition to other studies such as computer tomography to identify the location and size of renal and ureteral calculi. For this book, Ukimura and Gill have identified authors having expertise not only in intraoperative ultrasound but also in other applications such as therapeutics and intervention.

Ultrasound has been useful not only in identifying abnormalities such as stones or tumors in kidneys but also in monitoring therapies such as stone removal and renal tumor ablation, in assisting in prostate biopsy, and in studying blood flow to various structures. Applications such as the use of ultrasound contrast agents, elastrography, and tissue characterization are evolving and are expected to enhance diagnostic capabilities.

Many of the studies described in this book have proved to be valuable, and the examinations described have become an integral part of interventional and therapeutic applications. Other studies are also evolving, and more application by a large number of investigators is essential to determine their value. It is likely that a second edition of this book will be required to provide an up-to-date compilation of these new developments.

Martin I. Resnick
Hiroki Watanabe

Contents

Contributors

Richard J. Babaian
Prostate Cancer Detection Clinic, The University of Texas MD Anderson Cancer Centre, Houston, TX, USA

Patricia Beemster
Department of Urology, Academic Medical Center, University of Amsterdam, Amsterdam, The Netherlands

Fleur L. Broughton
Department of Urology, Creighton University Medical Center, Omaha, NE, USA

Christian Chaussy
Department of Urology, Krankenhaus München-Harlaching, Munich, Germany

Christopher R. Chiou
Department of Urology, Creighton University Medical Center, Omaha, NE, USA

Rei K. Chiou
Department of Urology, Creighton University Medical Center, Omaha, NE, USA

Antonio P. Ciardella, MD
Department of Ophthalmology, University of Colorado Health Science Center, Denver, Colorado

Jean J.M.C.H. de la Rosette
Department of Urology, Academic Medical Center, University of Amsterdam, Amsterdam, The Netherlands

Mingyue Ding
Imaging Research Laboratories, Robarts Research Institute, London, ON, Canada

Donal B. Downey
Imaging Research Laboratories, Robarts Research Institute, London, ON, Canada

Aaron Fenster
Imaging Research Laboratories, Robarts Research Institute, London, ON, Canada

Inderbir S. Gill
Department of Urology, Glickman Urological Institute, Cleveland Clinic, Cleveland, OH, USA

Srinivasa Kalidindi
Department of Cardiovascular Medicine, Cleveland Clinic, Cleveland, OH, USA

Kazumi Kamoi
Department of Urology, Kyoto Prefectural University of Medicine, Kyoto, Japan

Gert Karlsson
B-K Medical, Herlev, Denmark

Katharina Koenig
Department of Urology, University of Ruhr, Bochum, Germany

Pilar Laguna Pes
Surgery Unit, Academic Medical Center, University of Amsterdam, Amsterdam, The Netherlands

Anne Fung, MD
Pacific Eye Associates, California Pacific Medical Center, San Francisco, CA, USA

Surena F. Matin
Department of Urology, The University of Texas MD Anderson Cancer Center, Houston, TX, USA

Pierre Mozer
URobotics Program, Department of Urology, Johns Hopkins Medicine, Baltimore, MD, USA

Stephen J. Nicholls
Department of Cardiovascular Medicine, Cleveland Clinic, Cleveland, OH, USA

Steven E. Nissen
Department of Cardiovascular Medicine, Cleveland Clinic, Cleveland, OH, USA

Gary Onik
Prostate Cancer Research Centre, Celebration Health-Florida Hospital, Celebration, FL, USA

Doru Petrisor
URobotics Program, Urology Department, Johns Hopkins Medicine, Baltimore, MD, USA

Ulrich Scheipers
Department of Urology, University of Ruhr, Bochum, Germany

Dan Stoianovici
URobotics Program, Urology Department, Johns Hopkins Medicine, Baltimore, MD, USA

David D. Thiel
Department of Urology, University of Iowa Hospitals & Clinics, Iowa City, IA, USA

Stefan Thüroff
Department of Urology, Krankenhaus München-Harlaching, Munich, Germany

Osamu Ukimura
Department of Urology, Kyoto Prefectural University of Medicine, Kyoto, Japan

Bogdan Vigaru
URobotics Program, Urology Department, Johns Hopkins Medicine, Baltimore, MD, USA

Hiroki Watanabe
Kyoto Prefectural University of Medicine, Kyoto, Japan

Zhouping Wei
Imaging Research Laboratories, Robarts Research Institute, London, ON, Canada

Hessel Wijkstra
Department of Urology, Academic Medical Center, University of Amsterdam, Amsterdam, The Netherlands

Howard N. Winfield
Department of Urology, University of Iowa Hospitals & Clinics, Iowa City, IA, USA

Niels Wondergem
Department of Urology, Academic Medical Center, University of Amsterdam, Amsterdam, The Netherlands

Chapter 1
Historical Background

Hiroki Watanabe

Prologue

It was a dark evening in the late autumn of 1978. A middle-aged woman was urgently admitted to our hospital in Kyoto because of anuria for a few days. She had suffered from cancer of the right ureter and undergone nephro-ureterectomy. The anuria resulted from an obstruction of the contralateral ureter due to a recurrence of bladder tumor. An immediate catheterization from the left renal pelvis by nephrostomy was indicated.

Even now, senior urologists may remember very well what a dreadful surgery classic open nephrostomy was. The kidney was exposed after a large incision in the back, then a thick trocar was introduced blindly from the renal surface into the pelvis, because there was no means of guidance. Heavy bleeding often occurred. Since this was only a palliative treatment, there was a big imbalance between the risks of the invasion and the possible gains.

A week previously, we had taken delivery of a new machine direct from the manufacturer. It was the world's first mechanical sector scanner with a special attachment, which we had designed originally for real-time puncture guidance. After intense discussion among the staff of the risks involved, we made up our minds to introduce the machine in this case. None of us had yet used it, and only a few foreign reports on the procedure were available at the time, which was named later as percutaneous direct nephrostomy.

The patient was moved to the operating theater for general anesthesia. The scanner was positioned on her back, and a clear image of the hydronephrotic renal pelvis appeared on the oscilloscope. All the staff member of our department gathered and watched the operation, praying to God for success. At the first shot, puncture to the pelvis was achieved very easily and a catheter was placed correctly in a few minutes. Everybody was amazed and felt that this was a real innovation.

Only several months later, I found incidentally a young resident carrying out the same interventional operation at the bedside under local anesthesia. He was never nervous but was smiling, joking with the patient. Of course all the procedure was completed in safety. I understood that the technique had already been subsumed into everyday routine work.

The Period of the Central Canal Type Transducer

It is very difficult to determine who made the first application of interventional ultrasound, because ultrasound pictures were commonly used as reference images for puncture, even before the proposal of intervention techniques. Among the pioneers, Berlyne[1] in England is generally credited as the person who made the first trial intervention. He performed renal biopsy under the guidance of an A-mode chart recorded by an industrial flaw detector in 1961, only a few years after the first introduction of ultrasound in medicine.

In my opinion, however, the history of interventional ultrasound should start from the first development of a special apparatus designed purely for the puncture guidance.

A Danish urologist, Hans Herik Holm[2] (Fig. 1.1), and an American radiologist, Barry B. Goldberg[3] (Fig. 1.2), independently published the same idea of a "central canal" type transducer in the same month in different journals in 1972 (Figs. 1.3 and 1.4). Both transducers were designed to be attached to a "contact compound" B-mode scanner, which was the standard procedure for sonography at that time, to target the site by a needle inserted through the central canal of it.

Holm's group pioneered puncture to various organs with their transducer: the liver, pancreas, kidney, uterus, and so on. They used the term "ultrasonically guided puncture" for the procedure. On the other hand, Goldberg focused the object mainly on the aspiration of various fluids from within the body. "Ultrasound-aided needling" was his favorite term. However, a new term, "interventional ultrasound," which was derived from basic radiology terminology, has gradually become general at the international level since the 1980s, because this describes the technique compactly and sounds harmonious.

Though it is accepted that these two groups opened up the possibilities of ultrasound intervention, their idea of the transducer

O. Ukimura and I.S. Gill (eds.), *Contemporary Interventional Ultrasonography in Urology*,
DOI: 10.1007/978-1-84800-217-3_1, © Springer-Verlag London Limited 2009

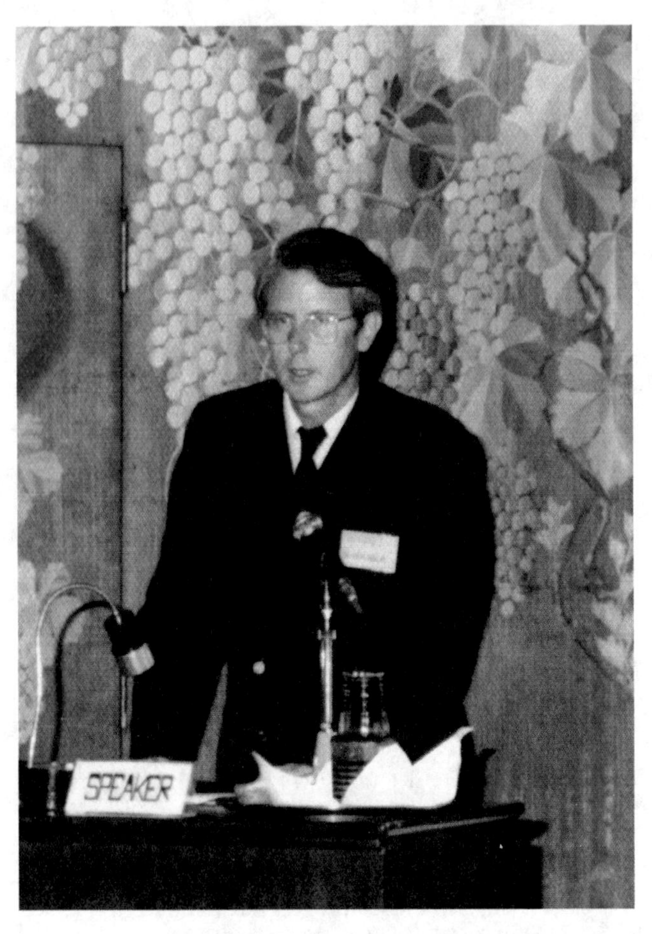

FIG. 1.1. A portrait of Hans Henrik Holm at the First International Workshop on Diagnostic Ultrasound in Urology and Nephrology, Kyoto, 1979. Hans Henrik has retired but is still active in good health

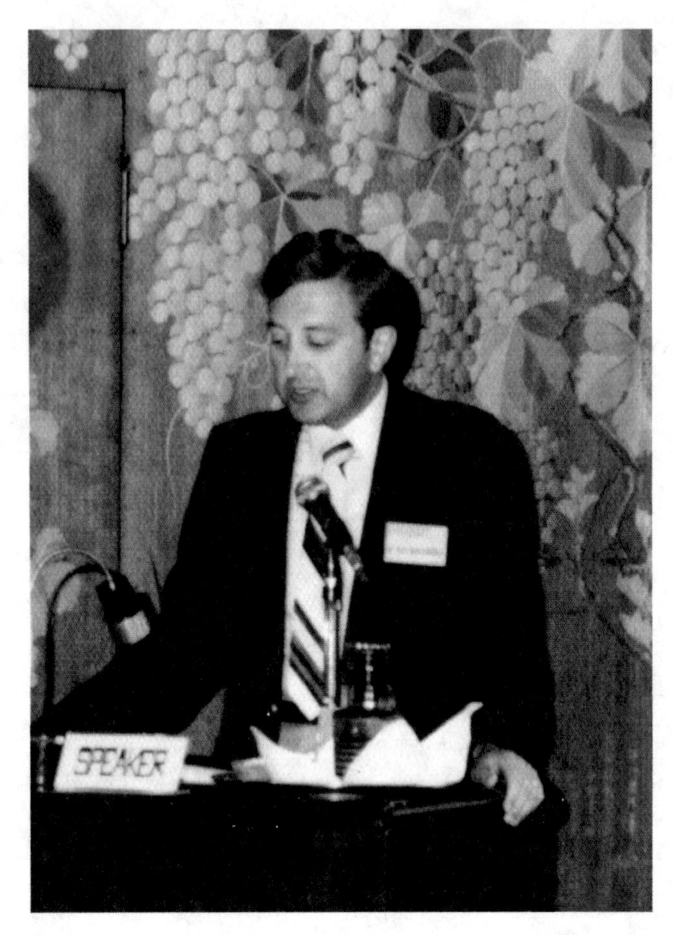

FIG. 1.2. A portrait of Barry B. Goldberg at the same occasion. Barry is hard at work as an academic researcher

having a central canal was not original. Earlier in 1969, an Austrian gynecologist, Alfred Kratochwil.[4] (Fig. 1.5), had already presented before a congress his trial on puncture to the amniotic cavity with a similar type of transducer developed by him, which was attached to an A-mode (only the intensity of the echo signals is shown on an *X–Y* graph) machine.

Anyhow, at this stage of the development, the procedure had not yet become very popular, because the imaging technique was inadequate for intervention. In the former "contact compound" scanning, a 2D image was constructed manually with the transducer being slid around the body surface. It took a considerable number of seconds to complete a cross-section picture. Although the target could be indicated on the picture, it vanished when the needle was inserted. No monitoring of the needle pathway was possible. Of course, A-mode gave far less information than B-mode.

The Period of Real-Time Intervention

The emergence of real-time scanners in the late 1970s eliminated the weak point mentioned. Only after this innovation did interventional ultrasound become accepted as an established technique for puncture guidance.

The first transducer for real-time intervention, though a kind of working model of electronic scan, was reported by a Danish group in 1977[5] (Fig. 1.6). Saitoh and Watanabe in Kyoto developed a commercially available puncture attachment for a newly developed compact mechanical real-time scanner (Fig. 1.7) in 1978[6] and started to seek out various indications of the puncture system in urology. The story described in the prologue happened in those days. Goldberg et al. also reported their new machine in 1980.[7] Since then many reports have followed from all over the world.

After the introduction of real-time intervention, various kinds of novel diagnostic and therapeutic means, which were never possible in the early days, have been realized. Among these innovations, the most important contributions to medicine, from the viewpoint of frequency of performance, must be selective renal biopsy and percutaneous lithotomy.

In nephrology, renal biopsy is an essential step in the differentiation of diseases. Open biopsy or blind percutaneous biopsy, which was generally performed in the early days, was invasive and risky. Unexpected bleeding occasionally caused a

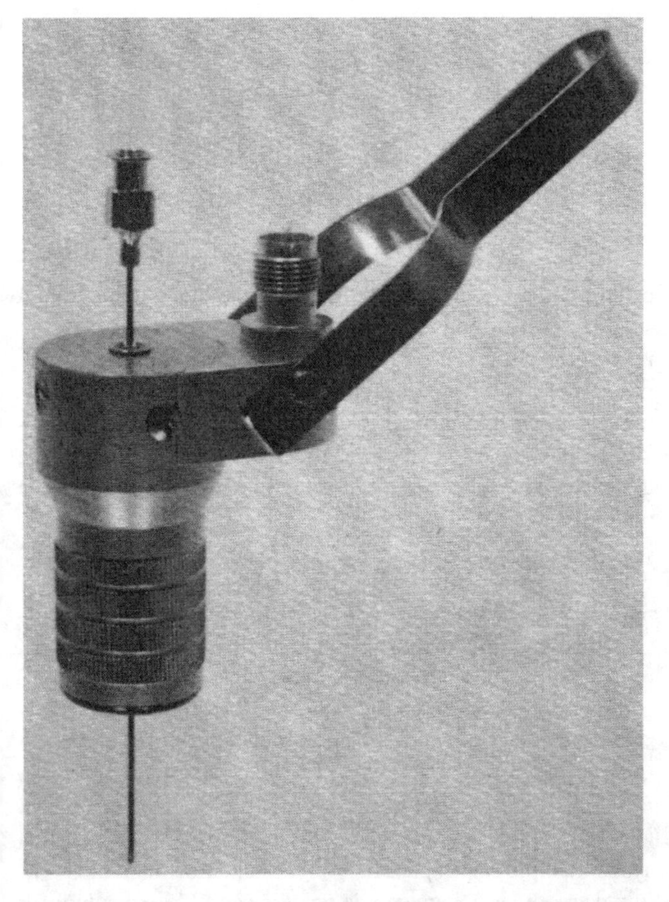

FIG. 1.3. The "central canal" type transducer developed by Holm et al.[2] Reproduced from Kristensen JK et al., Ultrasonically guided percutaneous puncture of renal masses, Scand J Urol Nephrol 1972; 6(Suppl): 15, 49–56

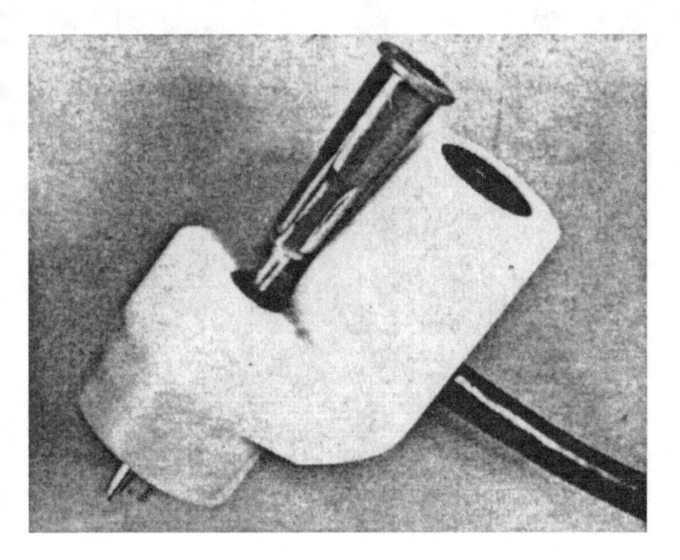

FIG. 1.4. A similar transducer developed by Goldberg et al.[3] Reproduced from Goldberg BB, Pollack HM[3]

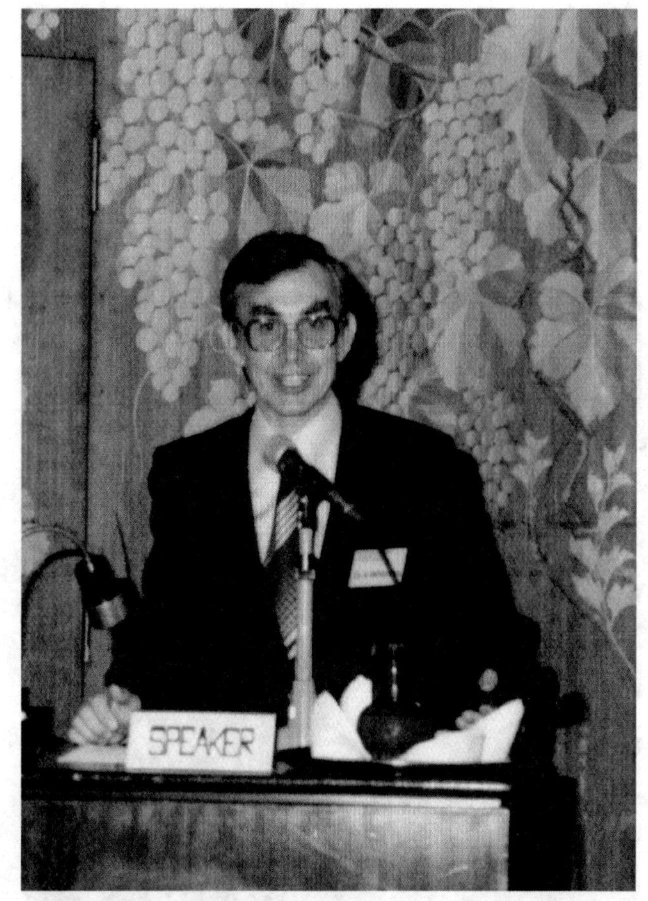

FIG. 1.5. A portrait of Alfred Kratochwil, on the same occasion as Figs. 1 and 2. Alfred occasionally gives fine lectures at meetings with his skilful computer presentation

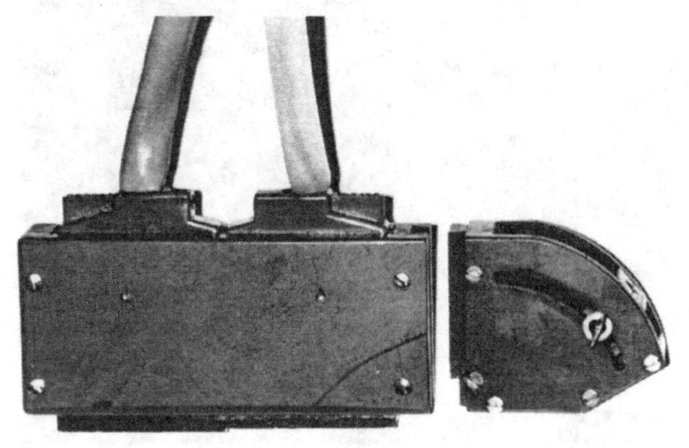

FIG. 1.6. An electronic real-time scanner with a puncture attachment by Pedersen.[5] Reproduced from Holm HH, Kristensen JK[24]

fatality. Selective renal biopsy under ultrasonic real-time guidance[8] brought a dramatic improvement of the technique, both in terms of on safety and accuracy. Today's professionals easily take a biopsy sample selectively from a target less than 1 cm in diameter in any portion in the kidney under local anesthetic.

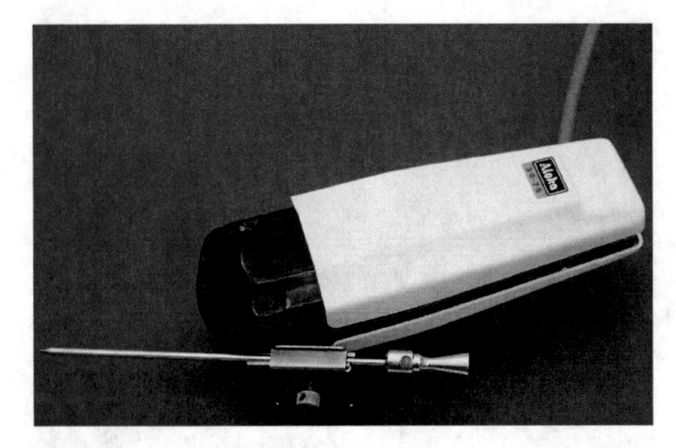

FIG. 1.7. A mechanical sector scanner with a puncture attachment by Saitoh et al.[6]

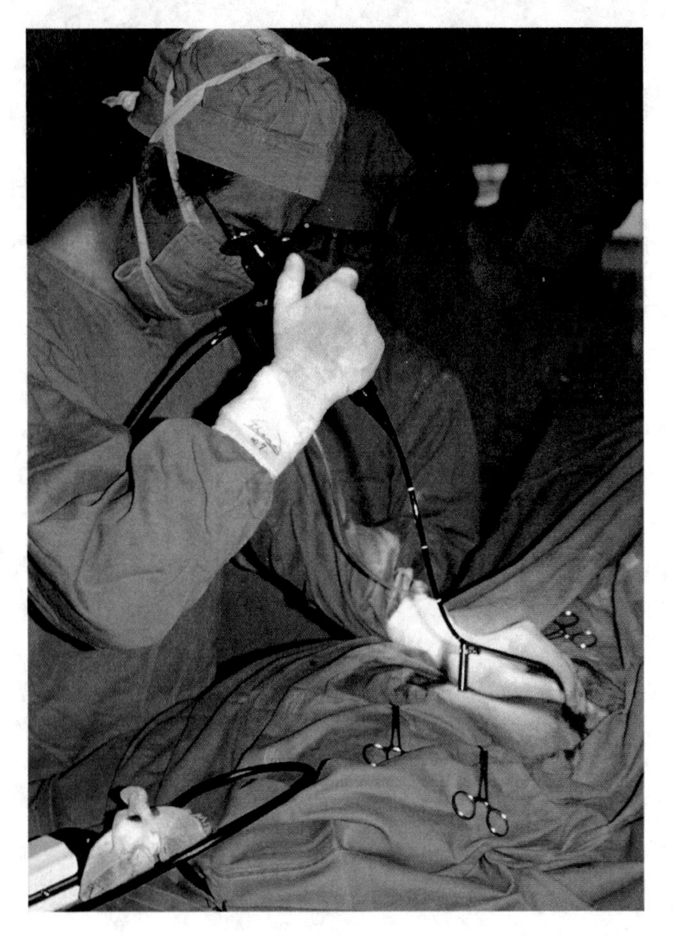

FIG. 1.8. A portrait of Masahito Saitoh, during his first successful surgery for single-stage percutaneous nephroureterolithotomy in 1981[9]

Percutaneous lithotomy was also revolutionary for the treatment of urinary calculi. This generated the vogue word, "Perc," among urologists in the late 1980s. Saitoh[9] (Fig. 1.8) first succeeded in percutaneous nephroureterolithotomy using a special ultrasonically guided pyeloscope in a single stage (several previous reports were available on lithotomy through an already-established nephrostomy channel by surgery) in 1981.

Intervention by Transrectal Ultrasound

Transrectal ultrasound[10,11] is a special technique developed for urology in 1967. In the early period of the method, horizontal sections were obtained by rotation of a single transducer inside the transrectal probe with an electric motor set outside the probe, while sagittal sections were made by manual pulling-down of the transducer. Even in this period, prostate puncture guidance was feasible, but the introduction of a real-time transrectal transducer encouraged the rapid distribution of the method at the worldwide level.

In this case again, the Danish group and the Japanese group were competing with each other. Holm and Gammelgaard[12] published a needle guidance system for puncture to the prostate and the seminal vesicles, monitored by ordinary transrectal ultrasound in 1981. On the other hand, Saitoh and Watanabe[13] had reported a puncture system using a newly developed transrectal electronic linear scanner with a needle guidance attachment in 1980 (Fig. 1.9). In this system, a longitudinal section of the prostate was delineated to monitor the advance of the needle directly in real time. Some authors[14–16] followed this system, employing Japanese probes, then ultrasound intervention came to be recognized as an indispensable procedure for prostatic biopsy. In recent days, the system has been modified to enable switching between two sections, horizontal and longitudinal, by using two different transducers fixed rectangular at the tip of the transrectal probe.

As is well known, the diagnosis of prostatic cancer is made by prostatic biopsy guided by interventional transrectal ultrasound

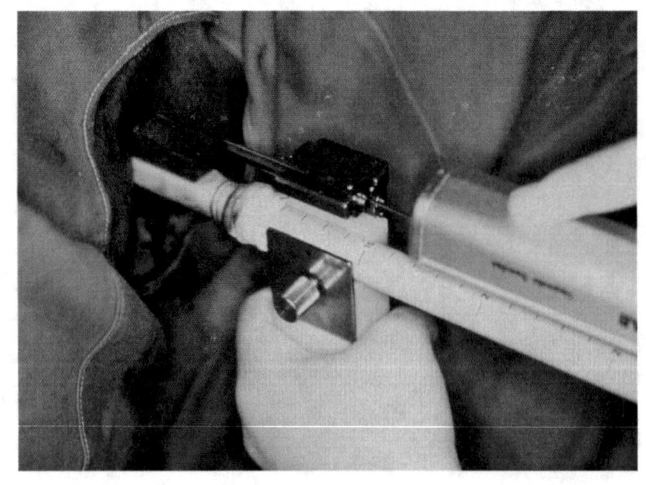

FIG. 1.9. Transrectal real-time linear scanner with a puncture attachment by Saitoh et al.[13]

alone today. Lee[17] and Cooner[18] promoted this routine in the late 1980s in the United States. Stamey and Hodge[19] established the concept of multicore biopsy, which is accepted as the gold standard worldwide.

Brachytherapy (radioisotopes' implantation) for prostatic cancer has become very common. Nowadays more than 60,000 patients a year undergo the procedure in the United States. Although originally conducted by retropubic open surgery,[20] the introduction of transperineal seeds insertion under interventional transrectal ultrasound by Holm[21] in 1981 greatly improved the technique. Presently available equipment for this therapy mostly benefits from his improvement.

References for Interventional Ultrasound

In the final part of this chapter, the titles of special books for interventional ultrasound published during the period described (Fig. 1.10) will be listed.

The first book for this purpose was *Ultrasonically Guided Puncture* written in Japanese language in 1979.[22] This was planned to publish the results of a special symposium with the same title, organized by the Japan Society of Ultrasonics in Medicine in December, 1978, in Kyoto. With the expanding demand in the field, another book written in English, *Interventional Real-Time Ultrasound* was published in 1985.[23]

The Danish group released two books for the same purpose in 1980[24] and in 1985.[25] They were based upon the two meetings of the International Conference on Ultrasonically Guided Puncture, held in Copenhagen in 1978 and 1983, sponsored by the Danish Society of Diagnostic Ultrasound. The first book dealt mainly with the central canal type transducer, while the second focused on real-time intervention.

Another essential book[26] and important articles on the history of interventional ultrasound[27–31] are also listed here.

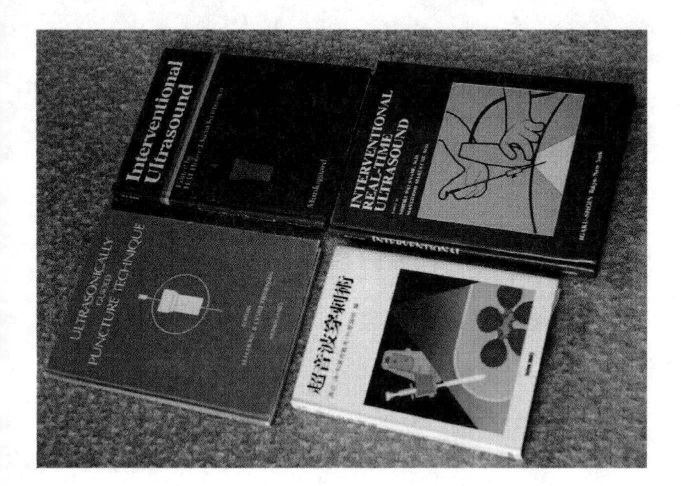

Fig. 1.10. Special books on interventional ultrasound

References

1. Berlyne GM, Ultrasonics in renal biopsy, Lancet 1961; I: 750–751.
2. Holm HH, Kristensen JK, Rasmussen SN, Northeved A, Barlebo H, Ultrasound as a guide in percutaneous puncture technique, Ultrasonics 1972; 10: 83–86.
3. Goldberg BB, Pollack HM, Ultrasonic aspiration transducer. Radiol 1972; 102: 187–189.
4. Kratochwil A, Ultrasonic localization of the placenta. Presented at the First Congress on Ultrasonic Diagnostics in Medicine, Wien (1969).
5. Pedersen JF, Percutaneous puncture guided by ultrasonic multitransducer scanning, J Clin Ultrasound 1977; 5: 175–177.
6. Saitoh M, Watanabe H, Ohe H, Tanaka S, Itakura Y, Date S, Ultrasonic real-time guidance for percutaneous puncture, J Clin Ultrasound 1979; 7: 269–272.
7. Goldberg BB, Cole-Beuglet C, Kurtz AB et al., Real-time aspiration-biopsy transducer, J Clin Ultrasound 1980; 8: 107–112.
8. Saitoh M, Selective renal biopsy under ultrasonic real-time guidance, Urol Radiol 1984; 6: 30–37.
9. Saitoh M, Watanabe H, Ohe H, Single stage percutaneous nephroureterolithotomy using a special ultrasonically guided pyeloscope, J Urol 1982; 128: 591–592.
10. Watanabe H, Kato H, Kato T, Morita M, Tanaka M, Terasawa Y, Diagnostic application of the ultrasonotomography for the prostate, Jpn J Urol 1968; 59: 273–279 (In Japanese).
11. Watanabe H, Kaiho H, Tanaka M, Terasawa Y, Diagnostic application of ultrasonotomography to the prostate, Invest Urol 1971; 8: 548–559.
12. Holm HH, Gammelgaard J, Ultrasonically guided precise needle placement in the prostate and the seminal vescles, J Urol 1981; 125: 385–387.
13. Saitoh M, Watanabe H, Inaba T, Giga K, Ultrasonically guided puncture in urology (3rd report) – Transrectal real-time linear scanner, Proc Jpn Soc Ultrasonics Med 1980; 37: 459–460 (In Japanese).
14. Rifkin MD, Kurtz AB, Goldberg BB, Sonographically guided transperineal prostatic biopsy: preliminary experience with a longitudinal liner-array transducer, Am J Roentgenol 1983; 140: 745–747.
15. Fornage BD, Touche DH, Deglaire M, Faroux MJ, Simatos A, Real-time ultrasound-guided prostatic biopsy using a new transrectal linear-array probe, Radiology 1983; 146: 547–548.
16. Abe M, Hashimoto T, Matsuda T, Saitoh M, Watanabe H, Prostatic biopsy guided by transrectal ultrasonography using a real-time linear scanner, Urology 1987; 29: 567–569.
17. Lee F, Littrup PJ, Torp-Pedersen S et al., Transrectal US of prostate cancer with use of transrectal guidance and an automatic biopsy system, Radiology 1987; 165 (Suppl): 215.
18. Cooner WH, Mosely BR, Rutherford CL Jr et al., Prostate cancer detection in a clinical urological practice by ultrasonography, digital rectal examination and prostate specific antigen, J Urol 1990; 143: 1146–1154.
19. Hodge KK, McNeal JE, Stamey TA, Ultrasound-guided transrectal core biopsies of the palpably abnormal prostate, J Urol 1989; 142: 66–70.
20. Whitmore WF, Hilaris B, Grabstald H, Retropubic implantation of iodine 125 in the treatment of prostate cancer, J Urol 1972; 108: 918–920.

21. Holm HH, Stroyer I, Hansen H, Stadil F, Ultrasonically guided percutaneous interstitial implantation of iodine 125 seeds in cancer therapy, Br J Radiol 1981; 54: 665–670.
22. Watanabe H, Wagai T, Takehara Y (edit), Ultrasonically guided puncture (238 pages) (In Japanese). The first special book on interventional ultrasound in various fields, Techno, Tokyo (1979).
23. Watanabe H, Makuuchi M (edit), Interventional real-time ultrasound (189 pages), The first book on realtime interventional ultrasound. Descriptions on what happens in the kidney tissue by puncture analyzed by biophysics are very important, Igaku-Shoin, Tokyo (1985).
24. Holm HH, Kristensen JK (edit), Ultrasonically guided puncture technique (128 pages), Munksgaard, Copenhagen (1980).
25. Holm HH, Kristensen JK (edit), Interventional Ultrasound (186 pages). The special book on realtime interventional ultrasound from the Danish group, Munksgaard, Copenhagen (1985).
26. van Sonnenberg E (edit), Interventional Ultrasound, Churchill Livingstone, New York (1987).
27. Holm HH, Skjodbye B, Interventional ultrasound, Ultrasound Med Biol 1996; 22: 773–789.
28. Holm HH, Interventional ultrasound in Europe, Ultrasound Med Biol 1998; 24: 779–791.
29. Watanabe H, History of ultrasound in nephrourology, Ultrasound Med Biol 2001; 27: 447–453.
30. Resnick MI, Ultrasonography of the prostate and testes, J Ultrasound Med 2003; 22: 869–877.
31. McGahan JP, The history of interventional ultrasound, J Ultrasound Med 2004; 23: 727–741.

Chapter 2
Laparoscopic Ultrasonography

Surena F. Matin

Introduction

For all the advantages of laparoscopic or robotic-assisted laparoscopic surgery, the absence of tactile sensation and haptic feedback (or the ability to mentally see what is touched) remains a major disadvantage for the novice as well as the experienced surgeon. With experience, laparoscopists can actually gain some sensation through the instruments, and both laparoscopic and robotic surgeons can visually sense the characteristics of tissue being manipulated. But, this is by no means a substitute for actual manual palpation and haptic sensation. Technological advances that allow for force-feedback are still in development and not yet a commercial or clinical reality. In this environment, laparoscopic ultrasonography (LUS) plays a critical and dominant role. Just as importantly, LUS uniquely provides internal visualization of the organ. Ultrasonography is used routinely even during some open operations when it is felt to be superior to manual palpation, such as for staging of upper-gastrointestinal malignancies, evaluation of hepatic malignancy, or in cases of complex partial nephrectomy.[1–4]

LUS has many advantages over transcutaneous ultrasonography. For one, transcutaneous ultrasonography is not effective through the pneumoperitoneum, and even for retroperitoneal organs, gas tracking in the soft tissues can significantly degrade the picture. Second, direct contact with the organ in question, such as the liver or kidney, allows the use of higher frequencies, which significantly improve image resolution. With higher frequencies, depth of penetration is lost, but this is usually not a concern due to the proximity of the organ.[5] Third, new probes that are actively steerable in two dimensions can be guided around the organ to provide visualization through a variety of angles and windows.

LUS does have some disadvantages. The direct contact does not allow for visualization of surface abnormalities because they are just within the focal zone. In these cases, a spacer is needed between the transducer head and the organ surface in order to bring the surface lesion within the focal zone. While guiding the laparoscopic ultrasound probe and interpreting the images, it may be difficult for the surgeon to also manipulate the machine settings because of the sterile field, and most operating-room circulators are not trained as ultrasound technicians. This adds a layer of complexity and potential frustration for the surgeon, but the concern is nullified when a radiologist is present with a dedicated ultrasonography technician. On the other hand, laparoscopic skills are required for steering the laparoscopic ultrasound probe, a skill that most radiologists do not have and may not be able to perform efficiently during surgery. It is therefore incumbent on our specialty to provide detailed instruction to urologists for performing and interpreting intraoperative LUS. And finally, it is difficult to visually guide the probe while simultaneously interpreting the ultrasound image; thus, having a picture-in-picture capability aids the process markedly (Fig. 2.1).

The first intraoperative LUS was performed in 1958, and one of the first practical uses of intraoperative ultrasonography was for localization of renal stones.[6–9] Dedicated laparoscopic probes became available in 1983.[10] Intraoperative ultrasonography in these early days was limited by poor imaging and limited image interpretation. These limitations dissipated with the advent of high-frequency real-time B-mode ultrasonography.[6] Only with the recent acceptance in the use of laparoscopy and the increasingly early detection of some malignancies, such as renal cell carcinoma, has LUS gained in popularity within the urology community.[5,11]*Clearly, the most important role of LUS at present is for renal surgery, where it is incorporated more and more in different types of renal procedures as will be described later.* Its use in miscellaneous other procedures, such as adrenalectomy, and other urology procedures is also described.

Laparoscopic Ultrasonography Technology

Medical ultrasound frequencies range from 1 to 30 MHz.[12] The transducer transmits ultrasound waves and receives the reflected echo. *Image resolution and tissue penetration are determined by frequency – the lower the frequency, the lower the resolution but the greater the tissue penetration.* Percutaneous

O. Ukimura and I.S. Gill (eds.), *Contemporary Interventional Ultrasonography in Urology,*
DOI: 10.1007/978-1-84800-217-3_2, © Springer-Verlag London Limited 2009

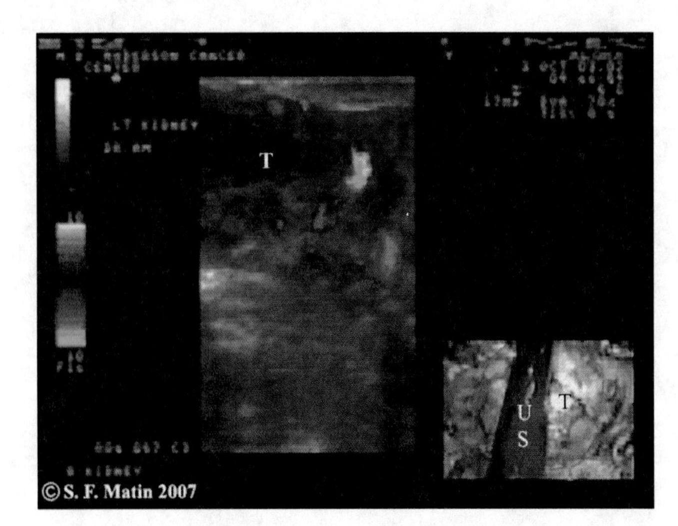

Fig. 2.1. Picture-in-picture (PIP) technology allows the surgeon to simultaneously visualize the laparoscopic view (seen in the lower right-hand corner) as well as the ultrasound image, facilitating guidance of the LUS probe around the tumor (*outlined in the laparoscopic view by a light gray broken line*) as well as facilitating image interpretation. The images can be switched to provide a larger laparoscopic picture and a smaller ultrasound picture (T, tumor; US, ultrasound probe) (used with permission, S.F. Matin 2007)

ultrasonography typically uses 5-MHz frequencies, whereas frequencies of 7.5–10 MHz are typically employed for LUS. A probe with a frequency of 7.5 MHz has the best image obtained between 1 and 4 cm. At this frequency, the ultrasound probe can detect tumors as small as 3 mm, cysts as small as 2 mm, and stones as small as 1 mm.[12,13]

Generally, different types of transducers are utilized for LUS (Fig. 2.2). The linear-array transducer has a series of multiple transducers placed longitudinally. This transducer works best for organs with a large flat surface, such as the liver. Another type of transducer has a convex array, which increases the field of view and works best for organs with a curved surface, such as the kidney, where only a small amount of surface contact is possible.[14] Recent advances to both types of transducer probes include an actively steerable, articulating tip, which enhances the flexibility of the entire unit and permits direct-contact scanning over irregularly shaped solid organs. *This author finds the convex array to be most ideal for use during renal laparoscopic surgery, because the surface of the kidney is curved and a linear probe does not always provide sufficient surface contact for adequate imaging.* Water or saline may be instilled via an irrigation device to eliminate any air pockets to optimize imaging.

Contrast-enhanced ultrasonography uses a contrast agent consisting of gas-filled microbubbles to provide vascular contrast enhancement. Its use during laparoscopic catheter ablation was investigated in an animal model, and its utility during transcutaneous ultrasonography for monitoring recurrence has also been evaluated.[15,16] This topic is covered in more detail elsewhere in this textbook.

The Radiologist, the Urologist, and Laparoscopic Ultrasonography

In some centers in the United States, a radiologist is present to perform LUS and provide image interpretation.[11,17,18] This radiologist is familiar with the operating room and with sterile procedures and is experienced with LUS technology, laparoscopic manipulation of instruments, and of course, sonographic interpretation. A technician typically accompanies the radiologist in manipulating the machine settings, troubleshooting, and making measurements. It is a reality, however, that many academic centers and most community hospitals either do not have the resources to provide for a dedicated radiologist to cover surgical cases or have no one on the staff that is able to or interested in performing LUS. As well, due to the logistics of scheduling, different radiologists with different skills may be available on different days, which results in inconsistent service. Thus, the radiologist's role is increasingly supplanted by the operating surgeon. At our center, routine cases are usually performed solely by surgeons, in both urologic and surgical oncology. While ultrasonography technique and image interpretation require considerable experience, this training is increasingly being incorporated into postgraduate and residency programs. *Diagnostic ultrasonography is currently a part of surgical training in many European and Japanese medical centers where, like a stethoscope, it is considered an extension of the physician's armamentarium.*[17,19] In fact, a survey by the European Society of Urological Technology found that nearly 80% of respondents performed ultrasonography themselves or they performed them in conjunction with a radiologist.[19] *It is important to note that if the urologist performs the intraoperative ultrasonography, the operative note must be adequately documented to facilitate proper coding and billing (see Fact Sheet).* Currently, the code is the same whether treatment approach is a laparoscopic or an open procedure.

Fact sheet

Code[a]	Charge	Title	Requirements
76,998	$878	Ultrasound guidance, intraoperative	In the Operative Note, dictate a separate paragraph documenting "Intraoperative Ultrasound Findings," such as: • Tumor appearance (hyper echoic, hypoechoic, or isoechoic to normal renal parenchyma; heterogeneous or homogeneous; circular or irregular; sharp or indistinct borders, etc.) • Size of tumor, stone, or cyst • Absence/presence of other tumors/cysts/other pathology • If use of US was critical for getting clear margins, if relevant

[a]Note that in 2007 the code was changed from 76,986, with no change in the amount of charge. Source: CPT® 2007 Professional Edition, published by the American Medical Association, Chicago, IL

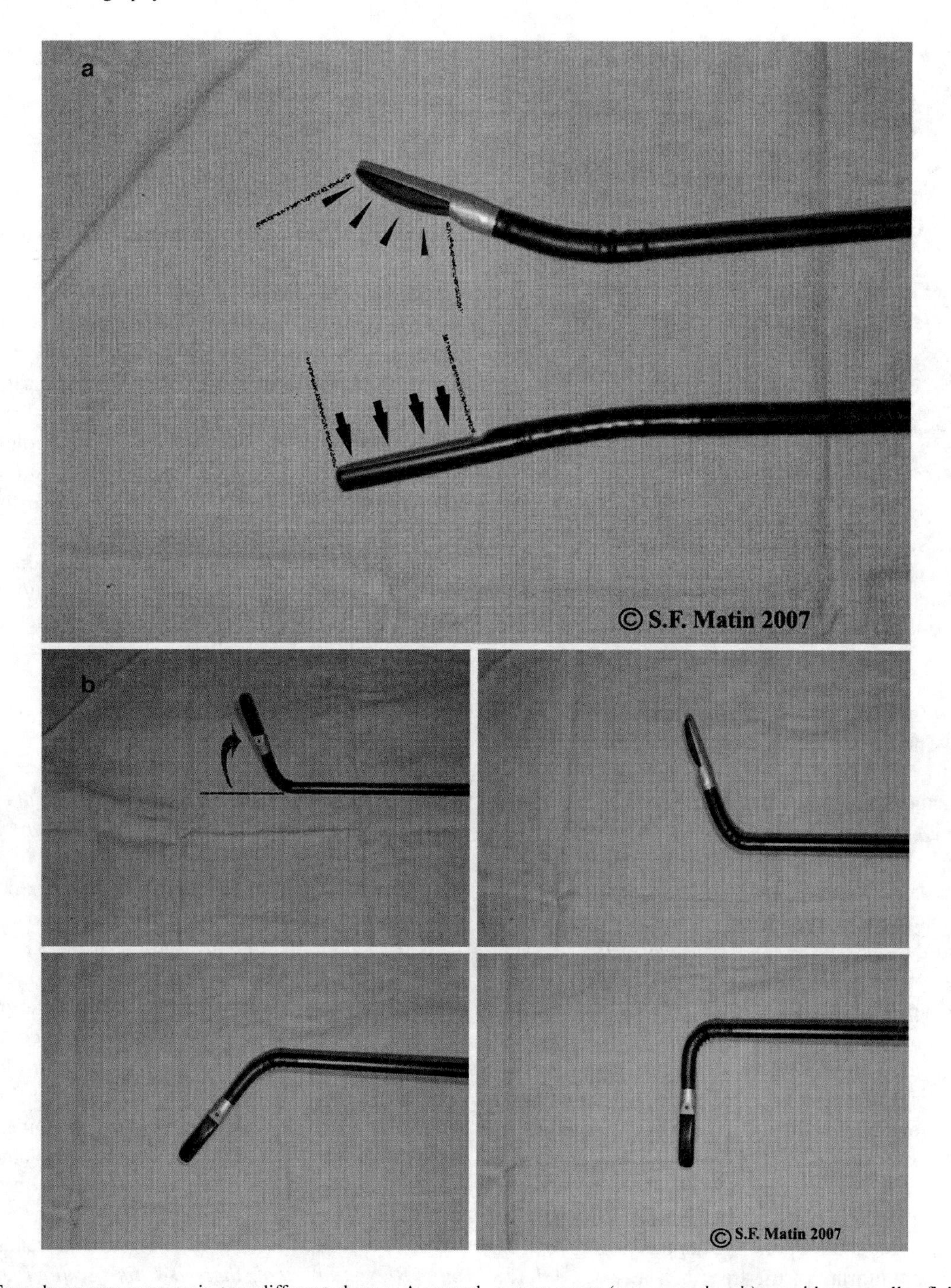

FIG. 2.2. (**A**) Transducer arrays come in two different shapes. A curved, convex array (*top, arrowheads*) provides a smaller field of view that expands with depth. However, it allows better surface contact with curved organs such as the kidney or exophytic renal tumors. A linear array provides a larger field of view that remains constant with penetration and is ideal for use with hepatic applications. When used to evaluate renal lesions such as an exophytic renal tumor, it may not allow good visualization due to poor contact from curved surfaces. (**B**). Some current probes such as the one in this figure actively deflect in two planes, right/left in angles close to 90° (*bottom panels*) and up/down (*top right panel*). Active deflection can be manipulated in both axes simultaneously to provide a variety of angles around organs of interest (*top left panel*) (used with permission, S.F. Matin 2007)

Lus During Renal Procedures

Probe Ablation: Cryotherapy

Uchida and associates first reported the use of percutaneous cryotherapy for renal cell cancer and angiomyolipoma in 1995, and their report was followed soon after by descriptions of open and laparoscopic approaches.[20–22] In all reports, ultrasonographic guidance and monitoring has been an essential adjunct for observing the evolving cryolesion. *Ultrasonography and cryoablation are well-matched technologies. The edge of the evolving ice ball is superbly visualized during*

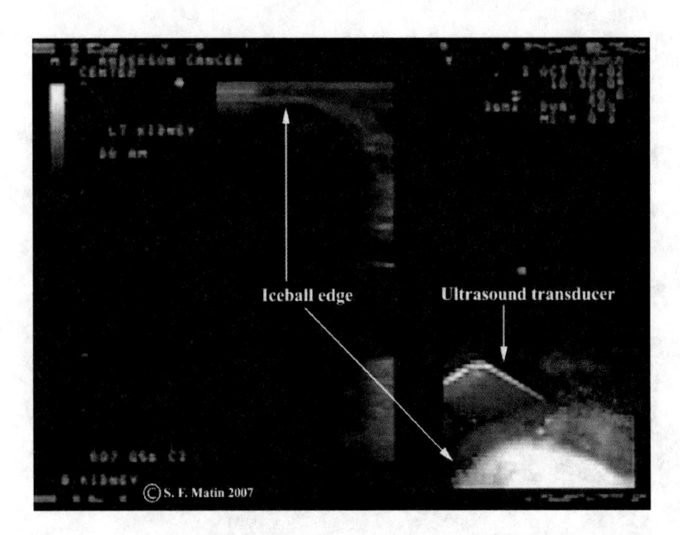

FIG. 2.3. A picture-in-picture view of the iceball edge is seen by LUS as well as visually (inset). The iceball itself is anechoic but its advancing edge, corresponding with 0-degrees Celsius, is well seen. Since the opposing iceball edge is not well seen, the surgeon drives the probe in opposing aspects around the kidney to confirm adequate treatment margins (used with permission, S.F. Matin 2007)

cryoablation, allowing real-time evaluation of the entire zone of treatment.[23] This advantage forms the central pillar supporting the use of cryoablation for the treatment of small renal masses, as no other form of ablative therapy can be monitored this well during treatment.

It is surprising to some that, despite the minimally invasive nature of the procedure, the degree of intracorporeal dissection required for laparoscopic cryoablation is actually quite extensive, as exposure of the entire renal surface as well as the side opposite the lesion is required. An articulating LUS probe with color Doppler capability is inserted through a 12-mm midaxillary port. Examination of the entire kidney is performed to evaluate tumor size, location of margins, and vascularity of the tumor and its proximity to the collecting system, as well as to rule out previously unidentified tumors. Needle biopsy of the lesion is carried out. The puncture site by the cryoprobe is determined by placing the steerable tip of the LUS probe directly on the opposite surface of the kidney, allowing real-time sonographic guidance of puncture depth by the cryoprobe and continuous monitoring of the freezing process.[18,21,24] The ice ball interface is seen as a hyperechoic, semilunar advancing edge.[23] The ice ball itself is anechoic (Fig. 2.3). Because transmission through the iceball is poor, the surgeon must manipulate the LUS probe to visualize the other advancing edges of the iceball, which usually requires significant previous dissection of the kidney to allow steering of the probe through multiple windows around the kidney. *Cryoablation is carried out beyond the tumor edge visually and ultrasonographically, by at least 5 mm in order to ensure an adequate treatment margin.*[25] The iceball edge corresponds to about 0-degrees Celsius, while 5 mm inside the edge the temperature is at about -20-degrees, which is the minimum temperature required for adequate cell kill. *Sonographic monitoring of the second freeze is suboptimal, as the ablated area is anechoic. However, continued monitoring ensures that the secondary ice ball does not advance beyond the initial boundary.*

Probe Ablation: Radiofrequency Ablation

Laparoscopic radiofrequency ablation (RFA) is generally carried out for anterior or lower-pole tumors that are inaccessible percutaneously or that are adjacent to visceral organs or the ureter (in case of a lower pole tumor) whereby a percutaneous approach may not be feasible. Alternatively, a laparoscopic approach may be favored by some, particularly if there is a limitation in accessing a skilled interventionalist.

Transperitoneal access is obtained and the colon is reflected. In the case of a lower-pole tumor, the ureter is mobilized away from the tumor and the lower pole of the kidney mobilized laterally. Similar to cryoablation, Gerota's fascia is opened surrounding the tumor and the surface of the kidney is exposed. Identification and characterization of the tumor is performed using LUS. Tumor size, enhancement characteristics, proximity to vessels, and the collecting system are all noted. Ultrasonography of the entire kidney is performed to rule out any other tumors that may not have been seen on preoperative imaging. *We also mark the treatment edge, located at least 5–10 mm beyond the tumor edge, with cautery. During RFA there is significant dessication and retraction of the tumor and surrounding parenchyma, making the treatment margins difficult to discern after treatment has begun. Having an anatomic landmark thus aids with establishing proper boundaries.* A needle biopsy is taken immediately prior to ablation. LUS is used to guide the initial insertion of the RFA probe to the deepest margin of treatment, because this is the most critical and most difficult area in which to obtain a margin. *Once RFA has been initiated, the ultrasound picture begins to degrade significantly due to interference from the radiofrequencies and also from microbubbles that form around the electrode* (Fig. 2.4). Several modern ultrasound machines have filters for minimizing this interference, but it is this author's experience that these filters do not work as well with renal RFA as they do with liver RFA, possibly because of the closer proximity of the electrode to the LUS probe with renal RFA. *Thus, after RFA is initiated, there is little use for LUS during the treatment. This emphasizes the importance of accurate initial guidance of the probe into the deepest margin of treatment by using LUS.* After the initial ablation, multiple sequential, overlapping, more superficial ablations are performed using a standard algorithm until complete ablation of the tumor and margin is achieved.

Laparoscopic Partial Nephrectomy

The technique described by the group at the Cleveland Clinic[26,27] has become the de facto standard for laparoscopic partial nephrectomy (LPN), with few modifications made at other centers. The routine use of LUS, cystoscopic placement

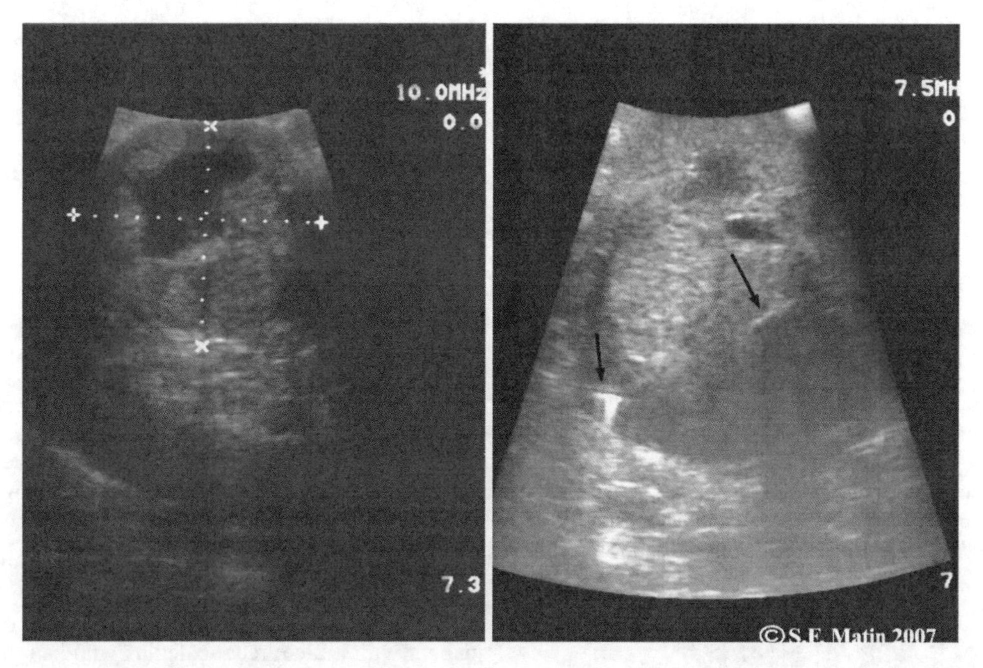

Fig. 2.4. LUS aids primarily with placement of the initial puncture for catheter-ablative therapy. In this case, an RFA electrode is placed at the deepest margin of treatment (*right panel*). *Arrows* indicate RFA electrode with deployable tines. After treatment starts, there is a progressive loss of image quality due to microbubble formation as well as frequency interference. Compare the quality of the image on the right, taken minutes after ablation has started, to the one on the left, before ablation. During RFA, this deep margin is treated first as a result of this phenomenon. Additional sequential ablations are performed as the probe is progressively withdrawn, then the catheter is redeployed more superficially and the procedure repeated (used with permission, S.F. Matin 2007)

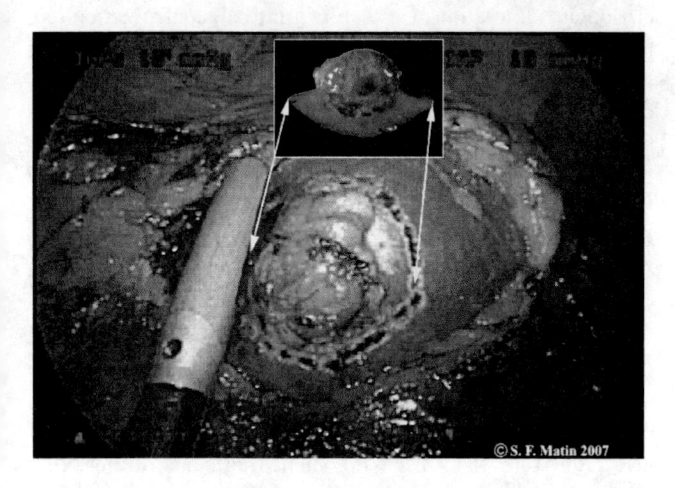

Fig. 2.5. LUS is critically necessary for demarcation of resection margins during laparoscopic partial nephrectomy. In this case the tumor is a conventional (clear cell) renal cell carcinoma resected with adequate margins (inset) (used with permission, S.F. Matin 2007)

of a ureteral catheter, suture repair of the collecting system, and renorrhaphy are used by most practitioners, but with growing experience, ureteral catheters can be omitted when tumors are completely exophytic and when resection is not expected to violate the collecting system.[28] Hilar clamping is routinely performed to obtain vascular control using bulldog clamping of the renal artery alone or in combination with the renal vein during a retroperitoneal approach or using a laparoscopic Satinsky clamp during a transperitoneal approach. This allows resection in a bloodless field with optimal visualization of the margins of resection. *Similar to any other form of nephron-sparing surgery for cancer, LUS allows evaluation of the entire kidney for lesions that may have been missed on preoperative imaging or lesions that may have progressed since the last preoperative imaging. As resection of an additional margin during LPN is difficult and to be avoided if at all possible, determination of the resection margins using LUS is critical* (Fig. 2.5). This is particularly true for deeper lesions, those with a significant intrarenal component, or those that are irregular in shape (Figs. 2.6 and 2.7). LUS has thus become a standard and expected adjunct to LPN for all tumors except maybe those that are obviously only cortical.

Renal Cyst Decortication

Laparoscopic decortication of symptomatic renal cysts is preferred over percutaneous aspiration due to the risk of recurrence with the latter, and certainly at this time is preferred to open surgery because it is a minimally invasive procedure.[29–31] Elashry and colleagues[29] reported two patients who underwent five LUS-guided cyst marsupialization procedures. A 10-MHz laparoscopic ultrasonic unit with an articulating tip was used to identify perihilar and hidden subcapsular cysts. Color Doppler imaging allowed discrimination of peripelvic cyst anatomy and surrounding vasculature, permitting safe

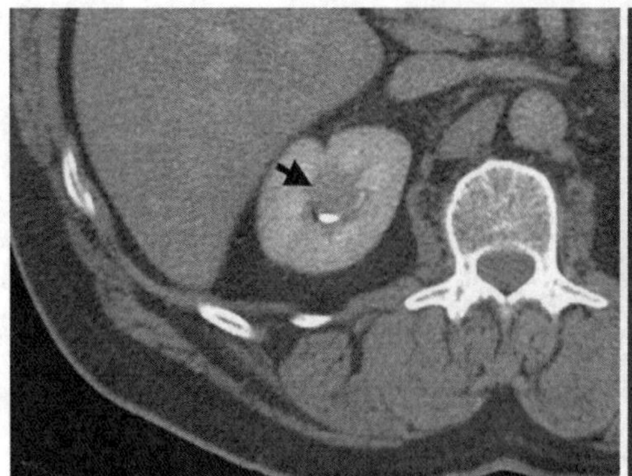

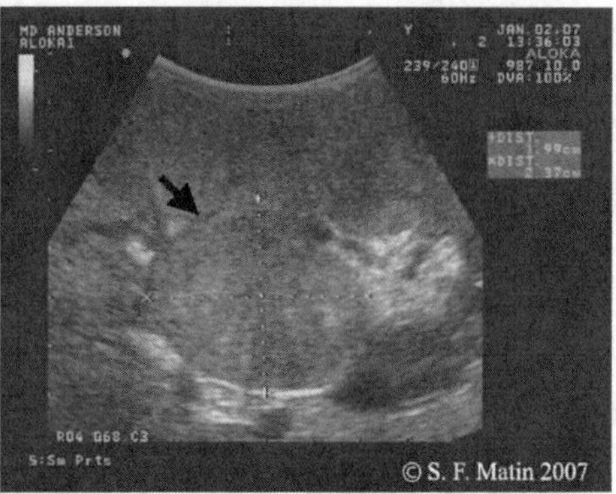

FIG. 2.6. Intraoperative ultrasonography is absolutely essential when tumors are completely intrarenal, and no surface landmarks exist to guide resection during laparoscopic or open partial nephrectomy. A computed tomography scan is shown of an upper pole, intrarenal, hilar renal tumor (*arrow*) in the *left panel*, and the corresponding intraoperative ultrasonography view is seen on the *right*. *Arrows* indicate similar perspective. The tumor was resected with clear margins by traditional open partial nephrectomy, showing a low-grade conventional (clear cell) renal cell carcinoma with negative margins. (used with permission, S.F. Matin 2007)

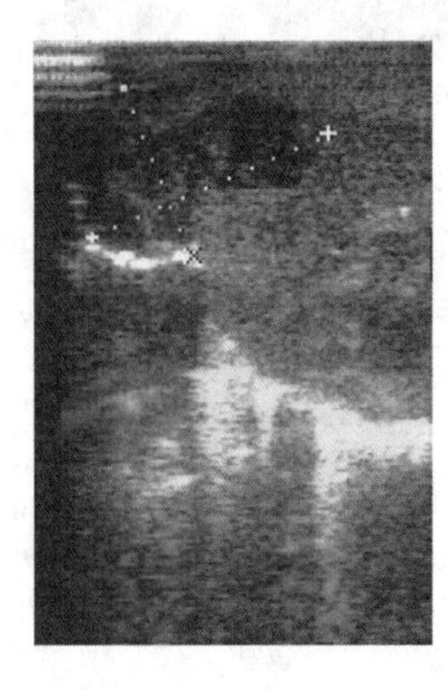

FIG. 2.7. Intraoperative ultrasonography is also critical when tumors are irregularly shaped, so that the visualized surface anatomy does not aid with prediction of the intrarenal anatomy, such as would be the case with a perfectly circular tumor. The figure shows the ultrasound appearance of a barbell-shaped renal cell carcinoma (used with permission, S.F. Matin 2007)

decortication of cysts adjacent to hilar vessels. McDougall has nicely described the laparoscopic approach to decortication of simple cysts and polycystic kidneys.[31]

Laparoscopic Renal-Stone Surgery

In 1977, Cook and Lytton[29] employed ultrasonography during an open nephrolithotomy using a 10-MHz probe that detected stones 2–3 mm in diameter, as judged by cadaveric studies. In their reports, ultrasonography was able to locate calculi in six patients who were otherwise difficult to identify.[7] The advantages observed during open renal-stone surgery prompted the use of LUS during laparoscopic nephrolithotomy and other laparoscopic renal-stone surgery. Van Cangh et al.[32] initially reported the technique of laparoscopic nephrolithotomy in a patient with a 2-cm renal calculus who had previously failed shock wave lithotripsy and was not a candidate for percutaneous therapy. LUS was felt to be critically important for accurate localization of the calculus. Additionally, the use of duplex ultrasonography assisted in the selection of a relatively thin, avascular site for the nephrotomy.

LUS appears to be eminently useful during laparoscopic calyceal diverticulectomy. Ruckle and Segura[33] reported laparoscopic obliteration of a stone-bearing calyceal diverticulum, but adjunctive ultrasonography was not employed because of the thin overlying cortex, which allowed ready visual identification of the diverticulum. *The use of LUS in the laparoscopic approach to calyceal diverticula has since shown great utility, as these lesions may not be readily identifiable by visual inspection of the cortex, even after complete exposure of the kidney.*[34] Miller et al.[35] have also described their technique in five patients, all of whom had complete stone clearance and obliteration of the diverticulum.

LUS may also aid in locating the calculus within the renal pelvis and may facilitate laparoscopic extraction.[36] Because the superior resolution of higher-frequency LUS probes allows detection of stones as small as 1–2 mm, the use of LUS may also reduce the risk of leaving small fragments during other types of laparoscopic stone surgery. *LUS during laparoscopic renal-stone surgery is a useful and dependable adjunct that can facilitate real-time localization of a calculus, can guide surgical planning, and identify residual calculi.*

Lymphocele Marsupialization

The definitive approach to symptomatic sterile pelvic lymphoceles involves drainage within the peritoneal cavity.[37] Open or laparoscopic marsupialization of the lymphocele into the peritoneal cavity is achieved by creation of a window in the common wall between the two cavities. Percutaneous treatment by simple aspiration is associated with significant recurrence, and although percutaneous sclerosis with various agents can be somewhat more effective, the resultant scarring can make future exploration difficult.[38,39] Laparoscopic marsupialization is considered standard therapy for sterile pelvic lymphoceles at many institutions. The safety and efficacy of laparoscopic marsupialization in comparison with open surgery has been shown in several series to be characterized by less blood loss and analgesic requirement and a shorter length of stay, more rapid recovery and by a similar ability to perform adjunctive measures such as omental interposition.[37,40,41] *LUS is a necessary adjunct to lymphocele marsupialization, especially if the lymphoceles are small or in proximity to important structures such as the iliac vessels, renal allograft, native ureter, bladder, or a combination of these.*[40,42] Transcutaneous ultrasonography can be used to provide real-time, dimensional operative guidance to locate the lymphocele and to facilitate safe creation of the peritoneal window, especially if the lymphocele does not share a wall with the peritoneum.[42] As Melvin et al.[43] have indicated, injury to the allograft ureter may occur and has been reported in 7% of patients undergoing laparoscopic lymphocelectomy. However, in a multi-institutional study of 87 patients, no allograft ureteral injury was noted during laparoscopic lymphocelectomy.[44] *The use of intraoperative ultrasonography, whether percutaneous, laparoscopic, or both, during laparoscopic lymphocele marsupialization is an important and useful adjunct.*

Fact sheet

- LUS is an indispensable, critically necessary adjunct during probe-ablative therapy
- LUS during LPN provides the surgeon with a view of the intrarenal anatomy and a guide for adequate resection margins at the surface level
- LUS should be considered as a necessary adjunct for laparoscopic calyceal diverticulectomy whenever renal surface anatomy may not provide sufficient landmarks
- Use of laparoscopic as well as transcutaneous ultrasonography during lymphocele marsupialization can increase the safety of the procedure and might prevent injury to surrounding structures

Miscellaneous Applications

Heniford et al.[45] reported using a 7.5-MHz LUS probe to locate the adrenal vein and detail the anatomy of the gland and tumor. The relations of the renal vessels, adrenal vein, tail of the pancreas, and inferior vena cava were carefully mapped using ultrasound. *Laparoscopic adrenalectomy has become such a standard for benign adrenal adenomas, however, that the use of LUS may be best reserved for those with challenging anatomy or unusual findings requiring further exploration.* During laparoscopic resection of pheochromocytomas, LUS can provide early identification of the adrenal vein and particularly aberrant venous drainage. Heniford used these techniques in 18 patients undergoing laparoscopic adrenalectomy and found that LUS facilitated the operative management in 68%.[45] The use of LUS expedited retroperitoneal dissection in obese patients, one of whom had previously failed an attempt at open resection, and also facilitated partial adrenalectomy in two patients with peripherally located tumors.[45] Lucas et al.[46] similarly utilized LUS to aid in the dissection of the adrenal vein in 36 patients, 35 of whom underwent successful laparoscopic adrenalectomy. Since these reports, the concept of cortical-sparing adrenalectomy has been proposed with those with familial syndromes or sporadic cases of pheochromocytoma and cortisol-secreting tumors.[47,48] Walther et al.[48] reported using LUS to perform partial adrenalectomy for eight pheochromocytomas in three patients. LUS was useful for localizing two tumors that were not seen visually. Pautler et al.[49] published their updated experience in 11 patients, all of whom managed to avoid steroid supplementation. *If cortical-sparing adrenalectomy is being contemplated, the use of LUS can make a critical difference for a favorable outcome.* In one of the more creative solutions for adrenalectomy in patients with a prohibitive abdomen, Gill et al.[50] used LUS for localization of the adrenal gland during a thoracoscopic approach to the adrenal.

LUS may have a role for evaluating a renal vein and vena caval tumor thrombus during laparoscopic nephrectomy.[51] We have also used it during laparoscopic-assisted radical nephrectomy with vena caval thrombectomy. As palpation is not possible or may be limited, accurate localization of the tumor thrombus can be performed using LUS during the laparoscopic portion of the procedure or by using the LUS probe via the mini-incision (Fig. 2.8). LUS has also been used during retroperitoneoscopic renal biopsy in extremely obese patients. Percutaneous ultrasonography was employed to identify bony landmarks prior to port placement in patients. The use of a laparoscopic probe can help identify the lower pole of the kidney in patients with excessive retroperitoneal fat.[52]

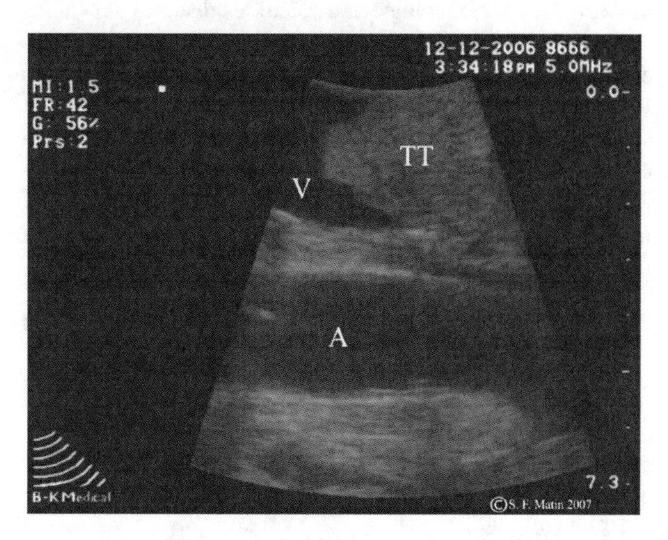

Fig. 2.8. LUS used during a laparoscopic-assisted nephrectomy and vena caval resection. LUS beautifully identifies the location of the tumor thrombus (TT), in this case located 2 cm below the hepatic veins. V, vena cava; A, aorta (used with permission, S.F. Matin 2007)

Future Directions

Undoubtedly, the role of LUS will continue to emerge. Nanotechnology and micromechanical systems have already had an impact in the evolution of this technology.[53] Areas of technology that will continue to improve the current state of the art include the improvement of directional steering, continued miniaturization of technology, and incorporation of multitask probes. The latter is already a reality within some disciplines, such as use of endobronchial ultrasonography (Olympus America, Inc., Center Valley, PA) for evaluation and diagnosis of pulmonary pathology. This technology incorporates a flexible videoendoscope, an ultrasonography examination, and a biopsy channel calibrated to the ultrasound view all within a single instrument. The surgeon can simultaneously visualize the anatomy, localize the approximate area of pathology by correlation with preoperative imaging, and then use the ultrasound located at the tip of the instrument to accurately localize the bronchial or extrabronchial pathology, such as an enlarged mediastinal lymph node.[54] An accurate biopsy of the lymph node is then simultaneously performed with the same instrument under ultrasound guidance. Three-dimensional ultrasonography capability is also currently available for some applications but has not yet reached full-scale clinical utility for LUS. This may hold the promise of allowing accurate treatment planning prior to any tumor manipulation and may improve geometric considerations of ablative therapies. The three-dimensional system has been explored for use with navigation systems to augment its utility.[55]

Overview

LUS has had a profound influence on the practice of minimally invasive urologic surgery, particularly on laparoscopic renal surgery for oncologic and calculous diseases as well as a variety of other miscellaneous procedures. LUS is a critical adjunct to probe-ablative therapy, whether cryoablation or RFA, as well as LPN. LUS advancements will enhance the surgeon's visual examination of disease and thereby play an ever-increasing role in advancing minimally invasive applications to urologic disease. Urologists have embraced the use of intraoperative ultrasonography and will continue incorporating this technology as a natural extension of patient care.

References

1. Torzilli G, Makuuchi M. Intraoperative ultrasonography in liver cancer. Surgical Oncology Clinics of North America. 2003;12(1):91–103.
2. Abdalla EK, Pisters PW. Staging and preoperative evaluation of upper gastrointestinal malignancies. Seminars in Oncology. 2004;31(4):513–29.
3. Choyke PL, Pavlovich CP, Daryanani KD, Hewitt SM, Linehan WM, Walther MM. Intraoperative ultrasound during renal parenchymal sparing surgery for hereditary renal cancers: a 10-year experience. Journal of Urology. 2001;165(2):397–400.
4. Remer EM, Herts BR, Veniero JC. Imaging for nephron-sparing surgery. Seminars in Urologic Oncology. 2002;20(3):180–91.
5. Kolecki R, Schirmer B. Intraoperative and laparoscopic ultrasound. Surgical Clinics of North America. 1998;78(2):251–71.
6. Makuuchi M, Torzilli G, Machi J. History of intraoperative ultrasound. Ultrasound in Medicine & Biology. 1998;24(9):1229–42.
7. Cook JHLB. Intraoperative localization of renal calculi during nephrolithotomy by ultrasound scanning. Journal of Urology. 1977;117:543.
8. Schlegel JUDP, Cuellar J. The use of ultrasound for localizing renal calculi. Journal of Urology. 1961;86:367.
9. Yamakawa KNS, Azuma K. Laparoscopic diagnosis of the intraabdominal organs. Japanese Journal of Gastroenterology. 1958;55:741.
10. Ohta Y, Fujiwara K, Sato Y, Niwa H, Oka H. New ultrasonic laparoscope for diagnosis of intraabdominal diseases. Gastrointestinal Endoscopy. 1983;29(4):289–94.
11. Abreu SC, Gill IS. Renal cell carcinoma: modern surgical approach. Current Opinion in Urology. 2003;13(6):439–44.
12. McIntyre RC, Jr., Stiegmann GV, Pearlman NW. Update on laparoscopic ultrasonography. Endoscopic Surgery & Allied Technologies. 1994;2(2):149–52.
13. Polascik TJMF. Intraoperative sonographic evaluation of the kidney. AUA Update Series. 1997;16(18):137.
14. Lirici MM, Caratozzolo M, Urbano V, Angelini L. Laparoscopic ultrasonography: limits and potential of present technologies. Endoscopic Surgery & Allied Technologies. 1994;2(2):127–33.
15. Slabaugh TK, Machaidze Z, Hennigar R, Ogan K. Monitoring radiofrequency renal lesions in real time using contrast-enhanced ultrasonography: a porcine model. Journal of Endourology. 2005;19(5):579–83.
16. Kawata N, Igarashi T, Ichinose T, Hirakata H, Hachiya T, Takimoto Y, et al. Usefulness of contrast-enhanced ultrasound for the diagnosis of recurrent renal cell carcinoma in contralateral kidney. International Journal of Urology. 2006;13(3):325–8.
17. Schirmer B. Laparoscopic ultrasonography. Enhancing minimally invasive surgery. Annals of Surgery. 1994;220(6):709–10.
18. Zegel HG, Holland GA, Jennings SB, Chong WK, Cohen JK. Intraoperative ultrasonographically guided cryoablation of renal masses: initial experience. Journal of Ultrasound in Medicine. 1998;17(9):571–6.
19. de la Rosette JJ, Gravas S, Muschter R, Rassweiler J, Joyce A, European Society of U-T. Present practice and development of minimally invasive techniques, imaging and training in European urology: results of a survey of the European Society of Uro-Technology (ESUT). European Urology. 2003;44(3):346–51.
20. Delworth MG, Pisters LL, Fornage BD, von Eschenbach AC. Cryotherapy for renal cell carcinoma and angiomyolipoma. Journal of Urology. 1996;155(1):252–4; discussion 4–5.
21. Gill IS, Novick AC, Meraney AM, Chen RN, Hobart MG, Sung GT, et al. Laparoscopic renal cryoablation in 32 patients. Urology. 2000;56(5):748–53.
22. Uchida M, Imaide Y, Sugimoto K, Uehara H, Watanabe H. Percutaneous cryosurgery for renal tumours. British Journal of Urology. 1995;75(2):132–6.
23. Onik GM, Reyes G, Cohen JK, Porterfield B. Ultrasound characteristics of renal cryosurgery. Urology. 1993;42(2):212–5.
24. Nadler RB, Kim SC, Rubenstein JN, Yap RL, Campbell SC, User HM. Laparoscopic renal cryosurgery: the Northwestern experience. Journal of Urology. 2003;170(4 Pt 1):1121–5.

25. Campbell SC, Krishnamurthi V, Chow G, Hale J, Myles J, Novick AC. Renal cryosurgery: experimental evaluation of treatment parameters. Urology. 1998;52(1):29–33.
26. Finelli A, Gill IS. Laparoscopic partial nephrectomy: contemporary technique and results. Urologic Oncology. 2004;22(2):139–44.
27. Gill IS, Desai MM, Kaouk JH, Meraney AM, Murphy DP, Sung GT, et al. Laparoscopic partial nephrectomy for renal tumor: duplicating open surgical techniques. Journal of Urology. 2002;167(2 Pt 1):469–7.
28. Brown GA, Matin SF. Laparoscopic partial nephrectomy: experience in 60 cases. Journal of Endourology. 2007;21(1):71–4.
29. Elashry OM, Nakada SY, Wolf JS, Jr., McDougall EM, Clayman RV. Laparoscopy for adult polycystic kidney disease: a promising alternative. American Journal of Kidney Diseases. 1996;27(2):224–33.
30. Rubenstein SC, Hulbert JC, Pharand D, Schuessler WW, Vancaillie TG, Kavoussi LR. Laparoscopic ablation of symptomatic renal cysts. Journal of Urology. 1993;150(4):1103–6.
31. McDougall EM. Approach to decortication of simple cysts and polycystic kidneys. Journal of Endourology. 2000;14(10):821–7.
32. Van Cangh PJ, Abi Aad AS, Lorge F, Wese FX, Opsomer R. Laparoscopic nephrolithotomy: the value of intracorporeal sonography and color Doppler. Urology. 1995;45(3):516–9.
33. Ruckle HC, Segura JW. Laparoscopic treatment of a stone-filled, caliceal diverticulum: a definitive, minimally invasive therapeutic option. Journal of Urology. 1994;151(1):122–4.
34. Wyler SF, Bachmann A, Jayet C, Casella R, Gasser TC, Sulser T. Retroperitoneoscopic management of caliceal diverticular calculi. Urology. 2005;65(2):380–3.
35. Miller SD, Ng CS, Streem SB, Gill IS. Laparoscopic management of caliceal diverticular calculi. Journal of Urology. 2002;167(3):1248–52.
36. Gaur DD, Agarwal DK, Purohit KC, Darshane AS. Retroperitoneal laparoscopic pyelolithotomy. Journal of Urology. 1994;151(4):927–9.
37. Gill IS, Hodge EE, Munch LC, Goldfarb DA, Novick AC, Lucas BA. Transperitoneal marsupialization of lymphoceles: a comparison of laparoscopic and open techniques. Journal of Urology. 1995;153(3 Pt 1):706–11.
38. Kay R, Fuchs E, Barry JM. Management of postoperative pelvic lymphoceles. Urology. 1980;15(4):345–7.
39. Bry J, Hull D, Bartus SA, Schweizer RT. Treatment of recurrent lymphoceles following renal transplantation. Remarsupialization with omentorplasty. Transplantation. 1990;49(2):477–80.
40. Gruessner RW, Fasola C, Benedetti E, Foshager MC, Gruessner AC, Matas AJ, et al. Laparoscopic drainage of lymphoceles after kidney transplantation: indications and limitations. Surgery. 1995;117(3):288–95.
41. Ishitani MB, DeAngelis GA, Sistrom CL, Rodgers BM, Pruett TL. Laparoscopic ultrasound-guided drainage of lymphoceles following renal transplantation. Journal of Laparoendoscopic Surgery. 1994;4(1):61–4.
42. Lucas BA, Gill IS, Munch LC. Intraperitoneal drainage of recurrent lymphoceles using an internalized Tenckhoff catheter. Journal of Urology. 1994;151(4):970–2.
43. Melvin WS, Bumgardner GL, Davies EA, Elkhammas EA, Henry ML, Ferguson RM. The laparoscopic management of post-transplant lymphocele. A critical review. Surgical Endoscopy. 1997;11(3):245–8.
44. Hsu TH, Gill IS, Grune MT, Andersen R, Eckhoff D, Goldfarb DA, et al. Laparoscopic lymphocelectomy: a multi-institutional analysis. Journal of Urology. 2000;163(4):1096–8; discussion 8–9.
45. Heniford BT, Iannitti DA, Hale J, Gagner M. The role of intraoperative ultrasonography during laparoscopic adrenalectomy. Surgery. 1997;122(6):1068–73; discussion 73–4.
46. Lucas SW, Spitz JD, Arregui ME. The use of intraoperative ultrasound in laparoscopic adrenal surgery: the Saint Vincent experience. Surgical Endoscopy. 1999;13(11):1093–8.
47. Diner EK, Franks ME, Behari A, Linehan WM, Walther MM. Partial adrenalectomy: the National Cancer Institute experience. Urology. 2005;66(1):19–23.
48. Walther MM, Herring J, Choyke PL, Linehan WM. Laparoscopic partial adrenalectomy in patients with hereditary forms of pheochromocytoma. Journal of Urology. 2000;164(1):14–7.
49. Pautler SE, Choyke PL, Pavlovich CP, Daryanani K, Walther MM. Intraoperative ultrasound aids in dissection during laparoscopic partial adrenalectomy. Journal of Urology. 2002;168(4 Pt 1):1352–5.
50. Gill IS, Meraney AM, Thomas JC, Sung GT, Novick AC, Lieberman I. Thoracoscopic transdiaphragmatic adrenalectomy: the initial experience. Journal of Urology. 2001;165(6 Pt 1):1875–81.
51. Hsu TH, Jeffrey RB, Jr., Chon C, Presti JC, Jr. Laparoscopic radical nephrectomy incorporating intraoperative ultrasonography for renal cell carcinoma with renal vein tumor thrombus. Urology. 2003;61(6):1246–8.
52. Chen RN, Moore RG, Micali S, Kavoussi LR. Retroperitoneoscopic renal biopsy in extremely obese patients. Urology. 1997;50(2):195–8.
53. Bernstein JJ, Bottari J, Houston K, Kirkos G, Miller R, Xu B, et al. Advanced MEMS ferroelectric ultrasound 2D arrays. The Proceedings of IEEE Ultrasonics Symposium. 1999;2(2):1145–53.
54. Herth FJ, Krasnik M, Vilmann P. EBUS-TBNA for the diagnosis and staging of lung cancer. Endoscopy. 2006; 38(1).
55. Ellsmere J, Stoll J, Rattner D, Brooks D, Kane R, Wells III W, et al. A navigation system for augmenting laparoscopic ultrasound. Lecture Notes in Computer Science. 2001;2208:1151–3.

Chapter 3
Ultrasound-Guided Prostate Cryosurgery: State of the Art

Gary Onik

Introduction

With the decision of the Centers for Medicare and Medicaid Services (formerly the Health Care Financing Administration [HCFA]) in 1999 to approve prostate cryosurgery for the treatment of primary prostate cancer, treatment options for patients were expanded.[1] Despite decades of investigation and incremental improvements in both radical prostatectomy (RP) and radiation therapy, neither treatment modality has distinguished itself as the procedure of choice for treating primary prostate cancer. Both modalities have limitations in treating patients with higher-stage and Gleason-grade disease. Also, the associated complications of RP and radiation therapy, while sometimes different in character, are not appreciably different in incidence to clearly recommend one treatment over the other. As a result, each approach can be justifiably recommended as the procedure of choice. These options, along with "watchful waiting"[2] or as it is now called "active surveillance," as possible strategies for prostate cancer management have led to patient confusion and frustration. Adding cryosurgery as still another treatment option to this already-confusing environment further complicates patient choices. As we will see, however, there have been major improvements in cryosurgical results gained in recent years due to the basic understanding of the thermal destruction of tissue and the advances in cryosurgical technique and equipment. Add to this its unique inherent advantages of being able to treat extensive local disease, be repeated, as well as form a platform for the focal therapy of prostate cancer, image-guided prostate cryosurgery (or perhaps another similarly image-guided ablative technology) has the potential to become the treatment of first choice for all stages and grades of localized prostate cancer.

Since the ultrasound-guided percutaneous transperineal approach for prostate cryosurgery is essentially identical to that of a radiation seed implantation, the potential advantages of cryosurgery can be well appreciated if freezing is viewed as another new implantable radiation source, i.e., ICE 101 (Fig. 3.1). Thus, like radiation seeds, the characteristics of the freezing probes are known and can be predicted, but unlike radiation seeds, freezing can be monitored and modulated in real time to ensure adequate therapy giving it a major advantage over seeds (Fig. 3.2). In addition, freezing creates a discreet lesion; it does not "scatter" as do radiation from seeds, affecting adjacent structures. In other words, when properly controlled and monitored, structures outside the target zone are not affected.

There is no "dose threshold" for the freezing allowing addition freeze-thaw cycles within a single procedure, or repeat treatment at a later sitting in the event of a local recurrence. Despite these advantages and the long history of thermal therapy (hyperthermia) in the field of radiation oncology, cryosurgery has been virtually ignored by the brachytherapy community. This review presents results suggesting that the advantages of freezing as a "radiation source" are finally being harnessed. This chapter reviews the background of prostate cryosurgery, its lackluster early performance that created a negative perception of the procedure, the changes in instrumentation and technique that have improved prostate cryosurgery results, and the patient selection criteria for prostate cryosurgery.

Background

The treatment of localized prostate cancer remains controversial. Although pathologic studies have shown that the prevalence of prostate cancer is high, many of these cancers are not clinically significant.[3] In addition, even clinically significant cancers – generally accepted as those of a volume of 0.5 mL or greater – have a variable biologic behavior. On the other hand, the treatments for prostate cancer include a substantial risk of lifestyle-limiting morbidity. With some recent studies showing minimal survival benefit between no treatment and RP, the concept of "watchful waiting," i.e., not treating the primary tumor at all, has gained acceptance by some as a viable management alternative in certain patient populations. The decision to treat prostate cancer with a particular therapy or with "watchful waiting" requires a careful assessment of

O. Ukimura and I.S. Gill (eds.), *Contemporary Interventional Ultrasonography in Urology*,
DOI: 10.1007/978-1-84800-217-3_3, © Springer-Verlag London Limited 2009

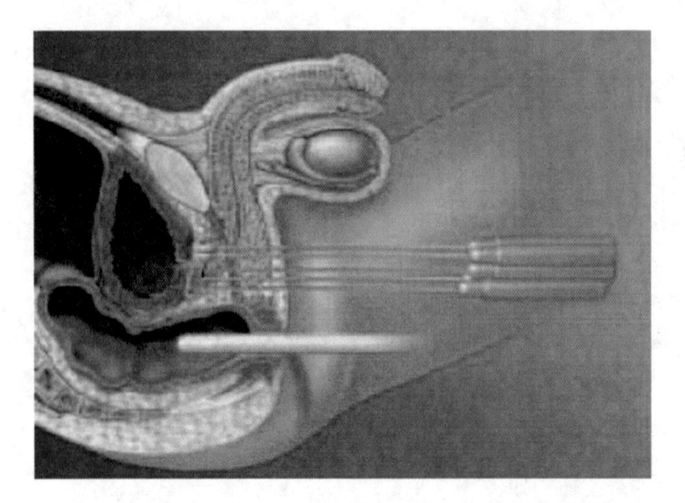

FIG. 3.1. Diagram showing the transperineal approach of prostate cryosurgery. The cryoprobes are placed percutaneously through the perineum using transrectal ultrasound for guidance. The approach is identical in concept to brachytherapy of the prostate. Reproduced with permission from Endocare, Inc, Irvine, California (1-888-236-3646; http://www.endocare.com)

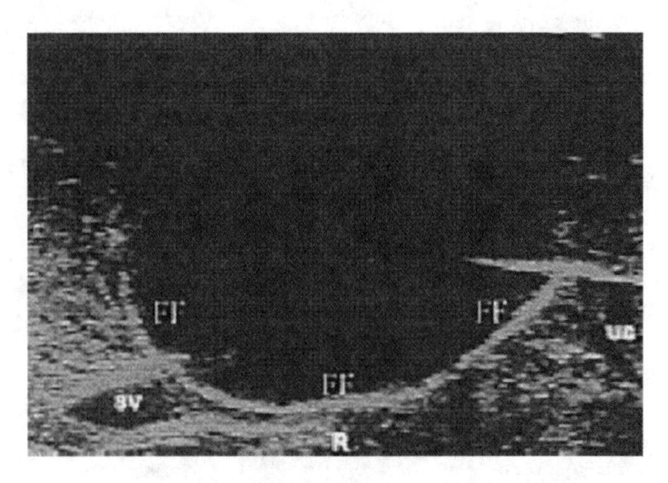

FIG. 3.2. US showing the ice as it extends toward the rectum. The freezing front (FF) is exquisitely seen as a hyperechoic (*white*) line extending toward the rectum (R). The seminal vesicle (SV) and urogenital diaphragm (UG) can be identified. The ability to visualize the freezing as it encompasses the prostate and approaches the rectum gives a "freezing radiation source" greater control than traditional brachytherapy

the risk vs. benefit for that patient. Obviously, as the complications and lifestyle-limiting side effects of treatments are reduced, these decisions become easier. The reintroduction of prostate cryosurgery using a percutaneous approach under ultrasound guidance was consistent with this concept of trying to decrease the morbidity of prostate cancer treatment. In 1966, Gondor et al.[4] first reported the concept of a cryosurgery procedure for the treatment of prostate disease. Subsequently, an open transperineal cryosurgery procedure was developed in which the freezing was carried out on the surface of the prostate with visual monitoring. Using this same approach, Bonney et al.[5] reported results of this procedure in 229 patients followed for up to 10 years. A comparison of patients who underwent RP and radiation therapy, showed equal survival among the treatment modalities. Although cryosurgery showed some advantages, such as being able to treat patients with large bulky tumors, poor monitoring of the freezing process resulted in major complications such as urethro-cutaneous and urethro-rectal fistula, thus limiting the acceptance of the procedure. In 1993, the first series of percutaneous ultrasound-guided and monitored prostate cryosurgery was reported by Onik et al.[6] which stimulated a resurgence of interest in this treatment modality. As with any new procedure, ultrasound-guided prostate cryosurgery went through a significant learning curve in which the goals of the procedure looked attainable but the reported results, in both cancer control and complications, were variable. A negative perception of the procedure was compounded by the fact that most early series predominantly treated patients in whom radiation therapy had failed, and these patients have higher complication rates, particularly incontinence, than those without a history of radiation therapy (73% vs. 3%).[7,8] The situation was also exacerbated by a high urethral complication rate caused by the use of an ineffective urethral warming catheter.[9] Despite these early obstacles, the long-term results from multiple institutions were examined, and in 1999 the Centers for Medicare and Medicaid Services removed cryosurgery from the investigational category and included it with radiation and RP as a treatment for primary prostate cancer. In a recently published article, Katz et al.[10] reviewed the 5-year biochemical disease-free survival of patients treated with brachytherapy, CT conformal radiation therapy, radical prostatectomy, and cryoablation for every article published in the last 10 years. The results were stratified based on whether the patients were low, medium, or high risk for biochemical failure. Based on this analysis the range of results for cryoablation was equivalent to all other treatments in low- and medium-risk patients and appeared to be superior in high-risk patients. Overall complications rates were similar with all the modalities. The only article directly comparing cryoablation with radical prostatectomy, published by Gould et al.,[11] showed cryoablation to be equivalent to RP in low-risk patients, but as patient's preoperative PSA increased, cryoablation results were superior to RP. The basis for this apparent superiority in high-risk patients may be the ability of cryoablation to treat extracapsular extension of cancer and to be repeated if needed. Based on these results one can conclude that cryoablation is a safe and effective treatment for treating prostate cancer.

Patient Selection

The extent and pathologic character of the patient's disease are importance factors in choosing a proper therapy for prostate cancer. Treatments such as RP and brachytherapy (without external boosting) have higher recurrence rates as the extent and aggressiveness (Gleason score) of the disease increases. *One of the great advantages of cryosurgery is the flexibility of the procedure to be tailored to treat both high- and low-risk patients, as well as patients in whom radiation therapy has failed.*

Patients at High Risk for Local Recurrence

The use of cryosurgery for the treatment of solid organ cancers made a resurgence with the advent of ultrasound monitoring of hepatic cryosurgery first proposed by Onik et al. in 1984.[12] Hepatic cryosurgery filled a unique place in the armamentarium of liver cancer treatment in that it successfully treated patients with multiple tumors or tumors that were unresectable due to proximity to major vasculature that could not be sacrificed[13,14] Due to its target patient population of previously untreatable patients with an expected mortality of virtually 100%, imaging-guided hepatic cryosurgery was readily embraced by the surgical oncology community.[15]

The situation with prostate cancer is similar to liver cancer in that a significant portion of prostate cancer patients have a risk of positive margins, based on the high proportion of patients who have capsular penetration at the time of definitive treatment. However, efforts at preoperative staging have been inadequate to identify this patient population. The difficulty is further compounded by the fact that at the time of RP, the surgeon's ability to appreciate capsular penetration and involvement of the neurovascular bundles is inadequate. Vaidya et al.[16] reported virtually no correlation between the surgeon's determination of tumor penetration into the periprostatic tissue with involvement of the neurovascular bundle and actual pathologic confirmation. The result is that in this study, as well as in other reports, positive margin rates of 30% associated with nerve-sparing RP are not uncommon. Using various clinical parameters such as Gleason score, clinical stage, and prostate-specific antigen (PSA) level, the statistical chance for capsular penetration can be reasonably predicted preoperatively.[17,18] This approach can lower the positive margin rate when rigorously applied, as demonstrated by Eggleston et al.[19] In actual clinical practice, however, most urologists believe that RP is still the "gold standard" of treatment. This leads to a natural reluctance, based on a statistical analysis, to deny a treatment that they believe may provide the best chance for cure. Based on the success of cryosurgery in treating unresectable liver cancer, it was hoped that the ability to freeze into the periprostatic tissue and encompass tumor capsular penetration could improve the treatment of prostate cancer patients at high risk of positive surgical margins. The preliminary data seem to support the potential success of this primary goal of prostate cryosurgery – improved treatment outcomes in patients at high risk of local recurrence. Numerous studies on ultrasound-guided prostate cryosurgery have demonstrated the ability of the procedure to successfully treat patients with stage T3 prostate cancer with demonstrated gross extracapsular disease.[20,21] (Fig. 3.3) Demonstration of this concept in

a

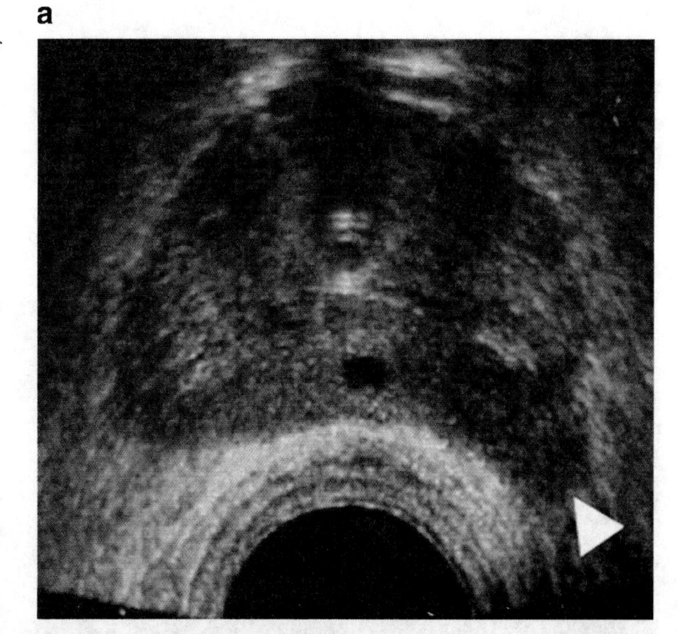

b

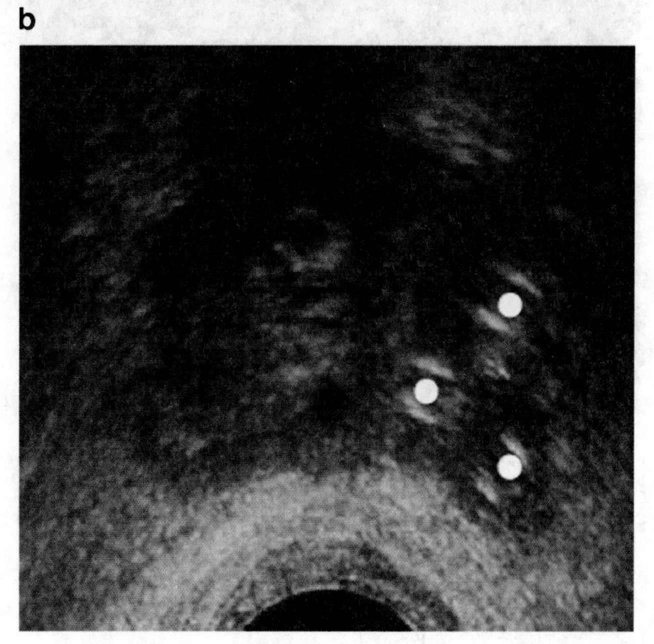

FIG. 3.3. (**a**) Ultrasound shows gross extracapsular extension of tumor through the area of the left neurovascular bundle (*arrowhead*). (**b**) Three cryoprobes have been placed to cover the area and destroy the extracapsular disease

patients with a "high likelihood" of capsular penetration, based only on statistical analysis, is more problematic since the exact margin status of the patient is not known preoperatively or postoperatively following a cryosurgical procedure. There is, however, some evidence to support excellent results in patients at high risk for positive margins. Onik et al.[22] have shown that aggressive periprostatic freezing was facilitated by separating the rectum from the prostate at the time of the operation by a saline injection into Denonvilliers' fascia (Fig. 3.4). No local recurrences were seen in 61 patients followed for

a

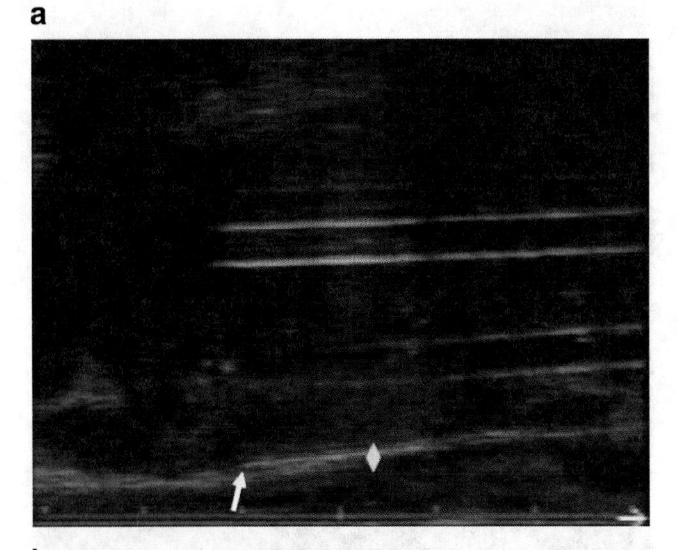

b

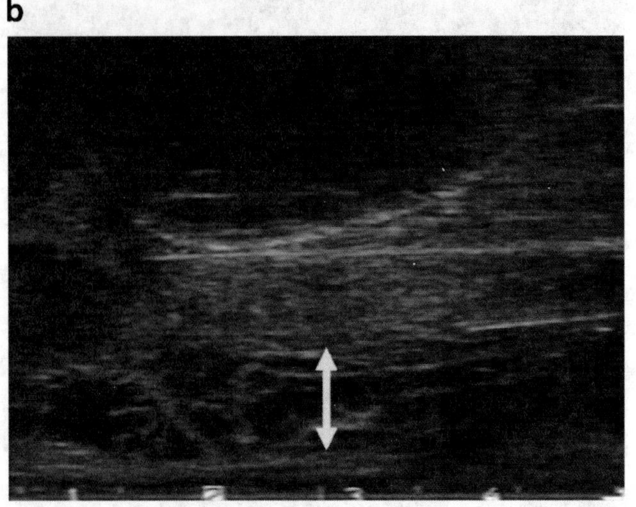

FIG. 3.4. (**a**) US shows the tip of a needle placed into Denonvillier's Fascia which appears as a *white line* between the rectum and the prostate (*arrow*). The width of the fascia is indicated by the diamond shape. (**b**) US after injection of saline into Denonvillier's Fascia. The *double-headed arrow* shows the increase in space between the prostate and the rectum. Downward traction on the rectum by the US probe keeps the space open

up to 4 years despite the fact that 68% of the patients were considered at high risk of capsular penetration and local failure, based on the factors of Gleason score of 7 or greater, PSA >10 ng mL^{-1}, already failed radiation, or extensive bilateral disease based on preoperative biopsies. These results were confirmed by Bahn et al.[23] in which 7-year results in over 500 patients showed that patients with medium and high risk had virtually identical results to low risk patients (88% BDF using the ASTRO criteria)

When cryosurgery is performed aggressively to achieve a negligible detectable PSA level, comparisons with RP should be possible. In the only published study comparing the outcomes between aggressive "total" cryosurgery and RP in one clinical practice,[11] cryosurgery had a 23% greater chance of resulting in a PSA level of less than 0.2 ng mL^{-1} than did RP (96% vs. 73%). When a 0.0 PSA was used as the success criteria, cryosurgery maintained its approximately 20% advantage over RP (66.9% vs. 48.2%). As patients became at greater risk for positive margins based on a PSA of 20 ng mL^{-1} or greater, cryosurgery maintained its results while the results of RP deteriorated further (86% vs. 36%). While this study was retrospective and included a relatively small number of patients, its results are consistent with the original cryosurgical treatment rationale of destroying extracapsular cancer by treating the periprostatic tissues. In addition, these findings are consistent with the other studies showing success in treating T3 disease and other high-risk patients, as well as the unequivocally successful results seen in treating unresectable liver tumors. These results, together with the relatively low morbidity of the procedure and its ability to be performed in older patients and repeated when needed, we believe make cryosurgery the procedure of choice in this patient population.

Adjuvant hormone therapy in high-risk patient populations is an important strategy. When combined with radiation, short-term hormone therapy appears to improve local regional control and distant metastatic in patients with bulky tumors (T2–T4).[24] Long-term adjuvant hormonal therapy in addition to radiation appears to significantly affect the survival of patients having a Gleason score of greater than 7.[25] Since adjuvant therapy in these studies also had a significant effect on local control of tumor, the question of the importance of local control of tumor on the incidence of subsequent metastatic disease still needs investigation. Based on these concepts, patients who are of medium to high risk of recurrence, we routinely place on 6 months of CHT prior to definitive cryosurgical treatment.

Patients with Organ-Confined, Low-Volume, Low Gleason Score Disease

Focal Cryosurgery

The use of breast-sparing surgery, i.e., "lumpectomy" to treat breast cancer revolutionized the local control of that disease. Lumpectomy experience showed that patient quality of life can successfully be integrated into the equation of cancer treatment without major treatment efficacy.[26] Men with prostate cancer face many of the same issues that breast cancer patients do. Focal therapy, in which just the known area of cancer is destroyed, appears to be a logical extension of the watchful waiting concept and very analogous to the lumpectomy in breast cancer. Focal therapy minimizes the risks associated with expectant management since the clinically threatening index cancer has been treated. Minimizing prostate trauma could, by treating only a portion of the prostate, decrease the risk of lifestyle-altering complications associated with morbid whole-gland treatments.

In 1992, Onik et al.[27] published the first article on the focal treatment of prostate cancer using cryosurgical ablation. Nine patients were reported who had been followed for an average of more than 3 years, all patients were BDF indicating that local control of prostate cancer was attainable with a focal approach. Morbidity was also low with seven of the nine patients retaining potency and none experiencing incontinence. A follow-up article is now in press describing our further experience with focal cryoablation, i.e., "Male Lumpectomy."[28] In this chapter, 51 patients, all of whom had at least 1 year follow-up, are reported in which the BDF rate using focal cryosurgery is 95%. In addition, no patient had evidence for a local recurrence in an area treated. Only four of the 51 patients had recurrences in areas not previously treated. All were retreated and were subsequently free of disease. Local control of cancer was 100% despite the fact that 50% of the patients were medium to high risk for local recurrence. Once again all patients were continent and potency was maintained in 85% of patients (Fig. 3.5).

The main conceptual objection to focal treatment of prostate cancer is that it is often a multifocal disease. Prostate cancer, however is a spectrum of diseases, some of which are may be amenable to focal therapy. The prostate cancer pathology literature shows that a significant number of patients have a single focus prostate cancer and that many other have additional cancer foci that may not be clinically significant.[29–32] Until now however, little attention has been paid in differentiating those patients with unifocal, from multifocal disease, since all treatments aimed at total gland removal or destruction.

In a study examining radical prostatectomy specimens Djavan et al.[29] showed that patients with unifocal disease constituted nearly one-third of the cases. In addition, Villiers et al.[30] showed that 80% of multifocal tumors are less than 0.5 cc, indicating they may not be of clinical significance. This study was confirmed by Rukstalis et al.[31] and Noguchi et al.[32] in which pathologic examination showed that unifocal tumors were present in 20 and 25% of patients, respectively, and using the size criteria of 0.5 cc or less as an insignificant tumor, an additional 60 and 39% of patients might be a candidate for a focal treatment approach. Based on this pathological evidence a significant opportunity exists to investigate a focal treatment approach for prostate cancer.

Newer biopsy techniques now being used, in which the gland is biopsied transperineally every 5 mm using a brachytherapy type grid, could have an impact on excluding patients with significant multifocal disease. A recent paper by Crawford et al.,[33] using computer simulations on RP and autopsy specimens, demonstrated that transperineal prostate biopsies, spaced at 5-mm intervals through the volume of a patients prostate had a sensitivity of 95% in finding clinically significant tumors. Our results in 110 patients undergoing what we call 3D Prostate Mapping Biopsies (3D-PMB), consistent with the protocol Crawford investigated, showed that cancer could be demonstrated in 50% of patients who previously had negative biopsies in the previously uninvolved prostate lobe on TRUS biopsy.[34] 3D mapping biopsy also provides superior localization of the tumor site than TRUS biopsies are able to provide. This information can therefore be used to guide the focally destructive agent to optimize destruction of the tumor while limiting the area that needs to be treated, hopefully minimizing the chance for side effects (Fig. 3.6).

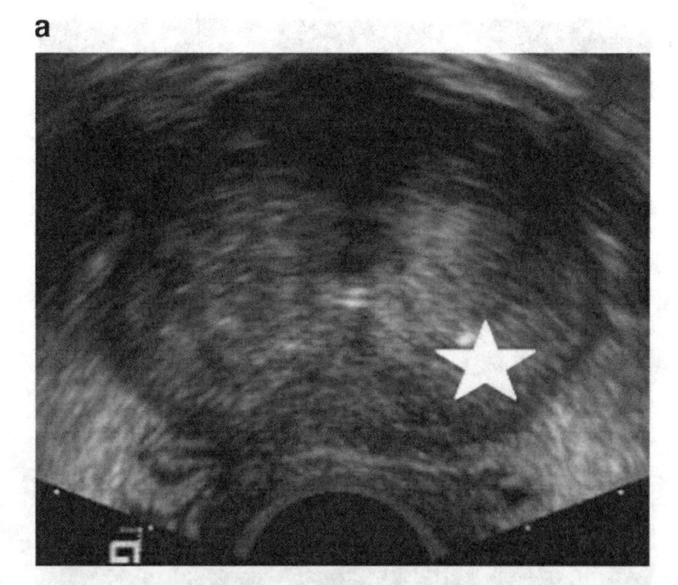

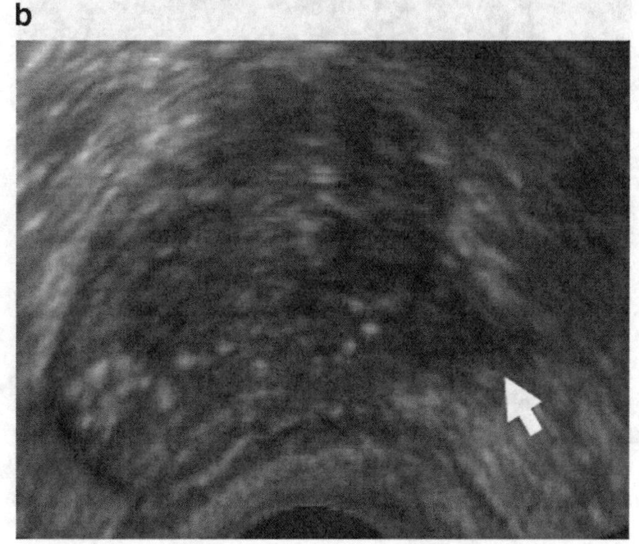

Fig. 3.5. (**a**) US shows the prostate of a 60-year-old male. The *star* indicates where his biopsy was positive for a Gleason 6 carcinoma. He was treated with focal cryosurgery. He was continent and potent immediately after the procedure. (**b**) Two years post cryosurgery the US shows that the area of previous cryosurgery has contracted to a small scar (*arrow*). The patient's biopsies were negative and his PSA remains stable 6 years after the procedure

Focal cryoablation is a unique blend of an aggressive yet minimal procedure, which accounts for its combination of excellent cancer control and lack of complications. Extensive freezing of the periprostatic tissue can still carried out on the side of the demonstrated tumor. In patients with a high

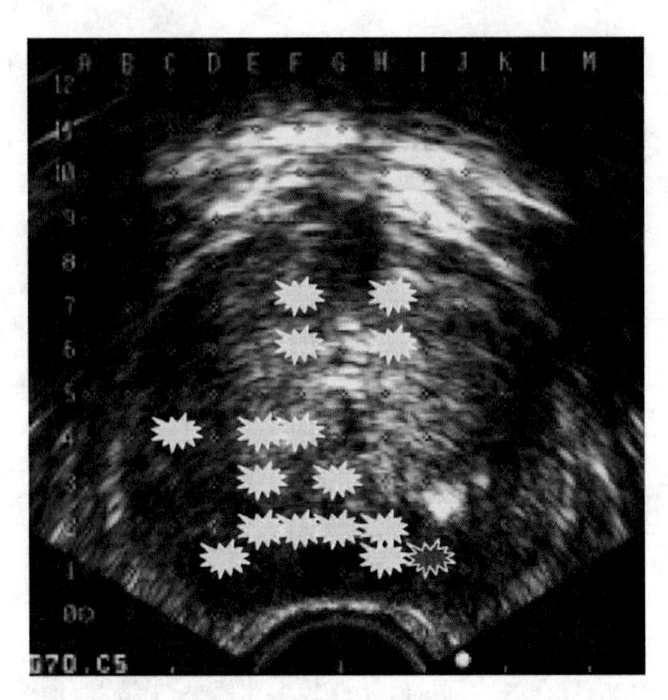

FIG. 3.6. US of a patient who presented with a single core positive, Gleason 6 on his TRUS biopsy on the left side of the gland. The *starburst patterns* indicate all the locations where he was positive on his 3D Prostate Mapping Biopsy (3D-PMB). The *pink starburst* indicates an area of extracapsular extension

Gleason score or in those with cancer demonstrated at the base of the gland, prophylactic freezing of the confluence of the seminal vesicles can also be carried out. The expected incidence of urinary and rectal complications is lower than that of total cryosurgery, RP, or brachytherapy. No patient in our series demonstrated persistent incontinence. Probably most important, however, is that an error in patient selection is correctable by retreatment without added morbidity, a situation unique to cryosurgery.

Patients with Local Recurrence After Radiation Therapy

Patients who received a maximal dose of radiation but suffer a local recurrence without evidence of metastatic disease are still theoretically curable. Unfortunately, radiation destroys the tissue planes needed for a safe and effective attempt at salvage RP. RP in a salvage situation has demonstrated positive margins in 40% of patients[35] with prohibitive morbidity demonstrating a 58% incontinence rate and an incidence of rectal injury as high as 15%.[36] Consequently, salvage RP is rarely performed in this setting with most patients being placed on palliative hormone ablation therapy.

Based on the successful application of cryotherapy in patients with liver cancer, percutaneous prostate cryosurgery was immediately applied to this difficult-to-treat patient population. The treatment of patients for salvage after radiation therapy was not without difficulties. Early findings showed poor cancer control results with less than 25% of patients reaching PSA levels of 0.2 ng mL^{-1} 33 or less, with positive biopsy rates as high as 35%. Also, complications in this patient population could be significant. While the incontinence rate for nonsalvage cryosurgery patients is less than 2%, significant incontinence for radiation salvage patients can be as high as 42%.[37] Advances in cryosurgical technique have improved these results, with an article by de la Taille et al.[38] demonstrating a 60% success rate at providing an undetectable PSA. The associated incontinence rate was 9%.

Based on these results, cryosurgery was approved by The Centers for Medicare and Medicaid Services as the only treatment specifically approved for the indication of recurrent local cancer after radiation failure. We are just gaining experience with treating these patients with focal therapy, and while the cancer control rates are yet to be determined it appears that the incidence of incontinence can greatly be reduced by this approach. We believe that based on its potential for cure, cryosurgery has become the procedure of choice in this difficult-to-treat patient population.

Technical Considerations in Cryosurgery

Saline Injection into Denonvilliers' Fascia

A major theoretical criticism of prostate cryosurgery involves the anatomy of the pelvis with the close proximity of the prostate capsule to the rectal mucosa. Inadequate space between the prostate and the rectum can result in freezing the rectal mucosa with resultant urethro-rectal fistula. Subsequently, fear of causing urethra-rectal fistula may result in stopping the freezing process prematurely and thus lead to a high incidence of tumor recurrence. Even for the experienced cryosurgeon, cryosurgery was at times a nerve-wracking balancing act between adequate treatment and rectal injury.

Probably the most important advance in the technique of prostate cryosurgery leading to the reproducibility of results involves the injection of saline into Denonvilliers' fascia at the time of freezing to temporarily increase the space between the rectum and prostate (Fig. 3.3). The success of this maneuver is dependent on a downward traction of the rectum by the transrectal ultrasound probe to keep the space open once the injection has been made. We have now utilized this saline injection technique in more than 400 patients, demonstrating that this maneuver virtually eliminates the risk of rectal freezing and the complication of urethro-rectal fistula without increasing morbidity. The elimination of the fear of rectal freezing has several consequences that improve the effect results of *cryosurgery.* First, with the rectum protected, free-zing can be sufficiently extended outside the prostate to bring the −35°C isotherm to the capsule of the prostate, thus ensu-ring adequate temperatures for cancer destruction everywhere within the prostate. The position of the −35°C temperature isotherm changes in relation to the freezing margin as the iceball grows, being closer to the freezing margin with smaller ice volumes. With more freezing room, cryoprobes can be placed farther into the peripheral zone of the gland, where 80% of cancers reside, making the destructive temperature zone easier to reach the capsule with less freezing volume. This also exposes these cancers to faster freezing rates and colder temperatures, both of which improve the cancer destruction. This has dictated the probe placement array that we now use for whole-gland destruction with probes 1 cm apart and within 5 mm of the capsule (Fig. 3.4). Second, freezing can be extended far enough outside the prostate to also include extracapsular extension of cancer, thereby improving the local control of cancer in high-risk patients. The arrangement of the cryoprobes can be placed into the posterior urethral region to encompass the confluence of the seminal vesicle, thus preventing recurrence in this region. Third, with this move of cryoprobes into the peripheral zone, the freezing of the periurethral tissue is adequate but less intense, which may decrease over time the rate of urethral sloughing.

Temperature Monitoring in Critical Areas and Improved Cryosurgical Protocols

For reliable destruction of cancer by freezing, temperatures must reach certain critical limits. Recent in vitro and in vivo studies have shown that at least two freeze-thaw cycles with temperatures reaching −35°C are needed to reliably destroy prostate cancer cells.[39] Clinical studies have confirmed these parameters as well as the improvement that can occur in clinical results when temperature is monitored by thermocouples placed in critical areas in the prostate and two full freeze-thaw cycles are carried out. We routinely place thermocouples at the capsule in the known area of the tumor and at the apex of the gland when whole-gland destruction is being carried out. In general, thermocouples should be placed equidistant between cryoprobes at the theoretically warmest location, in order to not give misleading results. Thermocouples are also very useful in monitoring temperatures in critical locations to prevent complications. We routinely place a thermocouple into the area of the external sphincter to keep that structure above freezing temperatures and in the area of the neurovascular bundle when nerve sparing is being attempted.

Role of US in Monitoring Prostate Cryosurgery

Modern cryosurgery would be impossible without transrectal US monitoring. *The imaging is needed to accurately place the probes and monitor the extent of freezing to prevent complication such as rectal freezing.* Only a biplane transrectal probe should be used to monitor prostate cryosurgery. All of the monitoring of the freezing process should be carried out by the longitudinal linear array probe because of the shadowing effect caused by the ice. Use of a sector probe overestimates the extent of the freezing, obscuring the margins of the ice in the shadow created by the freezing front, since the margin of the freezing front is at 0°C. The freezing front will not represent the area of reliably destroyed tissue, hence the need for thermocouple monitoring.

Argon-Based Cryosurgical Equipment

The original LN2-based freezing equipment has now been replaced by Joule-Thompson argon gas systems. These systems allow faster freezing rates, which improves the reliability of cancer destruction. The more precise control of the freezing process by gas systems also adds to the safety of the procedure by allowing the freezing process to be stopped in a more timely fashion. Increasing the number of probes from 5 to 8 has allowed a more uniform freezing temperature to be achieved throughout the gland, which also improves results. Increasing the number of probes beyond 8 could have a potentially negative effect. A "cryoseed system" (Galil Medical Inc, Haifa, Israel) that utilizes 17-gaugeneedle probes to create a 1-cm diameter ice ball was not able to totally ablate the prostate gland based on reported PSA results.[40] These poor results are probably the result of the short freezing length of these probes and the difficulty in accurately overlapping the freezing zones along the length of the gland. All the data currently used to gain acceptance of cryosurgery were developed with cryosurgical probes that freeze the length of the gland in one freeze; departing from this concept jeopardizes much of what has been learned about how to obtain consistent results using cryosurgery.

Future Technical Improvements

At the present time, the greatest improvements being made are those that have already been well established in the area of brachytherapy. Since the freezing capabilities of cryoprobes are predictable, planning software is already available to direct proper cryoprobe placement based on gland size and shape. Planning software has now been coupled to guidance software and hardware, which will simplify what was once a totally freehand approach to cryoprobe placement.

Conclusions

As we have seen ultrasound-guided cryoablation holds a unique place among prostate cancer treatments. It has the advantage of extending efficacious treatment to patients who are at particularly high risk for local recurrence and who have failed radiation therapy. With the advent of the concept of focal therapy for prostate cancer cryoablation may make its most important contribution to the care of the prostate cancer patient by offering excellent local tumor control without the attendant morbidity of previous whole-gland treatments.

References

1. Health Care Financing Administration. Medicare Coverage Policy: Decisions. Bagley GP. Cryosurgery ablation of the prostate (#CAG-00031). Available at: http://www.hcfa.gov/coverage/8b-f1 .htm. Accessed November 7, 2001.
2. George N. Therapeutic dilemmas in prostate cancer: justification for watchful waiting. *Eur Urol.* 1998;34(Suppl 3):33–36.
3. Villers A, McNeal JE, Freiha FS, et al. Multiple cancers in the prostate. Morphologic features of clinically recognized vs incidental tumors. *Cancer.* 1992;70:2313–2318.
4. Gondor MJ, Soanes WA, Shulman S. Cryosurgical treatment of the prostate. *Invest Urol.* 1966;3:372–378.
5. Bonney WW, Fallon B, Gerber WL, et al. Cryosurgery in prostatic cancer: survival. *Urology.* 1982;19:37–42.
6. Onik GM, Cohen JK, Reyes GD, et al. Trans-rectal ultrasound guided percutaneous radical cryosurgical ablation of the prostate. *Cancer.* 1993;72:1291–1299.
7. Pisters LL, von Eschenbach AC, Scott SM, et al. The efficacy and complications of salvage cryotherapy of the prostate. *J Urol.* 1997;157:921–925.
8. Wong WS, Chinn DO, Chinn M, et al. Cryosurgery as a treatment for prostate carcinoma: results and complications. *Cancer.* 1997;79:963–974.
9. Cespedes RD, Pisters LL, von Eschenbach AC, et al. Long-term followup of incontinence and obstruction after salvage cryosurgical ablation of the prostate: results in 143 patients. *J Urol.* 1997;157:237–240.
10. Katz A, Rewcastle JC. The current and potential role of cryoablation as a primary treatment for prostate cancer. *Curr Oncol Rep.* 2003;5:231–238.
11. Gould RS. Total cryoablation of the prostate versus standard cryoablation versus radical prostatectomy: comparison of early results and the role of trans-urethral resection in cryoablation. *J Urol.* 1999;162:1653–1657.
12. Onik G, Cooper C, Goldberg HI, et al. Ultrasonic characteristics of frozen liver. *Cryobiology.* 1984;21:321–328.
13. Onik G, Rubinsky B, Zemel R, et al. Ultrasound-guided hepatic cryosurgery in the treatment of metastatic colon carcinoma: preliminary results. *Cancer.* 1991;67:901–907.
14. Ravikumar TS, Kane I, Cady B, et al. A 5-year study of cryosurgery in the treatment of liver tumors. *Arch Surg.* 1991;126:1520–1524.
15. Steele GJr . Cryoablation in hepatic surgery. *Semin Liver Dis.* 1994;14:120–125.
16. Vaidya A, Hawke C, Tiguert R, et al. Intraoperative T staging in radical retropubic prostatectomy: is it reliable? *Urology.* 2001;57:949–954.
17. Partin AW,Yoo J, Carter HB, et al. The use of prostate specific antigen, clinical stage and Gleason score to predict pathological stage in men with localized prostate cancer. *J Urol.* 1993;150:110–114.
18. Tewari A, Narayan P. Novel staging tool for localized prostate cancer: a pilot study using genetic adaptive neural networks. *J Urol.* 1998;160:430–436.
19. Eggleston JC,Walsh PC. Radical prostatectomy with preservation of sexual function: pathological findings in the first 100 cases. *J Urol.* 1985;134:1146–1148.
20. Connolly JA, Shinohara K, Carroll P. Cryosurgery for locally advanced (T3) prostate cancer. *Semin Urol Oncol.* 1997;15:244–249.
21. Miller RJ Jr, Cohen JK, Merlotti LA, et al. Percutaneous transperineal cryosurgical ablation of the prostate for the primary treatment of clinical stage C adenocarcinoma, of the prostate. *Urology.* 1994;44:170–174.
22. Onik G, Narayan P, Brunelle R, et al. Saline injection into Denonvilliers' fascia during prostate cryosurgery. *J Min Ther Relat Tech.* 2000;9:423–427.
23. Bahn DK, Lee F, Bandalament R, et al. 7-year outcomes in the primary treatment of prostate cancer. Urology. 2002;60 (2 Suppl 1):3–11.
24. Pilepich MV,Winter K, John MJ, et al. Phase III radiation therapy oncology group(RTOG) trial 86–10 of androgen deprivation adjuvant to definitive radiotherapy in locally advanced carcinoma of the prostate. *Int J Radiat Oncol Biol Phys.* 2001;50:1243–1252.
25. Lawton CA,Winter K, Murray K, et al. Updated results of the phase III Radiation Therapy Oncology Group (RTOG) trial 85–31 evaluating the potential benefit of androgen suppression following standard radiation therapy for unfavorable prognosis carcinoma of the prostate. *Int J Radiat Oncol Biol Phys.* 2001;49:937–946.
26. Santiago RJ, Wu L, Harris E, Fox K, Schultz D, Glick J, Solin LJ. Fifteen-year results of breast-conserving surgery and definitive irradiation for Stage I and II breast carcinoma: the University of Pennsylvania experience. *Int J Radiat Oncol Biol Phys.* 2004;58(1):233–240.
27. Onik G, Narayan P, Vaughan D, et al. Focal nerve sparing cryoablation for the treatment of primary prostate cancer: A new approach to preserving potency. *Urology.* 2002; 60(1): 109–114.
28. Onik G, Vaughan D, Lotenfoe R et al. The "Male Lumpectomy", focal therapy for prostate cancer using cryoablation *Urology.* 2007;70(6 Suppl):16–21.
29. Djavan B, Susani M, Bursa B, et al. Predictability and significance of multi-focal prostate cancer in the radical prostatectomy specimen. *Tech Urol.* 1999;5(3):139–142.
30. Villers A, McNeal JE, Freiha FS, et al. Multiple cancers in the prostate. Morphologic features of clinically recognized vs. incidental tumors. *Cancer.* 1992;70(9):2312–2318.
31. Rukstalis DB, Goldknopf JL, Crowley EM, et al. Prostate cryoablation: a scientific rationale for future modifications. *Urology.* 2002;60(2):19–25.
32. Noguchi M, Stamey TA, McNeal JE, et al. Prognostic factors for multi-focal prostate cancer in radical prostatectomy specimens: lack of significance of secondary cancers. *J Urol.* 2003;170(2pt1):459–463.
33. Crawford ED, Wilson SS, Torkko KC, et al. Clinical staging of prostate cancer: a computer-simulated study of transperineal prostate biopsy. *BJU Int.* 2005;96(7):999–1004.
34. Onik GM. 3D Global mapping biopsies. A more efficacious method of determining the extent of prostate cancer. Presented at Consensus Conference on Focal Therapy of Prostate Cancer. Orlando, Florida February 24, 2006.
35. Neerhut GJ,Wheeler T, Cantini M, et al. Salvage radical prostatectomy for radiorecurrent adenocarcinoma of the prostate. *J Urol.* 1988;140:544–549.
36. Rainwater LM, Zincke H. Radical prostatectomy after radiation therapy for cancer of the prostate: feasibility and prognosis. *J Urol.* 1988;140:1455–1459.
37. Bales GT, Williams MJ, Sinner M, et al. Short-term outcomes after cryosurgical ablation of the prostate in men with recurrent prostate carcinoma following radiation therapy. *Urology.* 1995;46:676–680.
38. de la Taille A, Hayek O, Benson MC, et al. Salvage cryotherapy for recurrent prostate cancer after radiation therapy: the Columbia experience. *Urology.* 2000;55:79–84.
39. Tatsutani K,Rubinsky B,Onik GM, et al. Effect of thermal variables on frozen human primary prostatic adenocarcinoma cells. *Urology.* 1996;48:441–447.
40. Moore Y, Sofer P. Successful treatment of locally confined prostate cancer with the seed net system: preliminary multi-center results. Clinical Application Notes Feb 2001. Available through Galil Medical, Haifa, at http://Galilmedical.com. Accessed November 7, 2001.

Chapter 4
Recent Advance in TRUS-Guided Prostate Brachytherapy

Zhouping Wei, Mingyue Ding, Donal B. Downey, and Aaron Fenster

Introduction

The prostate, which is typically the size of a walnut, is a variable-sized gland that is located in the male pelvis. The urethra, which is surrounded by the prostate, travels through the center of the prostate and carries urine from the bladder to the penis.

Three potential problems can occur within a prostate: benign prostatic hyperplasia (BPH) (a nonmalignant enlargement of the prostate gland), prostatitis (inflammation of the prostate due to bacterial infection), and prostate cancer (an abnormal growth of malignant cells that usually starts in the peripheral zone of the prostate). Prostate cancer is the leading cause of death among men in North America. Autopsies have revealed small prostatic carcinomas in up to 29% of men 30–40 years of age and up to 64% of men 60–70 years of age.[1] In 2006, Canadian Cancer Statistics reports that 20,700 Canadians will be diagnosed with prostate cancer and 4,200 will die of prostate cancer.[2] In the United States, it is estimated that 218,890 new cases of prostate cancer will be diagnosed, and 27,050 American men will die from prostate cancer in 2007.[3]

Initially, cancer cells are confined within the prostate ducts and glands; however, in time, the cancer develops the ability to exit the ducts and migrates into the blood and lymphatic system. Prostate cancer can spread not only through lymphatic channels, producing metastases in pelvic lymph nodes, but also through the blood, producing metastases elsewhere in the body, particularly in the bones.

Currently, there are four standard treatments used for clinically localized prostate cancer, i.e., cancer that is still confined within the prostate: watchful waiting, radical prostatectomy (RP), external beam radiation therapy (EBRT), and brachytherapy.[4]

1. *Watchful Waiting*. During this period, the physician closely observes the cancer without initiating treatment. Watchful waiting represents a practical approach to those patients who are not at significant risk of dying from prostate cancer. Patients considered for this approach are typically men over the age of 70, or men at a lower risk of dying from prostate cancer.
2. *Radical prostatectomy (RP)*. This approach involves the surgical removal of the prostate gland, seminal vesicles, and a varying number of pelvic lymph nodes. RP offers the complete removal of prostate cancer within the patient. Patients who are considered candidates for RP are those who are in good health and those with a life expectancy of 10 years or more.
3. *External beam radiation therapy (EBRT)*. In EBRT, radiation is emitted from a linear accelerator. EBRT can potentially kill prostate cancer cells using a series of radiation treatments administered for a length of time. This approach has been recommended as a potential treatment option for patients who have localized cancer, who have a life expectancy of more than 10 years, and who are unable or unwilling to undergo RP.
4. *Brachytherapy*. Brachytherapy is a form of radiation therapy in which radioactive sources are implanted into the prostate permanently or temporarily. Candidates for the implantation of permanent radioactive sources are men with prostate volumes less than 60 cm^3, Gleason histologic scores <6, and PSA < 10 n ml^{-1}. However, candidates for the temporary implantation of radioactive sources are less limited. Patients with variably sized prostates, PSA levels, and Gleason scores are eligible to receive temporary implantations of radioactive sources.

Prostate Brachytherapy

While watchful waiting is an option for some low-risk patients, most North American patients expect, and may require, active treatment. However, although it has an excellent cure rate, RP may cause serious complications, such as incontinence, impotence, and contracture of the bladder neck. Compared with RP, EBRT has a lower risk for impotence and incontinence. Because the radiation beam passes through normal tissues on its way to the prostate, some healthy cells are killed. In addition, EBRT needs daily dose treatment, each of which requires realignment of the beams. A study has shown that for over half of the patients treated with EBRT, 5 mm or greater

O. Ukimura and I.S. Gill (eds.), *Contemporary Interventional Ultrasonography in Urology*,
DOI: 10.1007/978-1-84800-217-3_4, © Springer-Verlag London Limited 2009

realignment errors had occurred within EBRT treatments.[5] Therefore, EBRT can miss cancer cells, seriously damaging nearby normal cells.

Compared with RP, brachytherapy is minimally invasive: it involves no incisions or sutures; it essentially produces no blood loss. With accurate placement, brachytherapy can confine high dose of radiation to the prostate, dramatically limiting treatment-related complications by minimizing the radiation to nearby organs.[6] The results of treatment from the limited number of available comparative studies did not show any difference in the clinical effectiveness of RP, EBRT, or brachytherapy.[7] In addition, brachytherapy has the potential to achieve sharp demarcation between irradiated volume and healthy structures, achieving superior tumor control with significantly reduced morbidity and side effects in comparison to other treatment modalities and techniques.[8]

Currently, two different approaches to prostate brachytherapy are possible: temporary afterloading high dose rate (HDR) radioactive source (e.g., iridium-192) and permanent implantation of low dose rate (LDR) isotopes with low energy and short half-lives (e.g., iodine-125 and palladium-103).[9] An HDR procedure involves the placement of a hollowed catheter array into the prostate followed by the insertion of iridium-192. After the treatment has completed, iridium-192 (and the catheters) are removed and no radiation is left in the patient. In an LDR procedure, the radioactive seeds (iodine-125 or palladium-103) are permanently implanted into the prostate; therefore, over the course of their radioactive lives, the seeds will continuously emit low levels of radiation. Permanent seed implantation is technically easier to implement and perform. It, therefore, receives the most clinical interest. Since Holm et al. first described the use of transrectal ultrasound (TRUS) to guide transperineal insertion of needles into the prostate to permanently deposit iodine-125 sources into the gland,[10] two-dimensional (2D) TRUS-guided LDR prostate brachytherapy has become the standard approach to prostate therapy. This chapter will discuss the method of applying three-dimensional (3D) TRUS guidance with robot assistance in order to improve current LDR prostate brachytherapy procedures. LDR brachytherapy will be referred to simply as brachytherapy.

In an effort to achieve an optimal geometry of the implanted sources, a template is used in current prostate brachytherapy. With the patient in the lithotomic position, the template, which acts as a guide for each needle placement, is held rigidly in place over the perineum. This placement allows the physician to control the entire prostate target volume and to specify the placement of each radioactive source at any point within the gland. Within the pelvis, if the prostate is imaged in 3D, then any point within the prostate can be given a unique set of coordinates using the grid on the template to determine the X and Y coordinates and using the distance from the plane of the template at the perineum to define the Z coordinate. For every increment of 5 mm from the "zero plane" at the base of the prostate to the apex, TRUS can be used to map the area of the gland onto this grid. This mapping creates a series of 2D images that can be used to create a 3D target volume. Computers, which are used for treatment planning, can then use this planning target volume to develop a pattern for radioactive source placement that will deliver the desired dose. This treatment pattern is called the preimplant plan (or preplan). The position of each source is defined by the grid coordinate system that follows from the chosen template along with its depth or distance from the template.

Implantation is performed during a subsequent visit. The patient is positioned in a similar orientation to the preplanning position. Each of the needles is placed in the pattern that is determined by the preplan. The number of seeds to be placed in each needle and the spacing between seeds are determined by the preplan as well; however, the plan may be modified intraoperatively using real-time adjustments in the 2D TRUS image planes in order to improve the accuracy of the final distribution. These adjustments are made to compensate for the errors caused by the displacement of the prostate.

Among physicians, it is generally agreed that postoperative dosimetry must be performed to assess the adequacy of implantation and to determine the actual dose received by the prostate and normal tissues.[11] This process usually requires a postimplantation CT scan so that the position of the seeds in the prostate capsule (as well as critical tissues) can be outlined, and a full reconstruction of dose and volume can be made.[12]

Limitation of Current Brachytherapy

Although current prostate brachytherapy is widely accepted, it still suffers from limitations and variability due to the following four factors that have limited the full potential of prostate brachytherapy: pubic arch interference (PAI), geometric changes in the prostate, prostate trauma due to seed implantation, and prostate variations.

1. PAI with the implant path occurs in many patients with large prostates (>60 cm^3) and in some patients with a small pelvis. The PAI patients cannot be treated with current brachytherapy before their prostates have been shrunken using hormonal therapy – a separate process that typically takes 3–9 months,[13,14] because the anterior and/or the anterolateral parts of their prostate are blocked by the pubic bone using parallel needle trajectories guided by a fixed template.
2. Geometric changes occurring in the prostate between the preplan scan and the implantation scan will lead to incorrect seed placement. It has been shown that the prostate volume can change by as much as 50% in the time between the preplan and implantation.[15]
3. Seed implant procedures induce trauma and cause the prostate to swell due to edema.[16] Clearly, variations of prostate shape and volume during the procedure may result in "misplaced" seeds and lack of proper dose coverage. The AAPM TASK Group 64 has identified this as an issue that requires attention.[17]

4. Prostate variations and changes between seed implantation, postoperative dosimetry (and other factors such as TRUS imaging artifacts); migration of the seeds in the needle tracks, and needle deflection will lead to potential inaccuracies.[18] Discrepancies have also been reported between CT- and TRUS-based prostate volume measurements.[19] These factors could also incur wrong determination of dose coverage.

Potential Solutions

To solve several of the aforementioned problems, which are associated with current prostate brachytherapy, some researchers have proposed dynamic intraoperative procedure – an encompassing procedure that is carried out entirely in one session, including planning, monitoring of prostate changes, dynamic replanning, and optimal needle implantation (including oblique trajectories).[20]

TRUS-guided prostate planning and implantation are being used extensively in current prostate brachytherapy procedures; 2D TRUS imaging as well as 3D reconstruction provide a direct description of the 3D space. In recent years, many advances have been made in 3D ultrasound (US) imaging of the prostate,[21,22] US image processing for prostate boundary segmentation,[23–27] pubic arch detection,[13] needle segmentation,[28,29] and seed segmentation.[30] These advances have greatly enhanced the role of US in clinical diagnosis and image-guided surgery.

Because a robot can position, orient, and manipulate surgical tools along various trajectories in 3D space accurately and consistently, medical robotic systems have been achieving an increasing role in various image-guided surgical procedures. The mobility of the robot is important because it helps to free the insertion of the needle from the constraints of the parallel trajectory, allowing an oblique insertion of the needle to occur. Robotic systems can also be dynamically programmed, controlled, and effectively integrated with 3D imaging systems so that the robot can be instructed to target any point identified in the 3D image. Although they introduce more complex instrumentation and increased hardware costs, robotic approaches provide significant advantages and cost-saving techniques. As a result, medical robotic approaches are being extensively explored. Several research teams have already investigated the possibilities to use robot in prostate therapy.[31–33]

System Description

Before we describe the approach for robotic assistance, some consideration will be given to the tasks that are required for robot-assisted brachytherapy with 3D TRUS guidance. These tasks can be divided into two sections: preimplantation planning (or preplanning) and seed implantation. For the preplanning stage, the physician's tasks consist of positioning the patient, obtaining the 3D TRUS images of the prostate, and sending the 3D TRUS images to a medical physicist who determines the placement of the seeds. During seed implantation, needles, which implant seeds at various preplanned locations, are inserted into the prostate so that the total amount of preplanned radioactive dose is delivered. Therefore, before the implantation of seeds can begin, a method of registering the patient to the implantation system (i.e., the robot system) is required. This registration method differs among varying system designs.

Hardware Components

Figures 4.1 and 4.2 show the prototype of the robotic-assisted system with 3D TRUS guidance for prostate brachytherapy. The prototype consists of a 3D TRUS imaging system, which was developed in our laboratory,[21,22] and a robot with 6 degrees of freedom (dof). To evaluate the feasibility of the proposed approach, we used a CRS *A465* commercial robot system (Thermo-CRS, Burlington, Ontario, Canada); however, the software was developed to allow for the integration of the 3D TRUS imaging system with any robot with 6 dof.

The 3D TRUS imaging system consists of a Pentium III personal computer (PC) with a 1.2-GHz processor (for 3D image acquisition, reconstruction, and display), a Matrox Meteor II video frame grabber (for 30 Hz video image acquisition), a mover controller module (MCM), which controls the rotation of the transducer-mover assembly via the serial port of the computer, and a B-K Medical 2102 Hawk ultrasound machine (B-K, Denmark) with an *8558/S* 7.5 MHz side-firing linear array transducer. To produce a 3D US image, the *MCM* and the motor assembly rotate the transducer over an angle of approximately 120° about its long axis, while a series of 2D US images are digitized at 0.7° intervals by a frame grabber. These acquired images are reconstructed into a 3D image, which is available for viewing as the 2D images are being acquired. The 3D US image can be viewed using 3D visualization software,

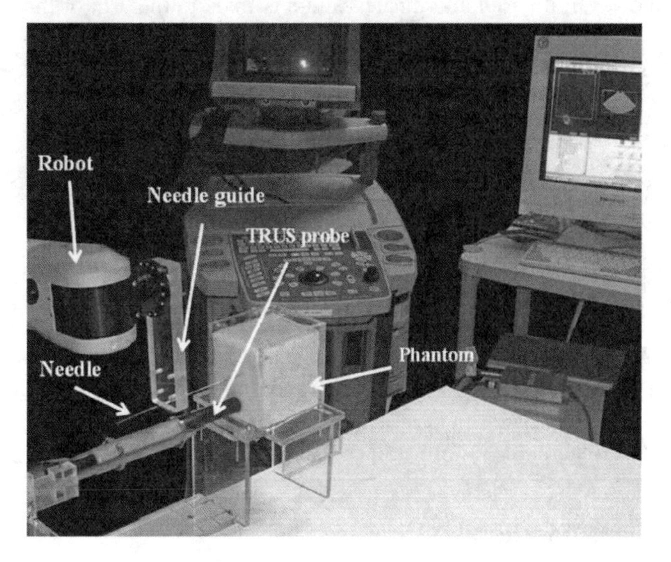

FIG. 4.1. The prototype of the robot-assisted and 3D TRUS-guided prostate brachytherapy system

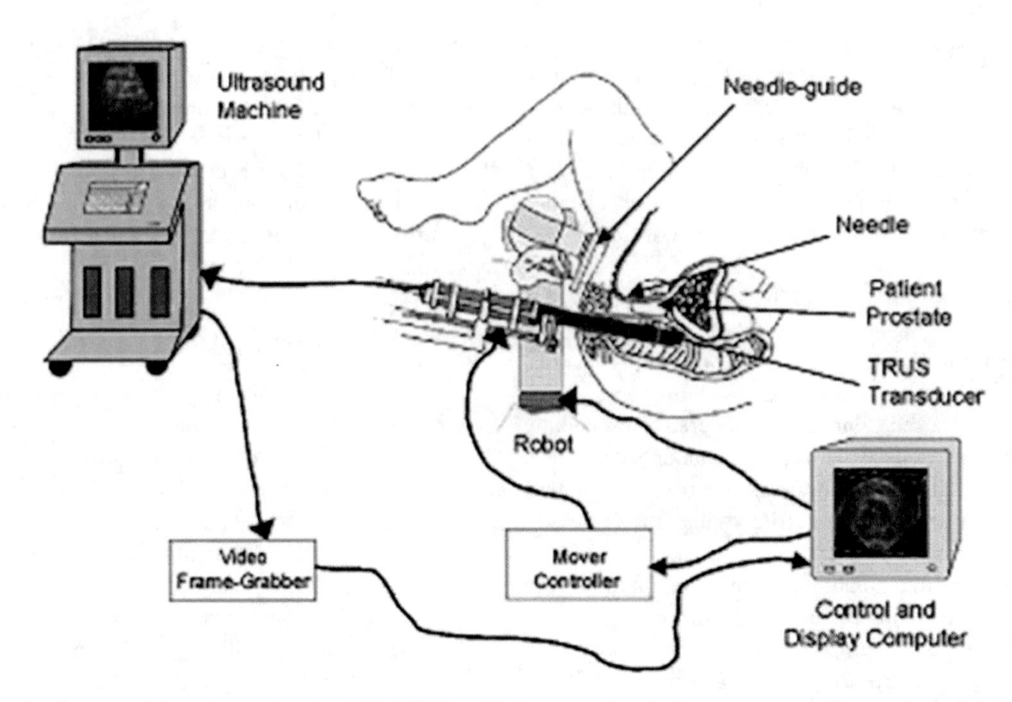

FIG. 4.2. Schematic diagram of the robot-assisted and 3D TRUS-guided prostate brachytherapy system. The rotation of the TRUS transducer is controlled by the mover controller. A video frame grabber is used for image acquisition. The acquired images are reconstructed into a 3D image and displayed in the computer. The robot is controlled to move to a position, so that the needle can be guided via the needle guide to a target identified in the 3D TRUS image

including multiplanar reformatting tools for viewing any plane in the 3D image, as well as measurement tools.[22]

The robot includes a robotic arm assembly with 6 dof (three translational, three rotational), a PC-based kinematics positioning software system, and a robot controller. The positioning software of the robot system can control the robotic arm assembly via the controller in terms of *world/tool* coordinate systems. The *world* coordinate system is fixed to the ground; however, the tool coordinate system is fixed to the arm of the robot. As the arms of the robot move, the position and orientation of the tool coordinate system change, as well. The robot control software has been integrated together with the 3D visualization software so that precise image-based planning of the robot path can be performed; multiple potential trajectories can also be viewed by using a graphical user interface. The needle guide for manually inserting the needle is attached to the arm of the robot, which has one hole for needle guidance. Because the needle guide is attached to the arm of the robot, the position and orientation of the needle guide hole (in the robot tool coordinate system) is known. A transformation is performed by a software module, calibrating the robot tool coordinate system to the world coordinate system so that the guidance hole can be described in the robot world coordinate system.

System Calibration

Integration of the 3D TRUS image-based coordinate system with the robotic coordinate system is required in order to allow for accurate needle target planning and insertion under 3D TRUS guidance. This approach involves two calibration steps: (1) calibration of the 3D US image to the coordinate system of the transducer (image calibration), and (2) calibration of the transducer to the coordinate system of the robot (robot calibration).

The transformation between any two different coordinate systems is found by solving the orthogonal Procrustes problem as follows[34]:

Given two 3D sets of points, $K = \{k_j\}$, $L = \{l_j\}$ for $j = 1, 2, \ldots, N$, we determine a rigid-body transformation such that F: $l_j = F(k_j) = \mathbf{R}\,k_j + \mathbf{T}$, where $\mathbf{R}$ is a 3×3 rotation matrix, and $\mathbf{T}$ is a 3×1 translation vector by minimizing the cost function:

$$C = \frac{1}{N}\sum_{j=1}^{N}\left\| l_j - (\mathbf{R}k_j + \mathbf{T})\right\|^2. \quad (4.1)$$

A unique solution to (4.1) exists if and only if the sets of points, K and L, contain at least four noncoplanar points.[35]

As shown in Fig. 4.3, the phantom used for the calibration of the image comprised seven 1-mm-diameter nylon strings positioned in a $14 \times 14 \times 14$ cm^3 Plexiglas box [**26a**]. The side of the Plexiglas box has a hole to simulate the rectum and to accommodate the TRUS transducer. The nylon strings were immersed in agar and were placed in three layers 1 cm apart. The strings were arranged with known separations, forming noncoplanar intersections. In the coordinate system of the transducer, the coordinates of these intersections were known

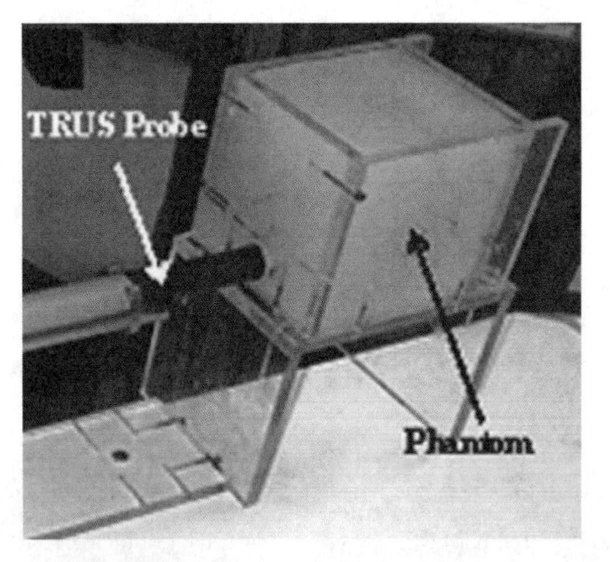

FIG. 4.3. Photograph of the image calibration phantom with the transducer inserted into the simulated rectum

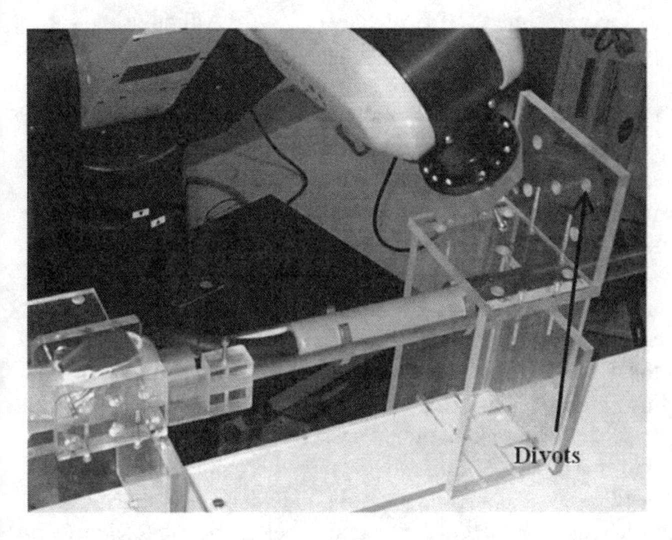

FIG. 4.4. The plates for robot calibration. The positions of the divots in the transducer coordinate system are all known through the phantom design. The positions of the divots in the robot coordinate system are determined by moving the robot to touch these divots as shown in this figure

from the phantom design; in the 3D TRUS coordinate system, the coordinates of the intersections were determined by scanning the intersections. Using the coordinates of the string intersections in both coordinate systems, we solved (4.1) in order to determine the transformation linking the two coordinate systems.

For the calibration of the robot, two orthogonal plates mounted on the transducer holder were used and drilled with ten hemispherical divots. Figure 4.4 shows these calibration plates along with the divots on each of the plates. Homologous points in the coordinate systems of the transducer and the robot are provided by the centers of the hemispherical divots on the two plates. The coordinates of these divot centers in the robot coordinate system were determined by moving the robot, sequentially touching the divots with a stylus tip, which was attached to the arm of the robot. Using the coordinates of the divots in the two coordinate systems, we solved (4.1) in order to determine the transformation linking the two coordinate systems.

Software Tools

Software tools are indispensable components in a 3D TRUS-guided robot-assisted system for prostate brachytherapy; they should include following items: prostate segmentation, needle segmentation, seed segmentation, and dosimetry.

Prostate Segmentation

Outlining the margins of the prostate manually is time consuming and tedious; therefore, an accurate, reproducible, and fast semi- or fully automated prostate segmentation technique is required. Because 3D US images suffer from shadowing, speckle, and poor contrast, fully automated segmentation procedures, at times, result in unacceptable errors. Our approach has been to develop a semiautomated prostate segmentation technique that allows the user to correct for errors.[25]

In our approach, the prostate is segmented as a series of cross-sectional 2D images obtained from the 3D TRUS image. The resulting set of boundaries is assembled into a single 3D prostate boundary. Our 3D prostate segmentation algorithm has been described in detail in previous publications.[25] As shown in Fig. 4.5, this algorithm consists of the following three steps:

(1) The operator manually initializes the algorithm by selecting four or more points on the prostate boundary (in one central prostate 2D slice). A curve passing through these points is then calculated and is used as the initial estimate of the prostate boundary (Fig. 4.5a).
(2) The curve is converted to a polygon with equally spaced points, which are then deformed using a Discrete Dynamic Contour algorithm until reaching equilibrium (Fig. 4.5b). If required, the polygon can be edited by manually repositioning selected vertices.
(3) The boundary of the 2D segmented prostate in one slice is extended to 3D by propagating the contour to an adjacent slice and repeating the deformation process (Fig. 4.5c). This process is accomplished by slicing the prostate in radial slices separated by a constant angle (e.g., 3°) intersecting along an axis approximately in the center of the prostate.[25]

Needle Segmentation

As described in sections "Hardware Components" and "System Calibration", 3D TRUS-guided robot-assisted prostate brachytherapy allows oblique needle insertion during seed implantation. Thus, the needle may be inserted in an oblique trajectory, which results in the image of the needle passing out

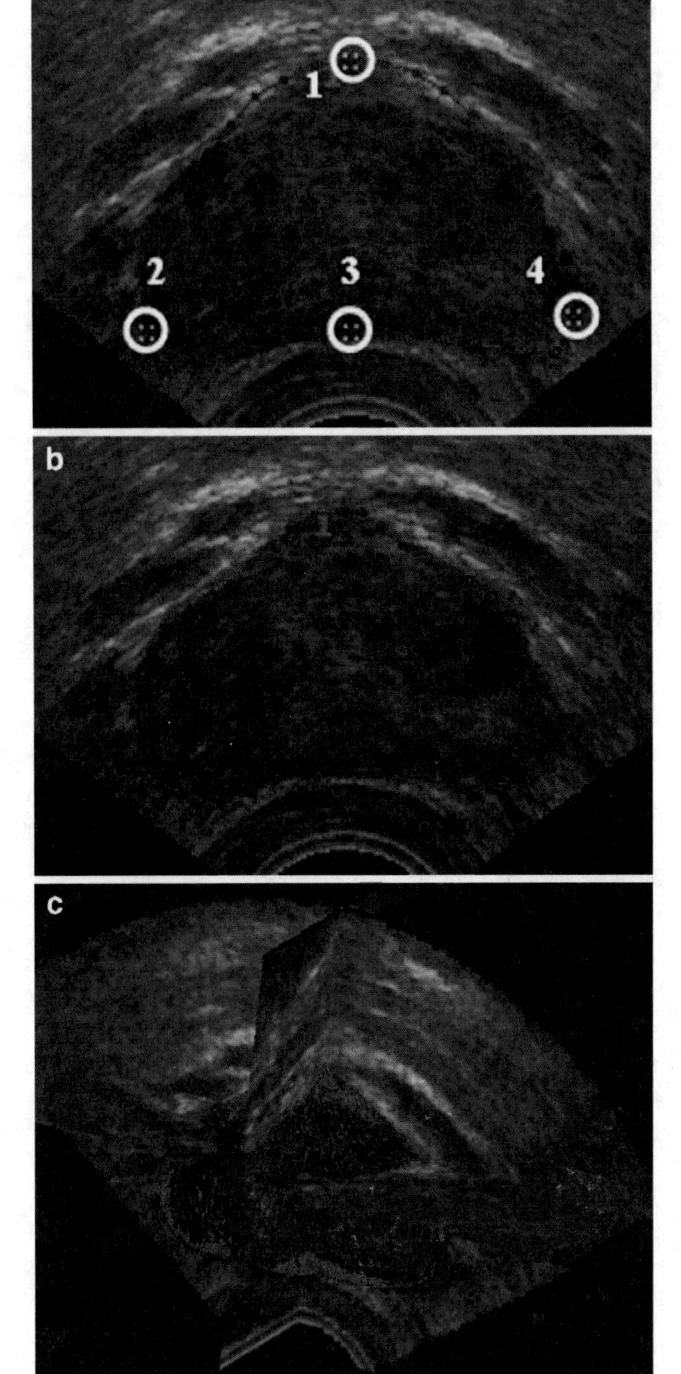

FIG. 4.5. Images showing the steps of the 3D prostrate segmentation algorithm. The 3D TRUS image is first resliced into 2D slices. (**a**) The user initializes the algorithm by placing four or more points on the boundary as shown. A model-based interpolation approach is used to generate an initial contour. (**b**) A deformable dynamic contour (DDC) approach is used to refine the initial contour until it matches the prostate boundary. (**c**) The contour is propagated to adjacent 2D slices of the 3D TRUS image and refined using the DDC. The process is repeated until the complete prostate is segmented as shown

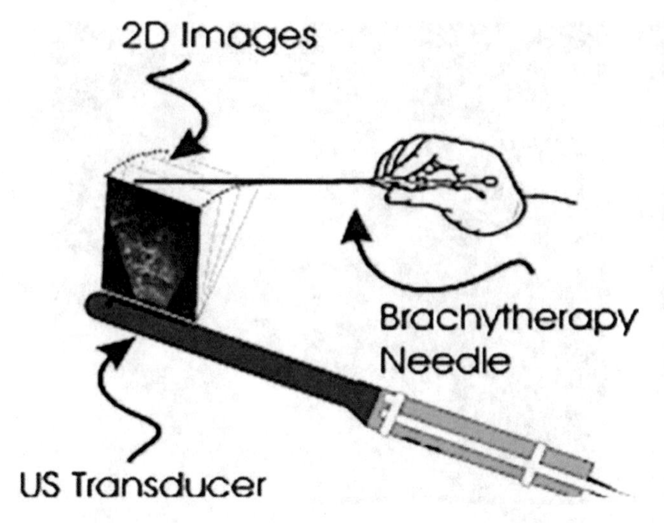

FIG. 4.6. The brachytherapy needle leaves the real-time 2D TRUS image for an oblique insertion, and the needle will only appear as a dot in the 2D US image, leading to suboptimal guidance

of the real-time 2D US image (Fig. 4.6). Although the robot possesses high positioning and angulation accuracies, and the robot and 3D US systems can be accurately related to each other through a careful calibration, the needle coordinates reported by the robot do not describe the actual needle trajectories due to needle deflection.[18] While the needle is being inserted into the prostate, visual tracking of the needle tip in an US image is necessary to ensure proper placement and to avoid implanting seeds outside the prostate. Automated segmentation of the needle during an oblique (as well as parallel) needle insertion would allow the position and orientation of the needle to be determined. As a result, rapid dynamic replanning could be performed based on the actual needle trajectory and seed locations to obtain an optimum 3D dose distribution within a prostate. Thus, we developed a technique to track the needle as it is being inserted obliquely.[36]

In our approach, we use gray-level change detection technique (i.e., values derived by comparing the gray-level values of the images before and after the need has been inserted and processed.). Because the needle may be angled, maximally, 20° from the orientation of the 2D US plane, and 2D images may be acquired at 30 images per second, a new 3D image may be formed in less than 1 s. From these 3D images, the needle may be segmented automatically, and the three planes needed to visualize the needle insertion may be displayed. The needle segmentation algorithm is composed of the following five steps:

(1) A 3D difference image of the gray-level change between the prescan and the live-scan is generated. The needle contrast in the difference image can be enhanced by suppressing the background noise caused by the implanted seeds and needle tracks.
(2) The needle candidate voxels from the background is segmented through a thresholding operation.
(3) Spurious needle candidate voxels are further removed.

(4) Linear regression of the needle candidate voxels is performed in order to determine the orientation of the needle in 3D space.
(5) The needle top position in 3D space is determined.

Figure 4.7 shows the result of the needle segmentation algorithm using a chicken phantom, which simulates the clinical environment. Figure 4.7a, b displays the needle in the reconstructed oblique sagittal and coronal planes. Figure 4.8 shows the result of the needle segmentation algorithm in a patient image that was obtained during a prostate cryotherapy procedure.

Seed Segmentation

Postimplant dosimetry is an important step in the treatment process. Thus, the American Brachytherapy Society (ABS) has recommended that postimplant dosimetry should be performed on all patients undergoing permanent prostate brachytherapy.[37] However, segmentation of the implanted radioactive seeds in US images of the prostate is made difficult by image speckle, low contrast, signal loss due to shadowing, and refraction and reverberation artifacts. To solve these problems, we proposed an algorithm,[30] which uses 3D TRUS

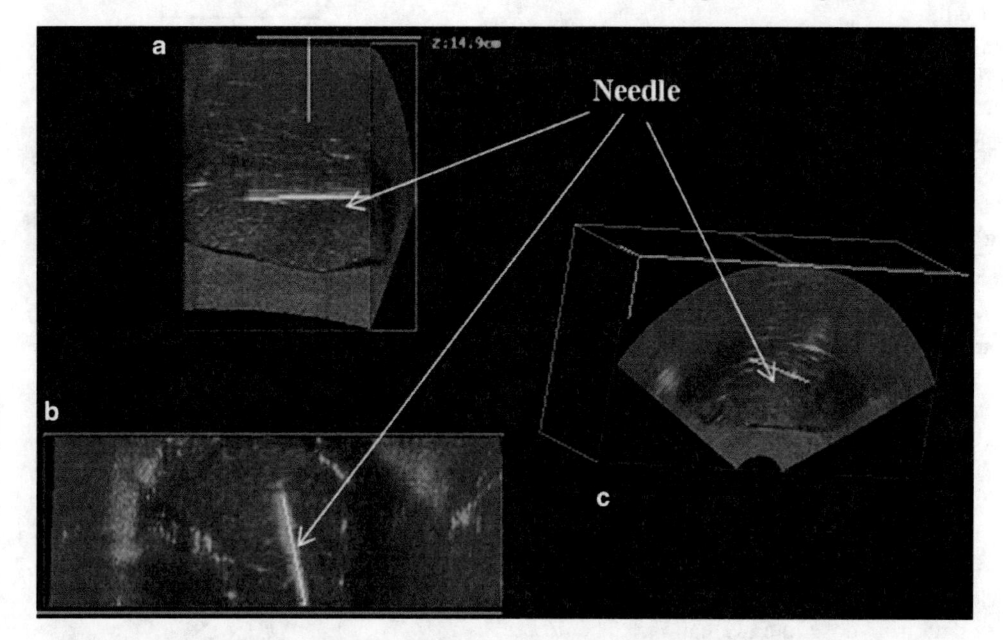

Fig. 4.7. A result of needle segmentation during insertion of a needle into a chicken phantom simulating clinical environment. (**a**) Oblique sagittal view; (**b**) oblique coronal plane; (**c**) transverse view with needle projected

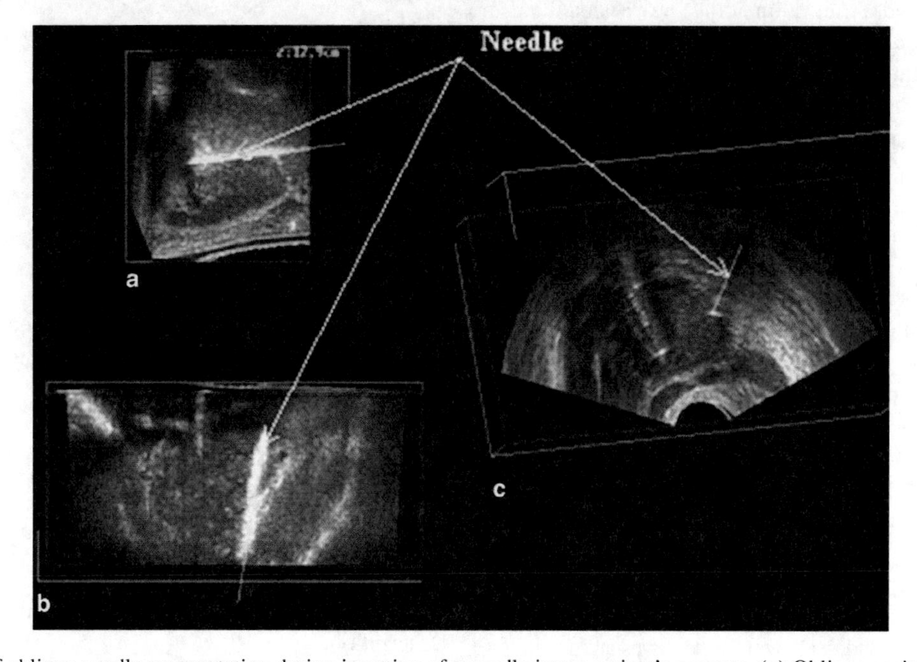

Fig. 4.8. A result of oblique needle segmentation during insertion of a needle into a patient's prostate. (**a**) Oblique sagittal view; (**b**) oblique coronal plane; (**c**) transverse view with needle projected

imaging and *prior* knowledge of the needle position described in the section "Dosimetry." The following six steps describe the algorithm as follows:

(1) A 3D difference image of the gray-level change is generated by subtracting the image before the needle has been inserted, from the image after the seeds have been implanted and the needle has been withdrawn from the prostate.
(2) The searching space from the whole 3D TRUS image is narrowed by the algorithm to contain a smaller cylinder around the needle.
(3) The seed candidate voxel is segmented from the background in the search cylinder using a thresholding operation.
(4) The seed candidate voxels are grouped to find the candidate seeds.
(5) The center location, orientation, and size of a seed are determined using 3D principal component analysis (PCA).
(6) Spurious seeds are further removed from the candidate seeds.

Steps (1)–(6) are repeated until all the seeds have been implanted and localized. Figure 4.9 shows the flowchart of the seed segmentation algorithm. Figure 4.10 shows an image of the segmented seeds in 3D TRUS images of chicken phantoms using the seed segmentation algorithm.

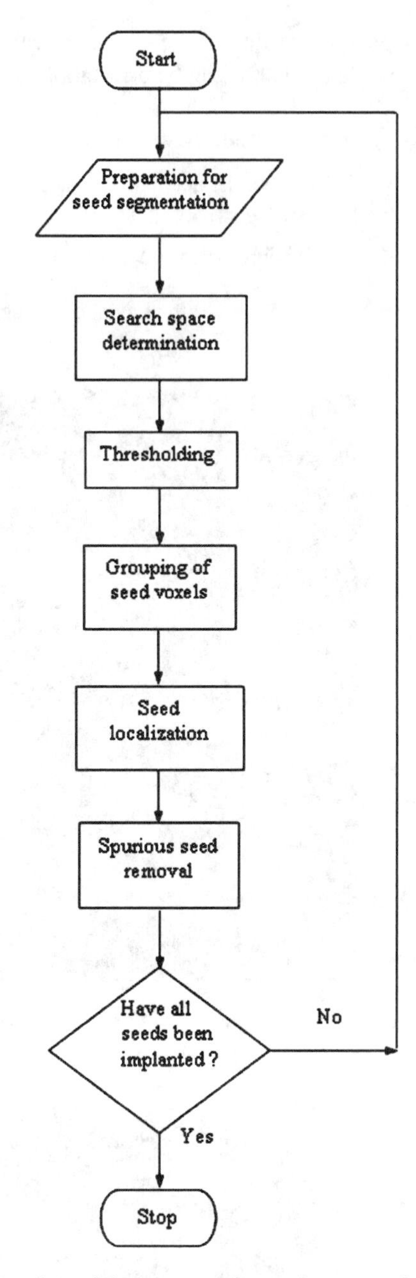

FIG. 4.9. Flowchart of the intraoperative seed segmentation algorithm

Dosimetry

We use the AAPM TG-43 formalism, which uses predetermined dosimetry data from dose rate evaluation.[38] The dose can be calculated by either considering the sources oriented in a line in any trajectory, or as point sources where source orientation is ignored. After delineating the organs, the user selects the type of source to be used and enters its calibration data. Considering the effects of PAI, the area of possible needle insertions is outlined and the preplan is produced. The preplan consists of about 20 needles, which can be oriented in oblique trajectories to avoid PAI. The isodose curves are displayed on the 3D TRUS image in real time as well as on a surface rendered view with the needles and the seeds. Each needle can also be activated and deactivated individually, and the modified isodose curves can be observed instantly. The user can evaluate the plan using dose volume histograms for each organ and make necessary modifications. Figure 4.11 shows an example of the use of the preplan software for oblique trajectory needle planning.

During a live planning procedure in the operating room (OR), after inserting each needle, the location of the actual needle is determined; the isodose curves are modified and displayed in real time. This procedure helps the user to decide whether the needle position is satisfactory. After retracting the needle, the actual seed locations are determined (currently we use assumed positions) and the new isodose curves are displayed. At this time, the user has the option of modifying the rest of the plan according to the "real" seed locations after the needle retraction.

System Evaluation

The following experiments were performed in order to evaluate our 3D TRUS-guided and robot-assisted prostate brachytherapy system, as described in the section "System Description."

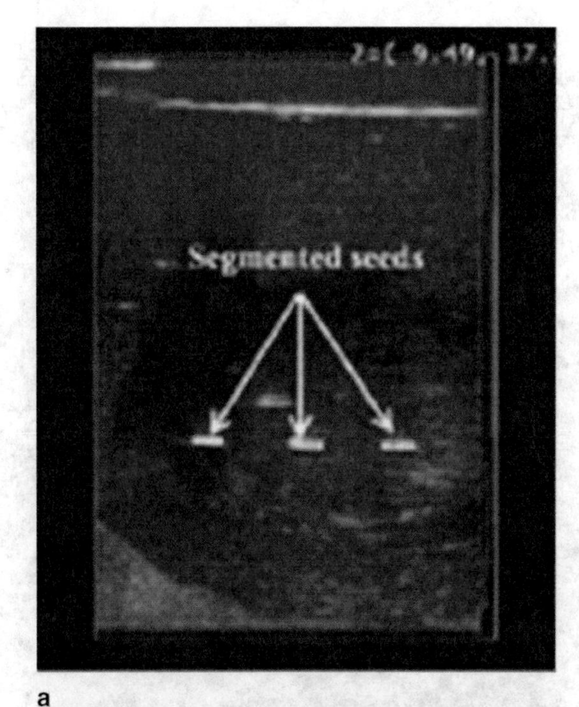

a

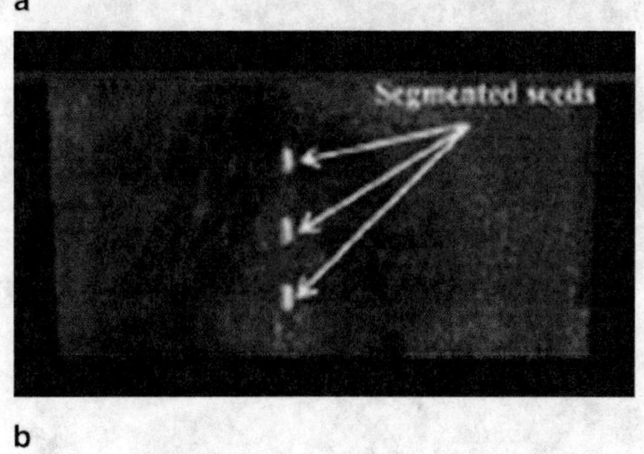

b

FIG. 4.10. An example image of the segmented seeds in a 3D TRUS image of the chicken phantom. (**a**) Saggital view; (**b**) Coronal view

Evaluation of Calibration

Method

Accuracy analysis of the image and robot calibrations was performed via the method for analyzing accuracy of point-based rigid-body registration.[39] This method involves the analysis of three errors: fiducial localization error (FLE), fiducial registration error (FRE), and target registration error (TRE).

FLE: The FLE is defined as the error in locating fiducial points used in the registration procedure.[40] We assumed that the mean value of the error in locating the fiducial points is zero and we calculated the root-mean-square (rms) distance between the exact and calculated fiducial positions[41]:

$$\begin{cases} \mathrm{FLE}_i^2 = \sigma_{ix}^2 + \sigma_{iy}^2 + \sigma_{iz}^2 \\ \mathrm{FLE}^2 = \dfrac{1}{N}\sum_{i=1}^{N} \mathrm{FLE}_i^2 \end{cases}. \tag{4.2}$$

The variances of the error in locating the fiducials points along the three orthogonal axes are σ_x^2, σ_y^2, and σ_z^2. Each of the terms in (4.2) is calculated as follows:

$$\sigma_{ij}^2 = \frac{1}{n-1}\sum_{k=1}^{n}(x_{ijk} - \overline{x}_{ij})^2 \tag{4.3}$$

The components (i.e., x, y, or z) are represented by $j = 1, 2, 3$, x_{ijk} is the kth measurement for ith fiducial point (for image calibration, $i = 1, 2, 3, 4$, and for robot calibration, $i = 1, 2, \ldots, 6$), and k is the number of measurements for each fiducial point. For both calibrations of image and robot, $n = 10$, and, $\overline{x}_{ij} = \frac{1}{10}\sum_{k=1}^{10} x_{ijk}$ is the mean measurement for the jth component of the ith fiducial point.

FRE: The exact positions of N fiducials in the transducer coordinate system, $\mathrm{P} = \{\mathbf{p}_j; j = 1, \ldots, N\}$, are known for either the image calibration phantom (Fig. 4.3) or the robot calibration plates (Fig. 4.4). For image calibration, we measured the positions of N fiducials (from the intersection of the nylon strings) in 3D TRUS image coordinate systems, $\mathrm{Q} = \{\mathbf{q}_j; j = 1, \ldots, N\}$. For robot calibration, we measured the positions of N fiducials (small divots), $\mathrm{Q} = \{\mathbf{q}_j; j = 1, \ldots, N\}$, in robot coordinate system by moving the robot to touch the small divots. The FRE is calculated as the *rms* distance between the corresponding fiducial positions, before and after registration:

$$\mathrm{FRE} = \sqrt{\frac{\sum_{j=1}^{N} \left\| q_j - F(p_j) \right\|^2}{N}}. \tag{4.4}$$

The rigid body transformation, F, registers the exact fiducial positions, P, with the measured fiducial positions, Q.

TRE: TRE is defined as the distance between the corresponding points (other than the fiducial points) before and after registration. The TRE is calculated by (4.4). We used four targets in the image calibration phantom to determine the TRE for image calibration; four other markers on the plates were used to determine the TRE for robot calibration.[33]

Results

Our ability to localize the intersections of the nylon strings in the 3D TRUS image for the calibration of the image was analyzed along the X-, Y-, and Z-directions; Table 4.1 shows the average fiducial localization error (FLE). From Table 4.1, it can be seen that the FLE for localizing the intersection of the strings is similar in the X- or Y-directions and larger in the Z-direction. This is attributed to the fact that the resolution in the X- and Y-directions (i.e., lateral and axial directions in the original acquired images) is best. The larger FLE in the Z-direction, which corresponded to the elevation (i.e., out-of-plane) direction of the acquired 2D images, is due to the poorer out-of-plane resolution in the 3D TRUS image.[22]

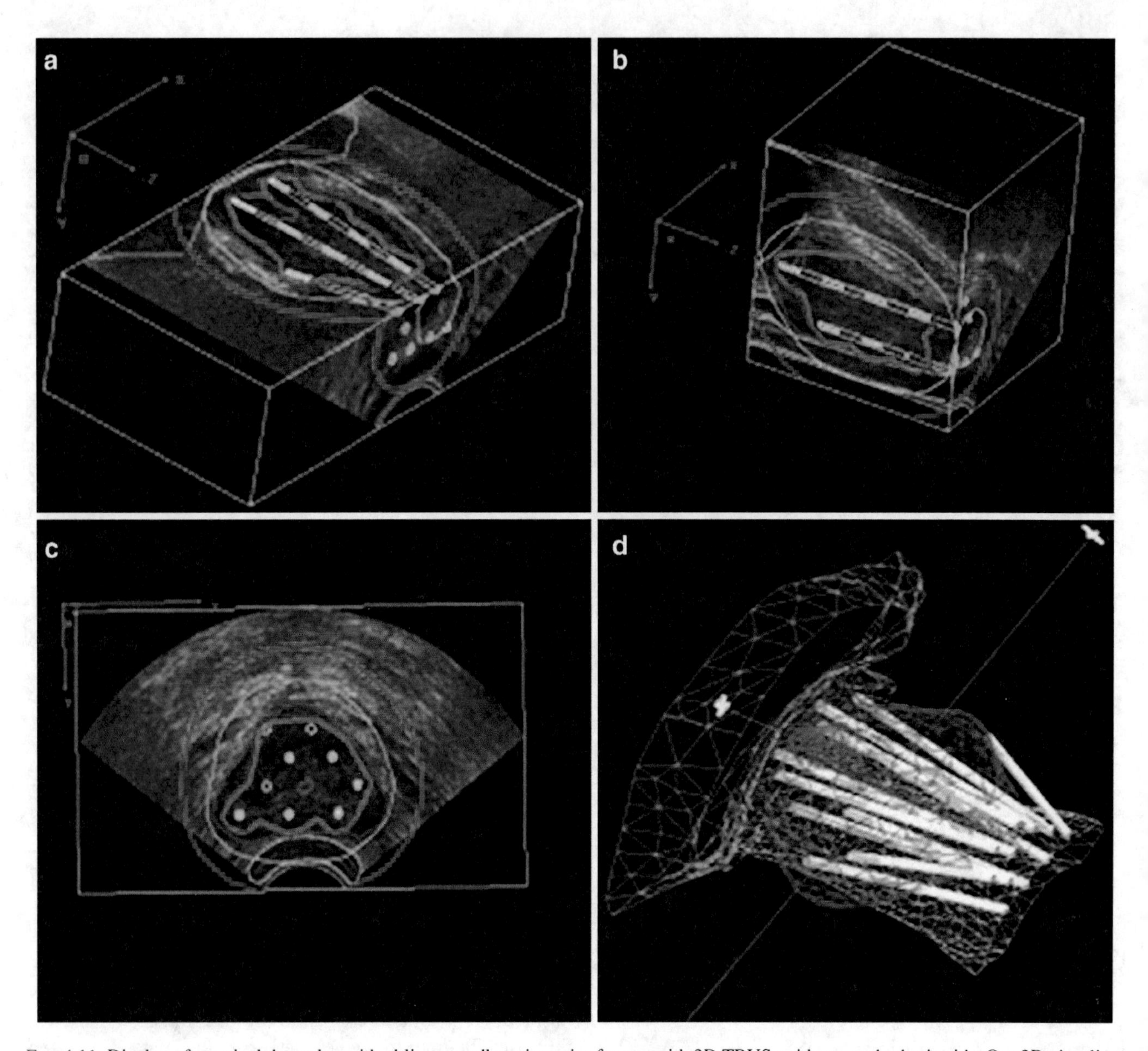

FIG. 4.11. Display of a typical dose plan with oblique needle trajectories for use with 3D TRUS guidance and robotic aids. Our 3D visualization approach allows display of a texture-mapped 3D view of the prostate, extracted planes, and graphical overlays of surfaces and contours. (**a**) Coronal view with delineated organs, needles, seeds, and isodose curves; (**b**) sagittal view; (**c**) transverse view; (**d**) surface rendered view showing the organs and needles with seeds

Table 4.2 shows the FLE for localizing the divots on the two orthogonal plates used for robot calibration. From Table 4.2, it can be seen that the FLE for the divot localization was approximately the same in the three directions. The measured error of the divots in the robot coordinate system is caused by such factors as the flexibility of the robot arm and the calibration plates, and the backlash in the robot arm joint. Comparing Table 4.2 with Table 4.1, it is seen that the FLE for the divot localization (i.e., robot calibration) is greater than that for the string intersection localization (i.e., image calibration). Therefore, the FLE for robot calibration will dominate the overall calibration errors affecting the accuracy of the whole system.

The FRE and TRE values for robot calibration are shown in Table 4.3. The mean FRE for the calibration of the robot was determined to be 0.52 mm ± 0.18 mm, and the mean TRE was determined to 0.68 mm ± 0.29 mm, which are greater than those for image calibration. As discussed, this results from the greater FLE for robot calibration. Because system errors will result from both the image and robot calibrations, the errors in robot calibration dominate the accuracy of integration of the two coordinate systems.

Needle Positioning and Orientation Accuracy by Robot

The accuracies of the needle position and orientation by the robot on the skin of the "patient" (i.e., before the needle has been inserted into the prostate) are described by the accuracy of the needle placement and the accuracy of the needle angulation.

Needle Placement Accuracy

We determined the needle placement accuracy by using the robot to move the needle tip to nine locations on a 5 cm × 5 cm grid that represented the skin of the patient (i.e., 3 × 3 grid of targeting points).[33] A three-axis stage (Parker Hannifin Co., Irwin, PA) with a measuring accuracy of 2 mm was then used to locate the tip of the needle. The displacement, ε_d, between the measured and targeted positions of the needle tip was found as follows:

$$\varepsilon_d = \sqrt{(x - x_i)^2 + (y - y_i)^2 + (z - z_i)^2}. \tag{4.5}$$

The coordinates for the targeted point are (x, y, z), where (x_i, y_i, z_i) are the coordinates for the ith measured point. The mean needle placement error, $\bar{\varepsilon}_d$, and the standard deviation (STD) from ten measurements at each position were found to be 0.15 mm ± 0.06 mm.

Needle Angulation Accuracy

To measure the accuracy of needle angulation using the robot, we attached a small plate to the needle holder and used the robot to tilt the plate in four angles vertically and laterally (0°, 5°, 10°, 15°). After each tilt, we measured the orientation of the plate using the three-axis stage and determined the angulation error by comparing the measured and planned plate angle.

Table 4.4 shows the mean angle differences between the measured and planned angulation by the robot and its STDs. As seen in Table 4.4, all mean angle differences were less than 0.12° with a mean of 0.07°. Because the angulation error will cause an increasing displacement error with increasing needle insertion distances, we estimated the displacement error after an insertion of 10 cm from the needle guide. Using the mean and maximum angulation errors, we determined the mean and maximum displacement errors for a 10-cm insertion to be ±0.13 mm and ±0.50 mm, respectively.[33]

Needle-Targeting Accuracy

The accuracy of the needle targeting reflects the accuracy of the needle tip after the needle has been inserted into the prostate under the guidance of 3D TRUS image with robotic assistance, as described in the section "System Description."

Method

We used tissue-mimicking phantoms made from agar,[42] which was contained in a Plexiglas box in order to determine the accuracy of needle insertion.[33] One side of the box was removable, allowing the insertion of the needle. As shown in Fig. 4.12, each of two phantoms contained two rows of 0.8-mm-diameter stainless beads.[43] This approach provided four different bead-targeting configurations: two different needle insertion depths and two different distances from the ultrasound transducer. These bead configurations formed a 4 × 4 × 4 cm^3 cube to simulate the approximate size of a prostate.

Results

Figure 4.13 shows a 3D ellipsoid representing the 95% confidence intervals for displacement errors of the needle insertion at one of the four targeting configurations, each of which is shown in Fig. 4.12. We plotted these ellipsoids using the axis that accounted for the least variation in needle targeting. Projections through the needle positions and 95% confidence intervals on the X–Y, X–Z, and Y–Z planes are also shown.

Table 4.5 lists the widths of the 95% confidence intervals along the primary, secondary, and tertiary axes plotted in Fig. 4.13. The 95% confidence interval is widest (i.e., the primary axis is greatest), for the predefined points on the top row – long penetration, and smallest for the bottom row – short penetration. The ellipsoid volumes (i.e., the volume encompassed by the 95% confidence intervals) were greater for the points farther from the ultrasound transducer than for those closer to the ultrasound transducer. As shown in Table 4.4 (and Fig. 4.13), the confidence widths were not centered at the origin of the coordinate system, (i.e., the positions of the predefined points), but, rather, at the average needle-targeting position for each of the four targeting configurations as shown in Fig. 4.12. The error of the needle targeting, which was obtained by averaging all 32 needle-targeting errors, was determined to be 0.79 mm ± 0.32 mm. The greatest targe-ting error was found to

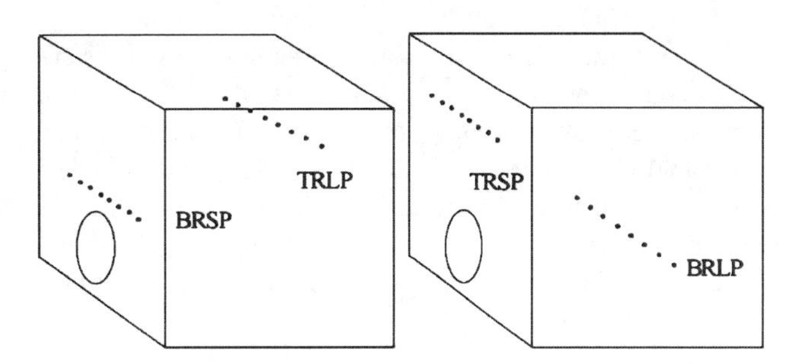

FIG. 4.12. Schematic diagram of the prostate phantom used for evaluation of needle-targeting accuracy. The *four rows of circles* represent the four different bead configurations. The needle entered the phantom from the front, parallel to the x-axis. TRLP = top row, long penetration; TRSP = top row, short penetration; BRLP = bottom row, long penetration; BRSP = bottom row, short penetration

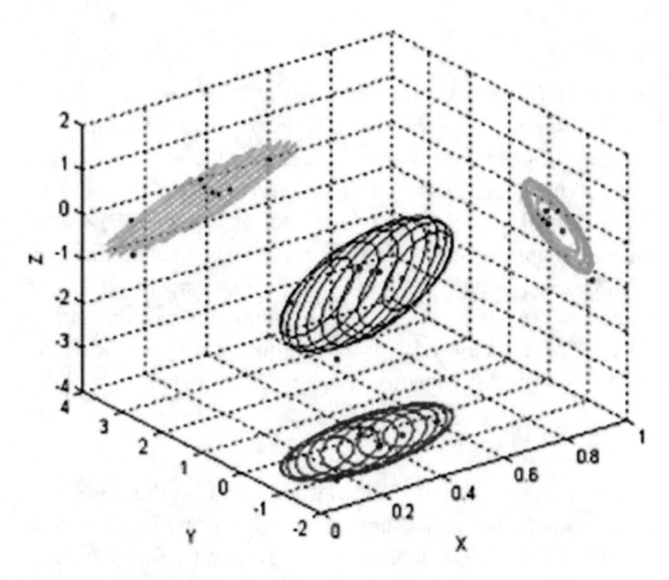

FIG. 4.13. Needle-targeting accuracy is displayed as the 95% confidence ellipsoid. The origin of the coordinate system represents the target and the needle tip positions after insertion (relative to the targets) are represented by the squares. The projections of the needle tip positions and the ellipsoid (on the three orthogonal planes) are also shown. These results are for the targets near the transducer and for a short penetration as shown in Fig. 4.12

be in *Z*-direction of the TRLP, and the smallest targeting error was found to be in the *X*-direction of the TRSP.[33]

Evaluation of the Prostate Segmentation Algorithm

Method

In order to evaluate the performance of the prostate segmentation algorithm, the surfaces we segmented using the algorithm were compared to the surfaces manually outlined by a trained technician. The technician is representative of users working in a radiological oncology department. Manual segmentation was performed using a multiplane reformatting image display tool.[44] The 3D prostate images were resliced into sets of transverse parallel 2D slices along the length of the prostate. 2-mm intervals were used at midgland and at 1-mm intervals near the ends of the prostate where the prostate shape changes more rapidly from one slice to the next. The prostate boundary was outlined in each slice, resulting in a stack of 2D contours; the contours were then tessellated into a 3D meshed surface. Manual outlining of the prostates from the 2D slices required about 30 min for each prostate.

Results

Figure 4.14 shows not only the quality of the fit of the algorithm but also the manually segmented meshes to the actual boundary of the prostate. Figure 4.14a shows the algorithm mesh in the 3D ultrasound image with (b) transverse, (c) coronal, and (d) sagittal cutting planes of the 2D cross-sectional images. Figure 4.14b shows a 2D transverse midgland slice of the 3D image with corresponding cross sections through the algorithm and manually segmented meshes superimposed. Figure 4.14c shows a coronal section with the corresponding cross section of the meshes, and Fig. 4.14d shows a sagittal section with the corresponding cross section of the meshes. The manual and algorithm contours in Fig. 14 are similar to each other. Each of the contours follows the prostate boun-dary well in regions where the contrast is high and the prostate is clearly separated from other tissues. In regions where the signal is low, the actual boundary is difficult to discern: the outlines generated by a manual segmentation differ from the outlines generated by the algorithm. As shown in Fig. 4.14d, these regions include images near the bladder (indicated by the white arrow) and the seminal vesicle (indicated by the black arrow).

Error analysis showed that the average difference between the boundaries generated by a manual segmentation compared to boundaries generated by the algorithm boundaries was 0.20 ± 0.28 mm; the average absolute difference was shown to be 1.19 ± 0.14 mm, the average maximum difference was shown to be 7.01 ± 1.04 mm, and the average volume difference was shown to be 7.16 ± 3.45%.[25]

Evaluation of the Needle Segmentation Algorithm

Method

The performance of the needle segmentation algorithm was evaluated using agar phantoms. To test the accuracy of the needle segmentation algorithm, we used a rigid rod with a 1.2-mm diameter, which is the same size of a typical 18-gauge prostate brachytherapy needle. The rigid rod was used in order to avoid the effect of needle deflection, allowing us to test the accuracy of the algorithm under ideal conditions. The position of the needle tip and the orientation of the needle were determined by the needle segmentation algorithm. Because the robot possesses high angulation accuracy, the position of the needle tip and the orientation of the needle were compared with the measurements of the robot (see the section "Needle Angulation Accuracy").

Results

The accuracy of the needle segmentation algorithm depends on the distance of needle insertion into the 3D TRUS images, angulations of the needle with respect to the TRUS transducer, and the distance of the needle from the TRUS transducer. Generally, the segmentation error and its standard deviation are larger at smaller insertion distances. Because more information about the needle can be obtained for segmentation (as the needle is inserted deeper into an image, resulting in a more accurate determination of the needle trajectory), the segmentation error and its standard deviation tend to decrease with increasing insertion distances. In addition, the errors appear to be larger at larger insertion angulations when the needle is angulated in both the horizontal and the vertical planes. In general, the segmentation error and its standard deviation

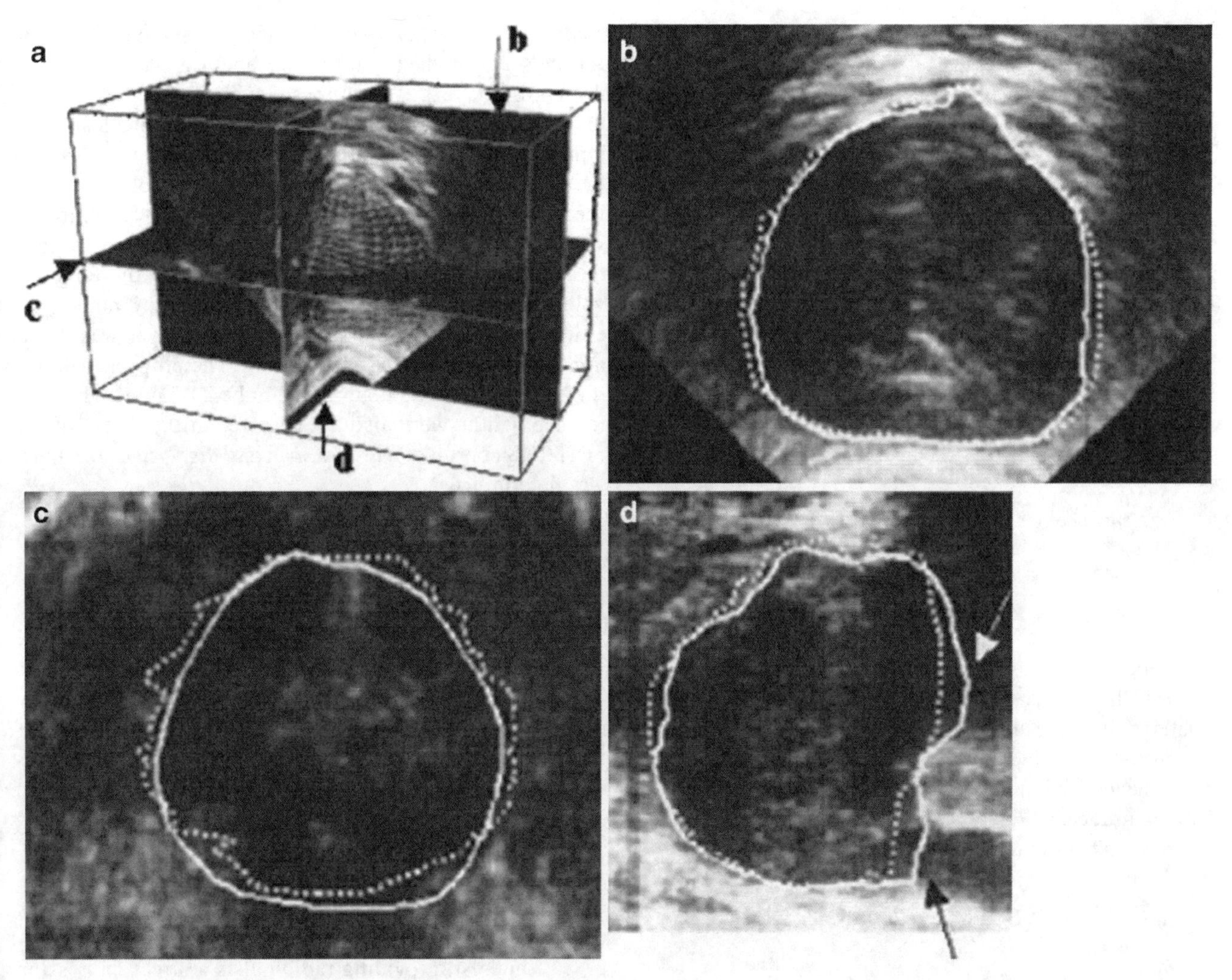

FIG. 4.14. Cross sections of a prostate showing the algorithm segmentation (*solid line*) and manual segmentation (*dotted line*). (**a**) 3D ultrasound image of the prostate with transverse, coronal, and sagittal cutting planes indicated by (**b**,**c**,**d**), respectively, to show 2D cross-sectional images. (**b**) Transverse cross section of the image and the boundaries corresponding to the plane shown in (**a**). (**c**) Coronal cross section of the image and the boundaries. (**d**) Sagittal cross section of the image and the boundaries

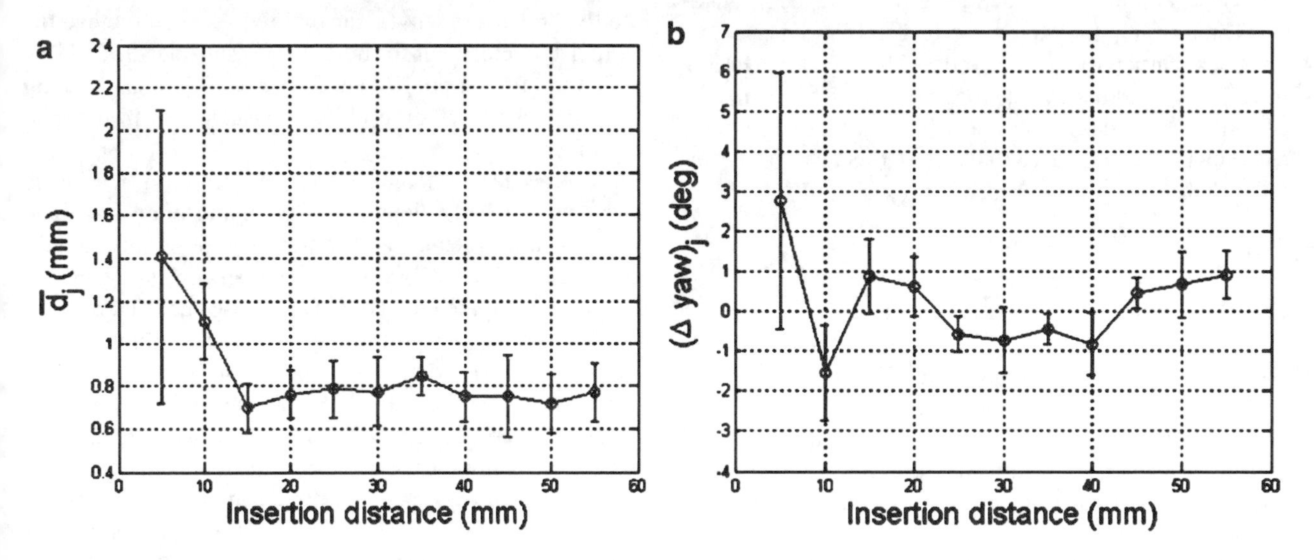

FIG. 4.15. Segmentation accuracy: effect of insertion distance. (**a**) Distance between the needle tip position derived from the algorithm and the robot, shown with respect to the preplanned insertion distance. (**b**) Difference in *yaw*, between the algorithm and robot data, shown with respect to the preplanned insertion distance. (**c**) Difference in *pitch*, between the algorithm and robot data, shown with respect to the preplanned insertion distance. In all three graphs, error bars represent one standard deviation

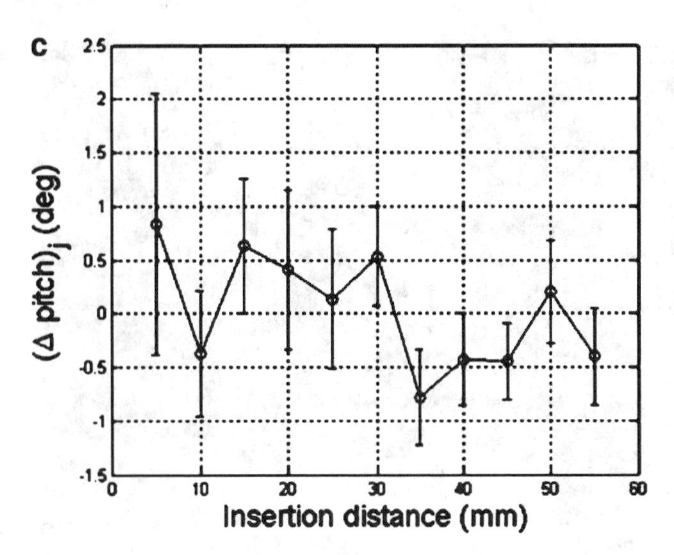

FIG. 4.15. (continued)

tend to decrease with decreasing insertion angulations. We also found that the mean errors (and their corresponding standard deviations) increase slightly with the increase of the distance of the needle from the transducer. This increase is due to the lower image resolution at larger distances away from the TRUS transducer.[36] Figure 4.15 shows the needle segmentation errors in respect to the different needle angulations.

Evaluation of the Seed Segmentation Algorithm

Method

We evaluated the seed segmentation algorithm by implanting 22 dummy iodine-125 seeds into a chicken phantom in three layers. The locations of those seeds were determined by the seed segmentation algorithm in 3D TRUS image first. We then scanned this phantom using the eXplore Locus Ultra Preclinical cone-beam CT scanner [GE Healthcare (Canada), London, Ontario, Canada], which possesses an isotropic voxel size of 154 μm. The seed positions were determined manually in the CT image. These seed positions were registered to the 3D TRUS image and compared with the algorithm-determined seed positions.[30]

Results

We evaluated the accuracy of registration by using the fiducial localization error (FLE), fiducial registration error (FRE), and target registration error (TRE). The FLE in the 3D TRUS image was determined to be 0.22 mm, and in CT image, the FLE was determined to be 0.15 mm. The FRE was determined to be 0.21 mm and the TRE was determined to be 0.35 mm. In our test, all 22 seeds were successfully segmented.[30]

Table 4.6 lists the widths of the 95% confidence intervals along the primary, secondary, and tertiary axes. The 95% confidence interval is widest (i.e., the primary axis is greatest for the seeds on the top layer and smallest for the seeds on the bottom layer). The ellipsoid volume for the seeds in the bottom layer was determined to be the smallest (0.68 mm^3), followed by the ellipsoid volume for the seeds in the middle layer (0.92 mm^3). The ellipsoid volume for the seeds in the top layer was largest at 1.15 mm^3. The ellipsoid volume for the seeds in the bottom layer was determined to be the smallest (1.07 mm^3), followed by the ellipsoid volume for the seeds in the middle layer (1.30 mm^3). The ellipsoid volume for the seeds in the top layer was determined to be the largest (1.40 mm^3). The ellipsoid volume for all the seeds was determined to be 2.07 mm^3. The confidence widths were also not centered at the origin of the 3D TRUS coordinate system. A mean distance of 0.30 mm was determined.[30]

Discussion and Conclusions

The prototype 3D TRUS-guided system with robotic assistance was developed for prostate brachytherapy. The fundamental motivation to apply robotic assistance in prostate brachytherapy originates from the motion features of a robot system. The motion features of a robot system include accuracy, consistency, and flexibility, i.e., a robot system that can be controlled to move to any position in any orientation along any trajectory at sufficiently high accuracies and consistencies within its 3D workspace. In addition, the 3D US image can provide a direct delineation of the volume of interest, providing radiologists a direct impression of the 3D anatomy and pathology of the prostate. It has also been reported that measurements of prostate volume in 3D are more accurate than that in 2D US images.[45] Therefore, by including 3D TRUS guidance and robotic assistance into the prostate brachytherapy system, we can remove the parallel trajectory constraints. As a result, needles can be guided to target a point identified in 3D US images along any trajectory (including oblique trajectories) in order to avoid PAI.

The procedures detailed in this chapter form a valuable precursor to the development of an intraoperative prostate brachytherapy system. The test results were promising, giving clinically relevant results in needle-targeting accuracy. We have shown that the prototype 3D TRUS-guided and robotic-assisted prostate brachytherapy system has the ability to target a location accurately and consistently. We believe that these results imply that the 3D TRUS-guided and robotic-assisted transperineal prostate brachytherapy – together with the progress in developing special software tools for prostate segmentation, dynamic replanning, needle, and seed segmentation – will soon provide a suitable intraoperative alternative, in which all steps of prostate brachytherapy procedure are carried out in one session.

References

1. Sakr WA, Grignon DJ, Crissman JD, Heilbrun LK, Cassin BJ, Pontes JJ, Haas GP. High grade prostatic intraepithelial neoplasia (HGPIN) and prostatic adenocarcinoma between the ages of 20–69: an autopsy study of 249 cases. In Vivo 1994; 8:439–443.
2. McLaughlin JR, Dryer D, Mao Y, Marrett L, Morrison H, Schacter B, Villeneuve G. Canadian cancer statistics 2006. National Cancer Institute of Canada, Toronto, Canada, 2006.
3. Jemal A, Siegel R, Ward E, Murray T, Xu J, Thun M. Cancer statistics, 2007. CA Cancer J Clin 2007; 57:43–66.
4. Bangma CH, Huland H, Schroder FH, van Cangh PJ. Early diagnosis and treatment of localized prostate cancer. Eur Urol 2001; 41:1–10.
5. Lattanzi J, McNeeley S, Donnelly S, Palacio E, Hanlon A, Schultheiss TE, Hanks GE. Ultrasound-based stereotactic guidance in prostate cancer: quantification of organ motion and set-up errors in external beam radiation therapy. Comp Aided Surg 2000; 5:289–295.
6. Ash D, Bottomley DM, Carey BM. Prostate Brachytherapy. Prostate Cancer Prostatic Dis 1998; 1:185–188.
7. Norderhaug I, Dahl O, Hoisater PA, Heikkila R, Klepp O, Olsen DR, Kristiansen IS, Wahre H, Johansen TEB. Brachytherapy for prostate cancer: a systematic review of clinical and cost effectiveness. Eur Urol 2003; 44:40–46.
8. Blasko JC, Mate T, Sylvester JE, Grimm PD, Cavanagh W. Brachytherapy for carcinoma of the prostate: techniques, patient selection, and clinical outcomes. Semin Radiat Oncol 2002; 12:81–94.
9. Butler EB, Scardino PT, Teh BS, Uhl BM, Guerriero WG, Carlton CE, Berner BM, Dennis WS, Carpenter LS, Lu HH, Chiu JK, Kent TS, Woo SY. The Baylor College of Medicine experience with gold seed implantation. Semin Surg Oncol 1997; 13:406–418.
10. Holm HH, Juul N, Pedersen JF. Transperineal 125iodine seed implantation in prostatic cancer guided transrectal ultrasonography. J Urol 1983; 130:283–286.
11. Prete JJ, Prestidge BR, Bice WS, Friedland JL, Stock RG, Grimm PD. A survey of physics and dosimetry practice of permanent prostate brachytherapy in the United States. Int J Radiat Oncol Biol Phys 1998; 40:1001–1005.
12. Roy JN, Wallner K, Harrington PJ, Ling CC, Anderson LL. CT-based evaluation method for permanent implants: application to prostate. Int J Radiat Oncol Biol Phys 1993; 26:163–169.
13. Pathak SD, Grimm PD, Chalana V, Kim Y. Pubic arch detection in transrectal ultrasound guided prostate cancer therapy. IEEE Trans Med Imaging 1998; 17:762–771.
14. Strang JG, Rubens DJ, Brasacchino RA, Yu Y, Messing EM. Real-time US versus CT determination of pubic arch interference for brachytherapy. Radiology 2001; 219:387–393.
15. Messing EM, Zhang JB, Rubens DJ, Brasacchio RA, Strang JG, Soni A, Schell MC, Okunieff PG, Yu Y. Intraoperative optimized inverse planning for prostate brachytherapy: early experience. Int J Radiat Oncol Biol Phys 1999; 44:801–808.
16. Badiozamani KR, Wallner K, Sutlief S, Ellis W, Blasko J, Russell K. Anticipating prostatic volume changes due to prostate brachytherapy. Radiat Oncol Investig 1999; 7:360–364.
17. Yu Y, Anderson LL, Li Z, Mellenberg DE, Nath R, Schell MC, Waterman FM, Wu A, Blasko JC. Permanent prostate seed implant brachytherapy: report of the American Association of Physicists in Medicine Task Group No. 64. Med Phys 1999; 26:2054–2076.
18. Wan G, Wei Z, Gardi L, Downey D, Fenster A. Brachytherapy needle deflection evaluation and correction. Med Phys 2005; 32: 902–909.
19. Bangma CH, Hengeveld EJ, Niemer AQ, Schroder FH. Errors in transrectal ultrasonic planimetry of the prostate: computer simulation of volumetric errors applied to a screening population. Ultrasound Med Biol 1995; 21:11–16.
20. Cheng G, Liu H, Liao L, Yu Y. Dynamic Brachytherapy of the Prostate Under Active Image Guidance. *Proc MICCAI 2001*, pp. 351–359, 2001.
21. Tong S, Downey DB, Cardinal HN, Fenster A. A three-dimensional ultrasound prostate imaging system. Ultrasound Med Biol 1996; 22:735–746.
22. Fenster A, Downey D, Cardinal N. Topic review: three-dimensional ultrasound imaging. Phys Med Biol 2001; 46:R67–R99.
23. Ladak MH, Mao F, Wang Y, Downey D, Steinman D, Fenster A. Prostate boundary segmentation from 2D ultrasound images. Med Phys 2000; 27:1777–1788.
24. Wang Y, Cadinal N, Downey DB, Fenster A. Semiautomatic three-dimensional segmentation of the prostate using two-dimensional ultrasound images. Med Phys 2003; 30:887–897.
25. Hu N, Downey D, Fenster A, Ladak H. Prostate boundary segmentation from 3D ultrasound images. Med Phys 2003; 30:1648–1659.
26. Ding M, Chen C, Wang Y, Gyacskov I, Fenster A. Prostate segmentation in 3D US images using the cardinal-spline-based discrete dynamic contour. *Proc SPIE*, Vol 5029, pp. 69–76, 2003
27. Shen D, Zhan Y, Davatzikos C. Segmentation of prostate boundaries from ultrasound images using statistical shape model. IEEE Trans Med Imag 2003; 22:539–551.
28. Ding M, Cardinal N, Fenster A. Automatic needle segmentation in 3D ultrasound images using orthogonal 2D image projections. Med Phys 2003; 30:222–234.
29. Ding M, Fenster A. A real-time biopsy needle segmentation technique using Hough Transform. Med Phys 2003; 30: 2222–2233.
30. Wei Z, Gardi L, Downey D, Fenster A. Automated localization of implanted seeds in 3D TRUS images used for prostate brachytherapy. Med Phys 2006; 33:2404–2417.
31. Fitchtinger G, Burdette EC, Tanacs A, Patriciu A, Mazilu D, Whitcomb L, Stoianovici D. Robotically assisted prostate brachytherapy with transrectal ultrasound guidance – Phantom experiments. Brachytherapy 2006; 5:14–26.
32. Yu Y, Podder TK, Zhang YD, Ng WS, Misic V, Sherman J, Fu L, Fuller D, Messing EM, Rubens DJ, Strang JG, Brasacchio RA. Robot-assisted prostate brachytherapy. MICCAI 2006, Copenhagen, Denmark.
33. Wei Z, Wan G, Mills G, Gardi L, Downey D, Fenster A. Robot-assisted 3D TRUS-guided prostate brachytherapy: System integration and validation. Med Phys 2004; 31:539–548.
34. Gower JC, Dijksterhuis GB. Procrustes problems. Oxford University Press, 2004.
35. Arun KS, Huang TS, Blostein SD. Least-square fitting of two 3-D point sets. IEEE Trans Pattern Anal Mach Intel 1987; 9: 698–700.
36. Wei Z, Gardi L, Downey DB, Fenster A. Oblique needle segmentation and tracking for 3D TRUS guided prostate brachytherapy, Med Phys 2005; 32:2928–2941.

37. Nag S, Bice W, DeWyngaert K, Prestidge B, Stock R, Yu Y. The American Brachytherapy Society recommendations for permanent prostate brachytherapy post-implant dosimetric analysis. Int J Radiat Oncol Biol Phys 2000; 46:221–230.
38. Nath R, Anderson LL, Luxton G, Weaver KA, Williamson JF, Meigooni AS. Dosimetry of interstitial brachytherapy sources: recommendations of the AAPM Radiation Therapy Committee Task Group No. 43. American Association of Physicists in Medicine, Med Phys 1995; 22(2):209–234.
39. Maurer CR, Jr., Maciunas RJ, Fitzpatrick JM. Registration of head CT images to physical space using a weighted combination of points and surfaces, IEEE Trans Med Imaging 1998; 17(5):753–761.
40. Fitzpatrick JM, West JB, Maurer CR, Jr. Predicting error in rigid-body point-based registration, IEEE Trans Med Imaging 1998; 17(5):694–702.
41. M Maurer CR Jr, McCrory JJ, Fitzpatrick JM. Estimation of accuracy in localizing externally attached markers in multimodal volume head images. *Proc SPIE*, Vol. 1898: pp. 43–54, 1993.
42. Rickey DW, Picot PA, Christopher DA, Fenster A. A wall-less vessel phantom for Doppler ultrasound studies, Ultrasound Med Biol 1995; 21(9):1163–1176.
43. Smith WL, Surry KJ, Mills GR, Downey DB, Fenster A. Three-dimensional ultrasound-guided core needle breast biopsy, Ultrasound Med Biol 2001; 27:1025–1034.
44. Fenster A, Downey DB. 3D ultrasound imaging: A review. IEEE Eng Med Biol Mag 1996; 15:41–51.
45. Tong S, Cardinal HN, McLaughlin RF, Downey DB, Fenster A. Intra- and inter-observer variability and reliability of prostate volume measurement via two-dimensional and three-dimensional ultrasound imaging. Ultrasound Med Biol 1998; 24:673–681.

Chapter 5
IntraOperative Real-Time Transrectal Ultrasound Monitoring During Energy-Free Nerve-Sparing Laparoscopic Radical Prostatectomy

Osamu Ukimura and Inderbir S. Gill

Abstract Ultrasound (US) guidance has been established as intraoperative image guidance to offset the disadvantage of the attenuated tactile feedback in minimally invasive surgery. The authors hypothesized that real-time "intraoperative" transrectal ultrasound (TRUS) guidance could increase the precision of nerve-sparing laparoscopic radical prostatectomy (LRP). Our clinical experience of TRUS-guided LRP provided initial proof of concept regarding the feasibility of real-time US navigation during radical prostatectomy to enhance intraoperative surgical performance in regard to both oncological and functional outcomes.

Introduction

The surgical management of localized prostate cancer continues to improve by refinements in surgical techniques, better understanding of anatomy, and using new imaging and endoscopic technologies. Laparoscopic radical prostatectomy (LRP) was first reported by Schuessler et al. in 1997.[1] Increasing numbers of laparoscopic or robotic radical prostatectomy are now becoming the procedure of choice.[2–4]

Tactile feedback is completely lacking during robotic surgery, and considerably attenuated during laparoscopic surgery, compared with open surgery. Ultrasound (US) guidance has been established as intraoperative image guidance to offset the disadvantage of such attenuated tactile feedback. Since real-time transrectal US (TRUS) allows visualizing prostate contour (such as difficult-to-see apical posterior protrusion (Fig. 5.1) and median lobe protrusion), a substantial percentage of cancer nodules (Figs. 5.2 and 5.3), and periprostatic anatomies such as the neurovascular bundles (NVBs) (Figs. 5.4 and 5.5), tented-up rectal wall (Fig. 5.6), and bladder neck (Fig. 5.7), the authors hypothesized that real-time "intraoperative" TRUS guidance could increase the precision of nerve-sparing laparoscopic radical prostatectomy.[5] The "intraoperative" performance of TRUS has the advantage for the ultrasonographer to have prior knowledge of systematic prostate biopsy-pathology outcome, which could improve the surgeon's understanding of the location, size, and Gleason score of the prostate cancer in order to determine appropriate decision making for nerve-sparing technique achieving negative surgical margin. Importantly, TRUS is the most popular imaging modality which can be handled by urologists in the operation room.

During TRUS-guided LRP, using gray-scale ultrasound (7.5 MHz) and power Doppler ultrasound, real-time US monitoring was performed preoperatively, intraoperatively, and immediately postoperatively in special reference to defining the prostate apex contour, evaluating the location and extent of any hypoechoic cancer nodules (Fig. 5.2), and identifying the neurovascular bundles in relation to the posterior-laterally located cancer nodule.[5] We revealed that intraoperative TRUS navigation appeared to be helpful for various specific technical aspects of LRP, including (1) identification of size and location of biopsy-proven hypoechoic cancer nodule, (2) staging of biopsy-proven cancer using Ukimura's nomogram (Figs. 5.8 and 5.9),[6] (3) calibrated, wider dissection at the site of suspected extracapsular extension of cancer nodules to achieve negative margins, (4) precision during lateral pedicle transaction and NVB release, (5) tailored dissection according to the individual prostate apex, and (6) facilitation of posterior bladder neck transaction especially for the novice.[7–9]

Improvement of Oncological Outcomes by TRUS Navigation

Approximately 25% of patients undergoing radical prostatectomy for clinically localized prostate cancer are estimated to suffer recurrence of their diseases, as a rising prostate specific antigen.[10] Both pathological extracapsular extension (ECE) and positive surgical margin have significant correlation with the biochemical recurrence after undergoing radical prostatectomy. In a recent large number (*n* 5,824) of LRP between 1999 and 2004, pathological ECE (pT3a) disease has still been reported in approximately one-fourth (*n*= 1,555, 27%) of clinically localized prostate cancers, revealing positive margin rates of 10.6% for pT2 and 32.7% for pT3a-tumors.[4]

O. Ukimura and I.S. Gill (eds.), *Contemporary Interventional Ultrasonography in Urology,*
DOI: 10.1007/978-1-84800-217-3_5, © Springer-Verlag London Limited 2009

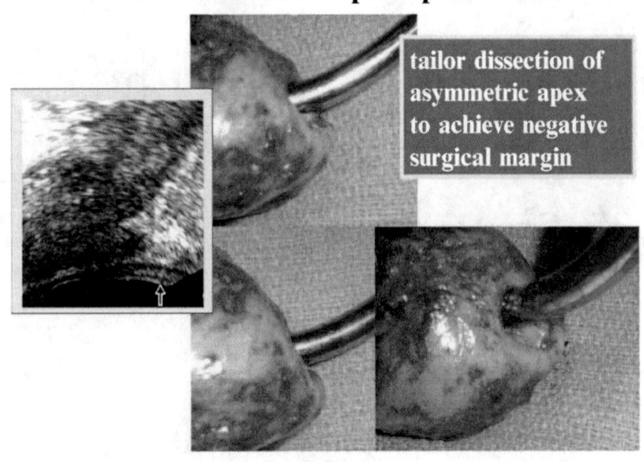

FIG. 5.1. Real-time TRUS monitoring of apical dissection, TRUS provided the characteristics of the distal protrusion of the prostate apex posterior to the membranous urethra. This real-time navigation allows the surgeon to appropriately tailor the apical dissection by maximizing the preservation of membranous urethral length, for achieving a negative surgical margin. Note: There were no thermal injuries on the surface of the prostate, especially along the posterolateral aspects, since cold sharp cutting and occasional gentle blunt dissection were performed in the interfascial plane between the prostatic capsule and the lateral pelvic fascia during entire release of the NVBs

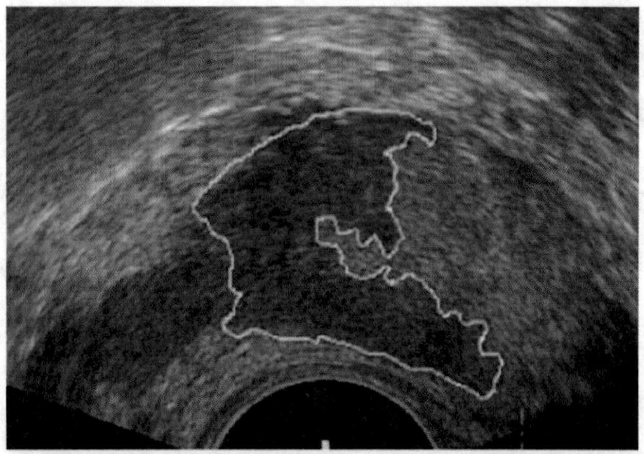

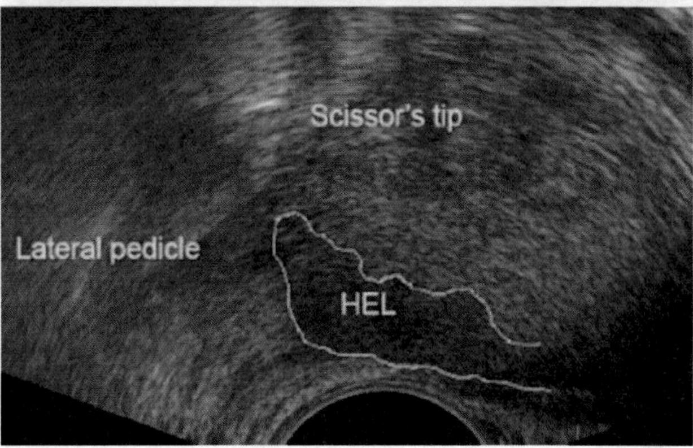

FIG. 5.2. Intraoperative TRUS-identified hypoechoic cancer lesion (HEL) (*yellow line*) occupying the relatively wide area of the base of the prostate. In this case, Ukimura's nomogram suspected ECE with greater than 80% and recommended the wider dissection for non-nerve sparing at the site of the high-risk cancer nodule. Pathology confirmed Gleason 7 (3+4) cancer with ECE of 0.3 mm and negative surgical margins (see Fig. 5.11)

Since ECE most likely happens at the locations of posterior-lateral aspects adjacent to the NVB, how to release the NVB is a controversial issue especially when clinical preoperative data (including systematic biopsy data, PSA, and DRE) suggested high risk of ECE,[11] or when ECE is intraoperatively suspected during nerve-sparing prostatectomy.[12] It is conceivable that the microscopic presence of ECE in clinically localized prostate cancer is not a contraindication to the nerve-sparing surgery, because cancer control is possible if the surgical margin is negative for cancer by a site-specific wide excision of the periprostatic tissues involving the ECE along with the NVB.[12] The surgeon's intraoperative knowledge regarding the presence and location of the high risk of ECE area close to the NVB will allow modifying the operation by performing a possible wider excision of periprostatic tissues at the site of the risk of ECE so that the tumor with ECE can be removed completely, while maximizing the preservation of the NVB.

The most potent men diagnosed with clinically localized prostate cancer could be considered candidates for complete or substantial partial preservation of NVBs. Although indications may be reported to modify the degree of nerve-sparing technique for use of preoperatively available clinical parameters,[11] the authors consider that a final determination to modify the degree of nerve-sparing technique should not be made until the extent of the tumor adjacent to the NVB has been intraoperatively assessed by intraoperative TRUS for LRP as well as by intraoperative direct palpation of prostate cancer nodule for open surgeon.[8,12]

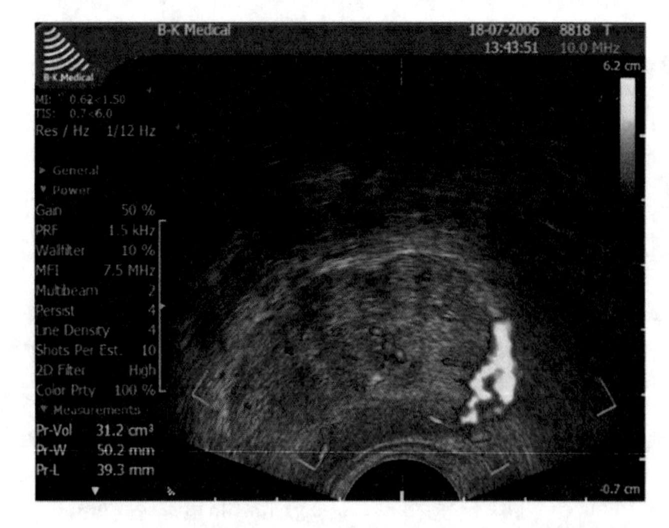

FIG. 5.3. Real-time TRUS (Power Doppler) demonstrating tumor neovascularity in the same patient as in Fig. 5.2

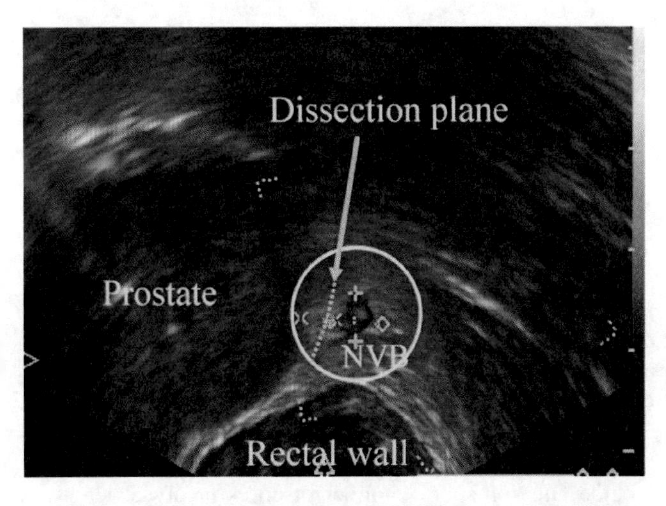

FIG. 5.4. Real-time monitoring of right NVB release. Note: Dissection line for energy-free nerve sparing

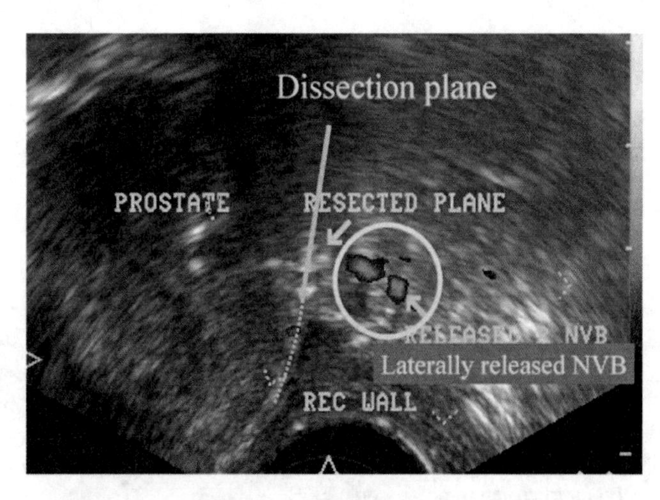

FIG. 5.6. Continued real-time monitoring of right NVB release and release of the rectal wall from the prostate. Note: the NVB in Fig. 5.2 is located at a slightly greater distance from the prostate edge compared to Fig. 5.1, indicating ongoing NVB lateral release and release of the prostate along the tented-up rectal wall

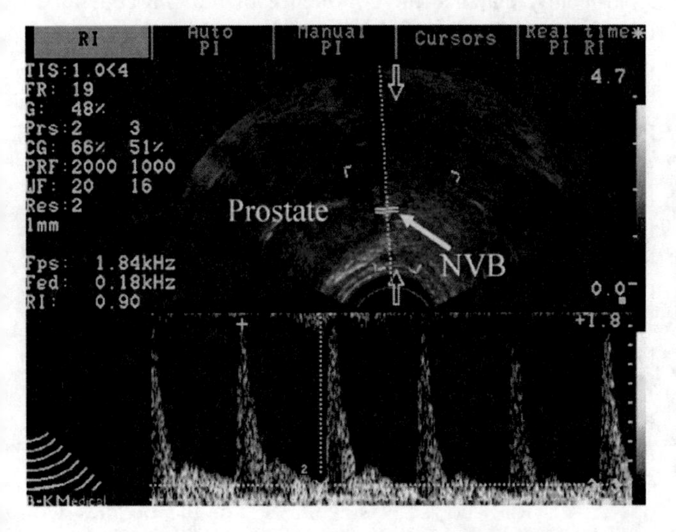

FIG. 5.5. Blood flow wave-form analysis of an arterial flow within the right NVB. Note: The TRUS cursor (*two parallel white lines*) is placed on the blood flow within right NVB to obtain Doppler measurements, including resistive index (RI = 0.90)

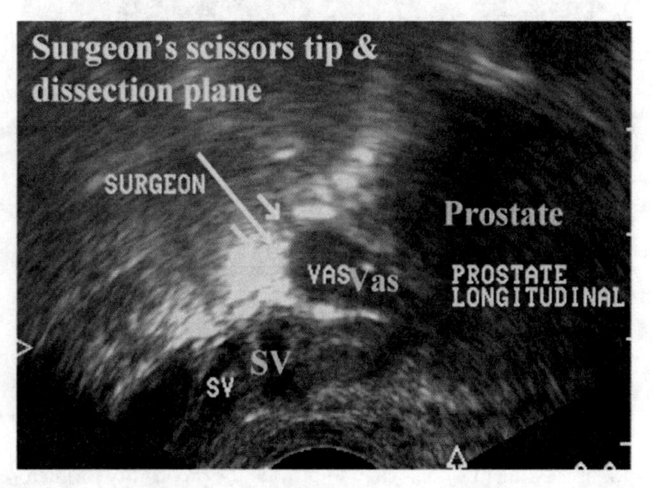

FIG. 5.7. Real-time TRUS monitoring of posterior bladder-neck transection. Herein, longitudinal TRUS view demonstrates the surgeon approaching between the vasa (VAS) and seminal vesicle (SV) in the correct plane using J-hook electrocautery

Real-time TRUS monitoring of the location of the laparoscopic scissors tip, which can be visualized as a hyperechoic spot, at the concerned anatomical site was feasible, during the safe releases of neurovascular bundle surrounding the hypoechoic cancer nodule. It will contribute to precision of the surgery to achieve negative surgical margin, by not only recommending wider dissection around the high-risk cancer with ECE but also avoiding to make iatrogenic positive surgical margin on the organ-confined cancer nodule (Figs. 5.10 and 5.11).

To predict the risk of microscopic ECE in hypoechoic cancer in clinically organ confined disease, Ukimura and associates defined a new quantitative TRUS staging criterion (i.e., US tumor contact length, the length of hypoechoic tumor contact with the boundary) (Figs. 5.8 and 5.9).[6] On the other hand, conventional TRUS criteria (such as bulging or discontinuity of boundary) correlate with macroscopic ECE, which is mainly related with clinically locally advanced disease.[13] Although the accuracy of staging for prostate cancer in conventional TRUS has been still critical,[14] the authors would like to point out an important distinction between conventional "screening" TRUS and new concept of "intraoperative" TRUS. Since biopsy-pathology datasets are not available to the ultrasonographer during "screening" TRUS, histopathologically naïve "screening" TRUS likely lacks accuracy for reliably identifying prostate cancer and detecting ECE. On the other hand, during "intraoperative" TRUS, the ultrasonographer has the clear advantage of being given prior knowledge of prostate biopsy-pathology dataset. Such biopsy-pathology dataset

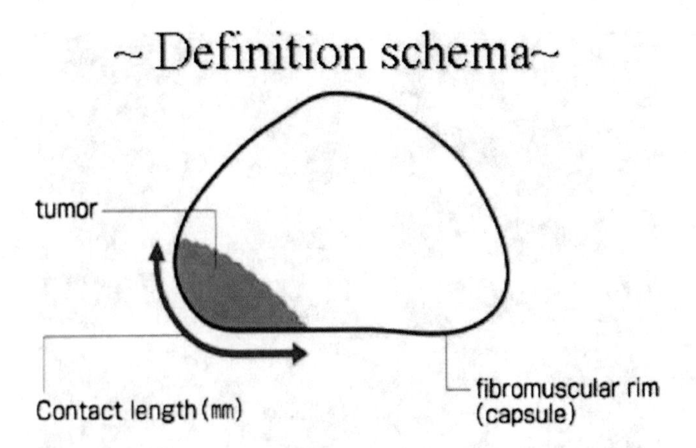

FIG. 5.8. Definition schema of tumor contact length for TRUS staging criteria for predicting microscopic ECE

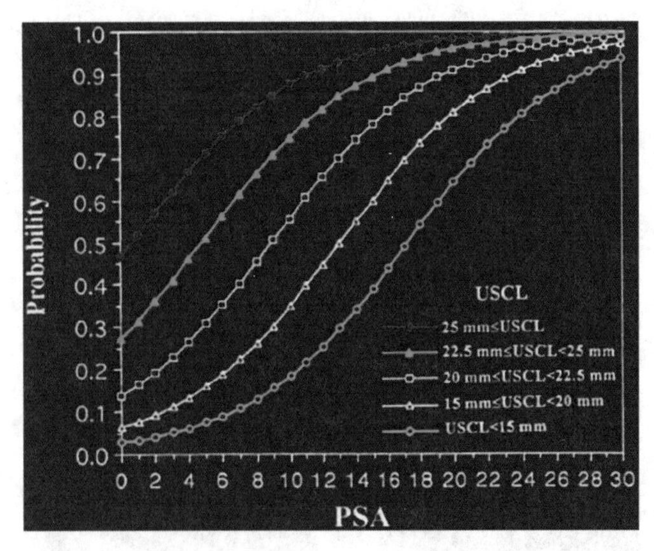

FIG. 5.9. Ukimura's nomogram to provide the probability of microscopic ECE, with combination of TRUS-measured contact length (USCL) and serum PSA value

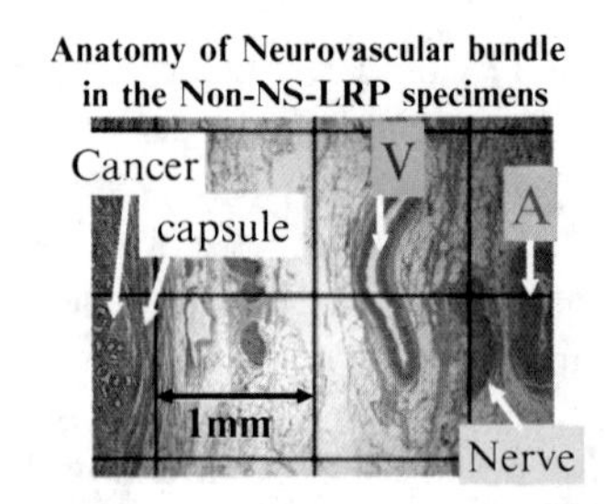

FIG. 5.10. Pathological specimen at the posterolateral aspects along the prostate cancer nodule, and the periprostatic tissues, which were widely dissected by intraoperative TRUS guidance. Note: TRUS-identified NVB was demonstrated as the complex of the nerve, artery, and vein with 0.3–1.0 mm in diameter. Each square of the grid is 1 mm × 1 mm in dimension

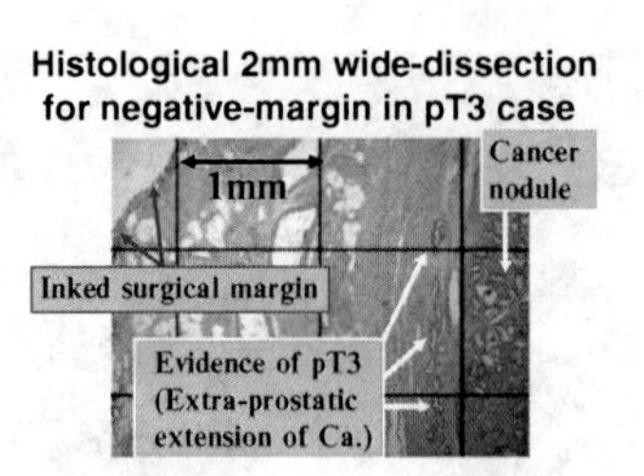

FIG. 5.11. Pathology confirms Gleason 7 (3+4) cancer with established 0.3-mm extracapsular extension (*white arrows*) with negative margin width of 1.5 mm, after performing the 2-mm wider dissection along the high-risk cancer nodule suggested by Ukimura's nomogram. Each square of the grid is 1 mm × 1 mm in dimension

include Gleason score, number of cores involved, length of cancer lesion, location of positive cores, and directed biopsy outcome. The preprovided, biopsy-proven, pathological information on the precise anatomical location of the cancer will significantly enhance the confidence of the "intraoperative" ultrasonographer in identifying and characterizing hypoechoic cancers during "intraoperative" TRUS. As such, using Ukimura's nomogram to predict microscopic ECE, intraoperative TRUS potentially contributes to the intraoperative assistance for identifying risky cancer. In our retrospective analysis to compare previously performed LRP between without versus with intraoperative TRUS, the incidence of positive margin rates improved from 29 to 9%.[8] In our initial experience of the 77 patients undergoing TRUS-guided LRP, intraoperative TRUS visualized a biopsy-proven cancer in 53% (41/77) of total 77 patients, in 45% of clinical T1c disease (29/65), in all 12 with clinical T2 disease (100%), in 40% of T2 disease (22/55), and in 86% of pT3 disease (19/22). Out of the 55 cases of pT2 disease, intraoperative TRUS overstaged 15% (8/55) as suspicious for ECE, using Ukimura's nomogram; while intraoperative TRUS correctly staged 88% of the nodules with pathologically confirmed ECE (23/26) and understaged 12% of them (3/26). Clearly, the greatest potential benefit of intraoperative TRUS is primarily in patients with a hypoechoic cancer with ECE (pT3a disease) (Fig. 5.11). The patients with higher-risk cancers (higher PSA, higher Gleason score, and prostate nodule on digital rectal examination) more likely have benefit from TRUS navigation.[8]

More recently our analysis on 215 consecutive patients undergoing TRUS-guided LRP revealed updated information. Intraoperative TRUS provided intraoperative information suggesting (1) hypoechoic lesion in 56% (120/215) and (2) suspicious for ECE in 28% (61/215). Multivariate logistic regression analysis to identify the variable to predict positive surgical margins demonstrated that the appearance of hypoechoic lesion was the only significant variable. Our data revealed that in patients with hypoechoic lesion, the chance of positive surgical margins was 23%, while only 1% were without hypoechoic lesion ($p < 0.0001$). Furthermore, in 61 patients with suspicion of ECE which was identified by intraoperative TRUS, 23% (14/61) unilateral and 27% (16/61) bilateral dissections of neurovascular bundles were performed to avoid positive surgical margins, resulting in successful achievement of negative surgical margin in 70% (43/61) of these high-risk patients. Importantly, negative intraoperative TRUS findings will make us confident of ensuring the safe posterolateral and apical dissection of the prostate. Since most of positive surgical margins arose in patients with the abnormal findings of hypoechoic lesion on TRUS, site-specific wider excision at the high-risk area of ECE should be considered to secure negative margins.

Recovery of Erectile Function After TRUS-Guided Nerve-Sparing LRP

Reported surgical hemostatic technique in LRP had typically involved the use of thermal energy (ultrasonic or electrical monopolar or bipolar). Such use of thermal energy had a risk to result in collateral damage to the NVB, compromising recovery of erectile function. In our attempt to eliminate such collateral thermal damage to the NVBs, we described an energy-free technique of nerve-sparing LRP.[7,15] Our recent analysis revealed that the TRUS-monitored energy-free nerve-sparing technique with elimination of any electrical and thermal energy during nerve-sparing LRP achieved superior and quicker potency recovery.[15]

In our experience of 200 cases of LRP from 2003 to 2006, initially 31 patients underwent conventional LRP with the use of an ultrasound-based energy source (harmonic scalpel) for hemostatical release of the NVB, while later 169 patients underwent our reported, energy-free nerve-sparing LRP. Of the 200, 110 consecutive potent patients with preoperative erections adequate for intercourse had reached 1 year of follow-up after LRP. Of these 110, 76 patients (69%) had returned paired preoperative and 1-year postoperative Sexual Health Inventory for Men (SHIM) questionnaires. Of these 76, we compared recovery of erectile function between the 22 patients undergoing the earlier thermal-energy based technique using an ultrasonic scalpel (group 1) and 54 patients undergoing the novel energy-free technique (group 2). We defined sexual intercourse ability as the ability to achieve erections sufficient for vaginal penetration with or without the use of phosphodiesterase-5 inhibitors. Intraoperative power Doppler TRUS monitored the pulsatile arterial flow in the NVB and the number of visible vessels. Intraoperative TRUS also measured the dimensions of NVB compared pre- and postoperatively.

Tables 5.1 and 5.2 presented time course recovery of SHIM scores (Table 5.1) and intercourse ability (Table 5.2). Interestingly, compared to energy-base technique, potency recovery appeared to be 6 months quicker in energy-free technique. Furthermore, energy-free technique significantly correlated with the better recovery of erectile function than energy-based technique.

Interestingly, intraoperative TRUS findings demonstrated the significant correlations between postoperative potency and the US-identified blood flow in the neurovascular bundles before, during, and after nerve-sparing LRP (Figs. 5.12 and 5.13). Postop SHIM scores significantly correlated with

TABLE 5.1. SHIM score recovery after nerve-sparing LRP.

	Group I (n= 22)	Group II (n= 54)	
	SHIM score (% of baseline)	SHIM score (% of baseline)	(p value, Group I vs. II)
Baseline preop	17.3 ± 5.4 (100%)	17.3 ± 4.9 (100%)	$p = 1.0$
3 months postop	4.3 ± 2.6 (24%)	7.5 ± 6.6 (43%)	$p = 0.03$
6 months postop	5.9 ± 4.5 (33%)	9.6 ± 6.1 (57%)†	$p = 0.01$
12 months postop	10.0 ± 8.4 (55%)†	13.4 ± 6.8 (73%)*	$p = 0.07$
18 months postop	12.6 ± 7.2 (76%)*	14.7 ± 7.2 (77%)	$p = 0.3$

Group I, energy-based technique using harmonic scissors; Group II, energy-free nerve-sparing technique. Potency recovered 6 months faster in Group II compared to Group I. Notice that SHIM scores (57% and 73%) in Group II at 6 and 12 months were similar to Group I outcomes (55% and 76%) at 12 and 18 months (†$p = 0.8$, *$p = 0.6$, respectively)

TABLE 5.2. Intercourse rates' recovery after nerve-sparing LRP.

	Group I (n= 22)	Group II (n 54)	
	Intercourse (%)	Intercourse (%)	(p value, Group I vs. II)
Baseline preop	22 (100%)	54 (100%)	$p = 1.0$
3 months postop	2 (9%)	13 (20%)	$p = 0.1$
6 months postop	3 (14%)	22 (42%)††	$p = 0.02$
12 months postop	8 (36%)††	33 (70%)**	$p = 0.04$
18 months postop	14 (64%)**	9/12 (75%)	$p = 0.4$

Potency recovered 6 months faster in Group II compared to Group I. Notice that Intercourse rates in Group II (42% and 70%) at 6 and 12 months were similar to Group I outcomes (36% and 64%) at 12 and 18 months (††$p = 0.5$, **$p = 0.5$, respectively)

Bilateral nerve-sparing LRP
Laparoscopy & TRUS findings

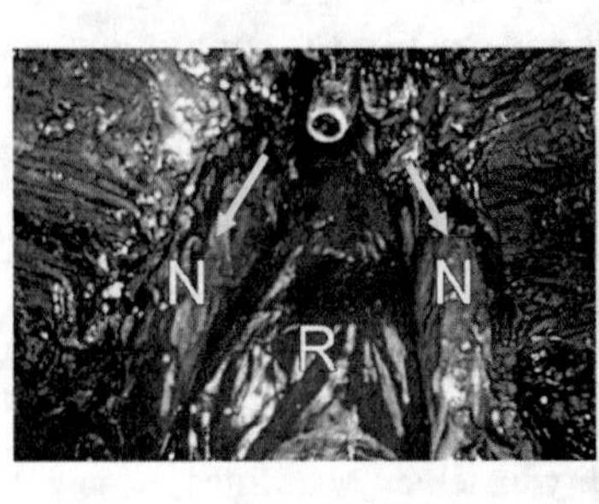

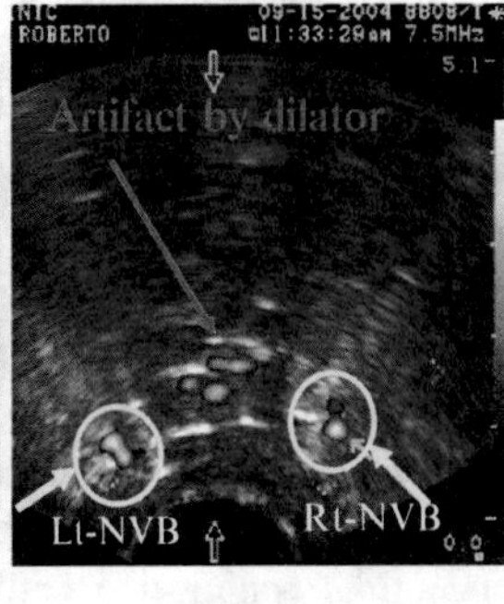

FIG. 5.12. Left, Intraoperative laparoscopic view of bilateral energy-free nerve sparing. Right, Intraoperative TRUS confirmation of bilateral preserved blood flows within the NVBs

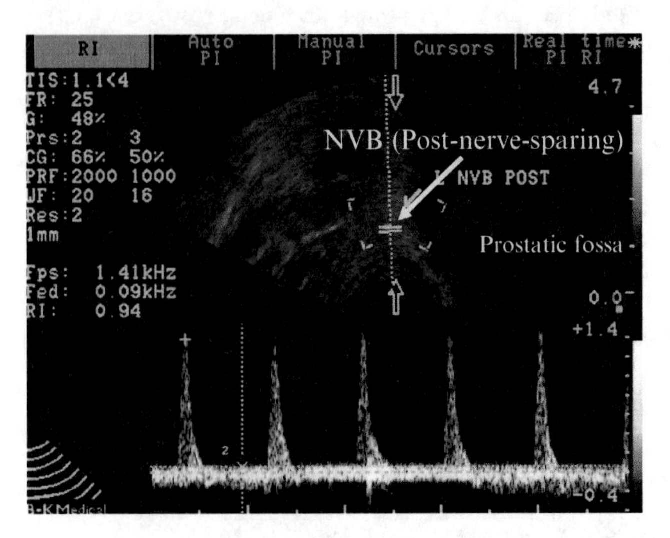

FIG. 5.13. Blood flow wave-form analysis within the preserved NVB after energy-free nerve sparing. Continued blood flow is documented, with Doppler wave-form measured arterial blood flow resistive index (RI: 0.94) within released NVB

TABLE 5.3. Spearman rank coefficient for assessing the correlation between postoperative SHIM score and pre-/intraoperative variables.

Variables	Co-efficient	*p* Value
Pulsatile arterial flow within NVB	Rs. 0.48	0.0001
No. of visible vessels within NVB	Rs. 0.34	0.003
Dimension of NVB	Rs. 0.21	0.07

US-identified pulsatile arterial flow within NVB (Rs. 0.48, $p = 0.0001$), and US-identified number of visible vessels within NVB (Rs. 0.34, $p = 0.003$), but were not significantly related to US-measured postop dimensions of NVB (Rs. 0.21, $p = 0.07$) (Table 5.3).[15] Power Doppler TRUS confirmed preserved pulsatile blood vessels within the NVB, which were more likely preserved by the energy-free LRP technique minimizing the

TABLE 5.4. Post-operative TRUS findings of NVB in patients undergoing complete bilateral nerve sparing.

	Group I NVB (*n*. 34)	Group II NVB (*n*. 76)	*p* Value (Group I vs. group II)
No. of visible vessels (%)	1.2 (40%)	1.8 (56%)	0.003
Pulsatile arterial flow (%)	18 (53%)	59 (78%)	0.01
Resistive index (%)	0.82 (95%)	0.83 (97%)	0.4
Max. NVB Dimension (mm) (%)	4.3 (74%)	4.5 (78%)	0.5

All percentages in this table represent percentages of preoperative baseline data

iatrogenic trauma against the cavernous nerve, and which could correlate with superior erectile function recovery (Table 5.4).[15] Multiple stepwise regression analysis revealed that optimal predictors for postoperative potency were a combination of preoperative SHIM score (*F*-value 27.9, $p < 0.0001$), US-confirmed pulsatile arterial flow within NVB (*F*-value 17.2, $p < 0.0001$), and US-identified number of visible vessels within the NVB (*F*-value 7.1, $p = 0.01$) (Figs. 5.12 and 5.13).[15]

Conclusion

Our clinical experience of TRUS guidance during LRP provided initial proof of concept regarding the feasibility of real-time US navigation during radical prostatectomy to enhance intraoperative surgical performance in regard to both oncological and functional outcomes. In this era of minimally invasive surgery with increasing number to use robot assistance in prostate surgery, in which the surgeon may lack completely tactile feedback, transrectal-based real-time imaging guidance will have a significant role to assist the precision of the surgery.

References

1. Schuessler WW, Schulam PG, Clayman RV, et al. Laparoscopic radical prostatectomy: initial short-term experience. Urology. 50: 854–857, 1997
2. Guillonneau B, el-Fettouh H, Baumert H, Cathelineau X, Doublet JD, Fromont G, et al. Laparoscopic radical prostatectomy: oncological evaluation after 1,000 cases at Montsouris Institute. J Urol. 169: 1261, 2003
3. Menon M, Tewari A, Peabody JO, et al. Vattikuti Institute prostatectomy, a technique of robotic radical prostatectomy for management of localized carcinoma of the prostate: experience of over 1100 cases. Urol Clin North Am. 31: 701–717, 2004
4. Rassweiller J, Stolzenburg J, Sulser T, Deger S, Zumbe J, et al. Laparoscopic radical prostatectomy – the experience of the German Laparoscopic Working Group. Eur Urol. 49: 113–119, 2006
5. Ukimura O, Gill IS, Desai MM, Steinberg AP, Kilciler M, Ng CS, et al. Real-time transrectal ultrasonography during laparoscopic radical prostatectomy. J Urol. 172: 112–118, 2004

6. Ukimura O, Troncoso P, Ramirez EI, and Babaian RJ. Prostate cancer staging: correlation between ultrasound determined tumor contact length and pathologically confirmed extraprostatic extension. J Urol. 159: 1251–1259, 1998
7. Gill IS, Ukimura O, Rubinstein M, Finelli A, Moinzadeh A, Singh D, et al. Lateral pedicle control during laparoscopic radical prostatectomy: refined technique. Urology. 65: 23–27, 2005
8. Ukimura O, Magi-Galluzzi C, and Gill IS. Real-time transrectal ultrasound guidance during nerve-sparing laparoscopic radical prostatectomy: Impact on surgical margins. J Urol. 175: 1304–1310, 2006
9. Ukimura O, and Gill IS. Pictorial essay: real-time transrectal ultrasound guidance during nerve-sparing laparoscopic radical prostatectomy. J Urol. 175: 1311–1319, 2006
10. Bianco FJ Jr, Scardino PT, Eastham JA. Radical prostatectomy: long-term cancer control and recovery of sexual and urinary function ("trifecta"). Urology. 66(5 Suppl): 83–94, 2005
11. Partin AW, Kattan MW, Subong EN, Walsh PC, Wojno KJ, Oesterling JE, Scardino PT, Pearson JD. Combination of prostate-specific antigen, clinical stage, and Gleason score to predict pathological stage of localized prostate cancer. A multi-institutional update. JAMA. 277: 1445–1451, 1997
12. Hernandez DJ, Epstein JI, Trock BJ, Tsuzuki T, Carter HB, and Walsh PC: Radical retropubic prostatectomy.How often do experienced surgeons have positive surgical margins when there is extraprostatic extension in the region of the neurovascular bundle? J Urol. 173: 446, 2005
13. Purohit RS, Shinohara K, Meng MV, and Carroll PR. Imaging clinically localized prostate cancer. Urol Clin North Am. 30: 279, 2003
14. Rifkin MD, Zerhouni EA, Gatsonics CA, Quint LE, Paushter DM, Epstein JI, Hamper U, Walsh PC, McNeil BJ. Comparison of magnetic resonance imaging and ultrasonography in staging early prostate cancer. Results of a multi-institutional cooperative trial. N Engl J Med. 323: 621–626, 1990
15. Gill IS, and Ukimura O. Thermal energy-free laparoscopic nerve-sparing radical prostatectomy: 1 Year potency outcomes. Urology. 70: 309–314, 2007

Chapter 6
Contemporary TRUS-Guided Prostate Biopsy for Screening and Staging

Kazumi Kamoi and Richard Babaian

Introduction

Historically, the diagnosis of the prostate cancer (PCa) has been limited to digital rectal examination (DRE) and digitally directed biopsy only for patients with symptoms suspicious for PCa. Introduction of prostate-specific antigen (PSA) measurement and advances in PCa screening have led to an increasing number of patients who undergo prostate biopsy. Currently, transrectal ultrasound (TRUS)-guided prostate biopsy is the gold standard to take pathological specimens for the diagnosis of PCa. Initial studies found that random systematic sextant biopsies provided superior detection compared with biopsies directed only at specific hypoechoic defect.[1] However, more recent studies have suggested that standard sextant biopsies may underestimate the incidence of cancer, with reported false-negative rates of 20–30%.[2,3] Several investigators have altered the biopsy scheme in an effort to enhance the detection rates.[4–8] Despite modification of standard biopsy techniques, urologists frequently face the dilemmas in men at risk of PCa, thus candidate for TRUS-guided biopsy. What is optimal timing and PSA cutoff for biopsy? What is optimal number and location of cores at the initial biopsy? How should patients be prepared for the biopsy? When and how to repeat the biopsy? How do we use the information from biopsy specimens for staging of PCa? This chapter describes the technical details of TRUS-guided systematic sampling, its evolution, its accuracy, and associated morbidity.

Indications and Contraindications

The indication for biopsy should be individualized depending on the risk assessment of each patient. The factors most consistently shown to increase risk of PCa are early age of onset, baseline PSA levels, and number of affected family members. According to the recommendations of the American Cancer Society,[9] both PSA test and DRE should be offered annually beginning at age of 50 years to men who have a life expectancy of at least 10 years. Men at high risk, including men of sub-Saharan African descent and men with a first-degree relative diagnosed before age 65 years, should begin testing at age 45 years. Men at even higher risk of prostate cancer due to more than one first-degree relative diagnosed with prostate cancer could begin testing at age 40 years, although if PSA is less than 1.0 ng ml^{-1}, no additional testing is needed until age 45. If PSA is greater than 1.0 ng ml^{-1} but less than 2.5 ng ml^{-1}, annual testing is recommended. If PSA is 2.5 ng ml^{-1} or greater, further evaluation with biopsy should be considered.[9] Among men older than 50 years with baseline PSA ≤1.0 ng ml^{-1} and normal DRE, PCa screening could be safely performed every 3 years, while men with baseline PSA levels >1.5 ng ml^{-1} will need annual testing.[10] In men older than 65 years with PSA value ≤1.0 ng ml^{-1}, it is presumable that further follow-up can be omitted.[11]

The specificity of PSA is limited because of its fluctuation due to prostatitis, benign prostatic hyperplasia (BPH), or gland manipulation; therefore, the optimal upper limit of normal is also a matter of debate. In a large recent study, 15% of patients with PSA value ≤4.0 ng ml^{-1} and normal DRE had prostate cancer.[12] There is accumulating evidence that the detection rate of PCa among men in the 2.6–4.0 ng ml^{-1} range is similar to that found in the 4.1–10.0 ng ml^{-1} range,[13–15] that most of these cancers are clinically significant,[16,17] and, lastly, that more than 80% of them are organ confined, thus candidates for curative treatment.[18,19] These data suggest that 2.5 ng ml^{-1} may be a more appropriate cutoff point than 4.0 ng ml^{-1}, particularly in younger men for those elevated PSA levels that are less associated with BPH.

Conversely, lowering the PSA cutoff for biopsy indication to 2.5 ng ml^{-1} in all men will most probably increase the overdiagnosis of nonlife-threatening PCa for the following reasons: moderately elevated serum PSA is more related to BPH than to cancer;[20] most early-stage PCa have an indolent course at least for the first decade;[21] and, lastly, there is no convincing evidence that men with PCa treated when their PSA levels of 4.0 ng ml^{-1} or less have better outcomes than men treated when their PSA is more than 4.0 ng ml^{-1}.[22]

Percent free PSA can yield greater specificity in order to select which patients are necessary for biopsy. In a systematic

O. Ukimura and I.S. Gill (eds.), *Contemporary Interventional Ultrasonography in Urology,*
DOI: 10.1007/978-1-84800-217-3_6, © Springer-Verlag London Limited 2009

review,[23] percent free PSA >25% in men with serum PSA between 4.0 and 9.9 ng ml^{-1} avoided about 18% of unnecessary biopsies (allowing 5% of cancers to be missed). When applied in the PSA range of 2.0–3.9 ng ml^{-1}, percent free PSA >28% avoided only 6% of unnecessary biopsies while missing 5% of cancers. Newer agents (PSA isoforms) are also under investigation to identify high-risk patients for PCa and reduce the number of unnecessary biopsies.

In summary, the indication for biopsy is an area of a continuing debate and shifting consensus, but currently an abnormal DRE and/or elevated PSA (greater than 4.0 ng ml^{-1} or the age-corrected level) is taken as suggestive of an increased risk of prostate cancer. Other than the screening purpose, current indications for prostate biopsy include prior to intervention in symptomatic BPH or orthotopic urinary diversion as well as post to external beam radiotherapy, brachytherapy, cryotherapy, or radial prostatectomy for rising serum PSA level.

Contraindications for prostate biopsy include acute painful perianal disorder, severe immunosuppression, acute prostatitis, and coaglopathy. There is no proven increase in hemorrhagic complications with aspirin or nonsteroidal anti-inflammatory drug NSAID use.[24,25] A recent study has suggested that warfarin therapy may not increase bleeding rates,[26] though this finding may be due to the small sample size and possible reporting bias.[27,28] Our policy is to continue aspirin, but to stop warfarin (to achieve INR <1.3 on the day of biopsy) following consultation with the clinician. These are restarted after 24 h, as all major recorded bleeds took place within 24 h of biopsy. If anticoagulation/antiplatelet agents cannot be safely discontinued, the patient should be converted to heparin and biopsied as an inpatient.

Patient Preparation

Antibiotics

Transrectal prostate biopsy involves a tiny perforation of the rectal mucosa to reach the prostate. This procedure has a slight risk of complications including infections. Therefore, most centers routinely administer antibiotic prophylaxis to all patients undergoing transrectal prostate biopsy. In fact, Shandera et al.[29] reported that as many as 99% of urologists in the United States administer antibiotic prophylaxis for prostate biopsy. However, antibiotic prophylaxis cannot eliminate the possibility of infection. There are currently no standard rules on antibiotic prophylaxis for transrectal prostate biopsy and extensively different regimens are employed. Several studies have demonstrated a significant decrease in infectious complications when prophylactic antibiotics were used.[30–32] Recently the use of only 1-day prophylaxis medication with fluoroquinolone has been shown to be safe for prostate biopsy. Shigemura et al.[33] demonstrated that there is no statistically significant difference between levofloxacin at 600 mg for 1 day and levofloxacin at 300 mg for 3 days regarding the elevation of WBC and CRP. Briefly, infectious complications after prostate biopsy are rare and oral therapy is sufficient.[34] Thus, cost issues need to be considered when selecting the type of antibiotic prophylaxis to be used.

Enemas

Some urologists believe an enema is effective to empty the rectal cavity because stool may obstruct the image of the prostate. Others believe that it decreases the risk of infection. One of the first preventive measures introduced in transrectal prostate biopsy was local antisepsis applied to the rectal mucosa with povidone-iodine. Rees et al.[35] observed that bacteremia decreased from 76 to 17% after prostate needle biopsy when no rectal cleansing was done versus phosphate enema administration followed by proctoscopy with rectal flushing with povidone. Lindert et al.[36] randomized 50 men without prophylactic antibiotics to receive a prebiopsy enema or no enema. Of the patients 28% who did not receive an enema had bacteremia, although it was asymptomatic, while 4% given an enema had a positive blood culture. They concluded that an enema decreases the amount of bacteria from the rectum as well as the amount introduced by the biopsy. Contrarily, Sharpe et al.,[37] in a randomized study of 80 patients who underwent transrectal prostate biopsy without antibiotic prophylaxis, found no significant differences in infectious complications between the group receiving povidone-iodine local antisepsis and the placebo group. Carey et al.[38] reported a retrospective review of patients with identical antibiotic prophylaxis comparing who received enemas before biopsy and not. Overall, clinically significant complications developed in 4.4% (10 of 225) of patients who had versus 3.2% (6 of 185) of those who did not have an enema. They concluded that enema before biopsy provides no clinically significant outcome advantage, and potentially increases patient cost and discomfort.

Accumulating complication rates between studies performed without enema before biopsy have been similar to those performed with enema before biopsy.[25,39–41] A retrospective review of 4,439 biopsies with no prebiopsy enema and antibiotic prophylaxis using ciprofloxacin showed a symptomatic infection rate of 0.1%.[34] No consensus in the literature exists in regard to the impact of a bowel-cleansing enema before biopsy on transrectal prostate biopsy complication rates. Davis et al.[42] surveyed urologists in community and academic practice regarding their standard approach to patient preparation for transrectal prostate biopsy. They mailed 110 surveys to community urologists in Florida and urological oncologists at academic centers across the United States. Overall 79% of respondents prescribe an enema in preparation for biopsy and 81% administer an oral fluoroquinolone before biopsy. A current preparation for transrectal biopsy at M.D. Anderson Cancer Center consists of the use of enema at 1–2 h prior to procedure and the administration of Levofloxacin 500 mg p.o. 1 h prior to procedure. For patients with prosthetic joint, 1 dose of Gentamicin 80 mg i.m. is given 30 min prior to procedure. For patients with valvular heart disease, Gentamicin 80 mg and Ampicillin 2 gm i.v. are given 30 min prior to procedure.

Anesthesia

Urologists frequently experience anxiety in men presenting for TRUS-guided biopsy. Reducing patient discomfort becomes more important as increasing numbers of patients require repeat biopsy. There is strong evidence in the current literature that anesthesia and/or analgesia improves patient tolerance and comfort. Therefore, urologists should be aware of introducing it in clinical practice as a routine part of the procedure whatever the patient characteristics and biopsy scheme.

The most popular approach is the periprostatic nerve block. Prospective randomized trials have proven its efficacy when compared with placebo or rectal anesthetic gel.[43,44] The nerves can be blocked with either unilateral or bilateral injection, around the apex or base of the gland. Our technique is described in Fig. 6.1, but no single technique or drug combination demonstrated superiority and all methods appear safe with no additional infective and hemorrhagic complications.[45,46]

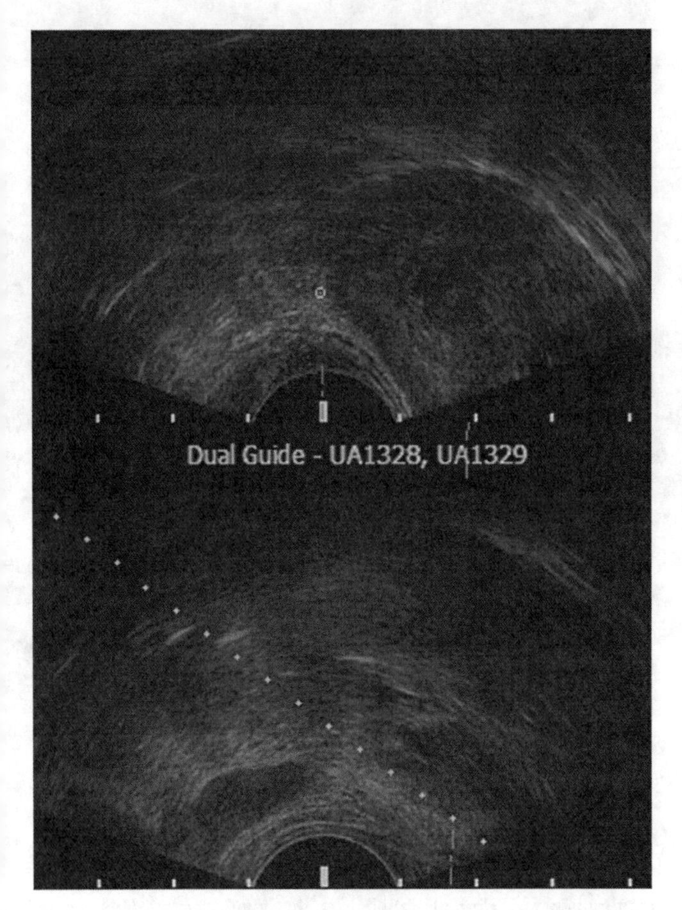

Fig. 6.1. Periprostatic nerve block before biopsy. Our technique to reduce the discomfort of TRUS-guided biopsy is through the use of: (1) intrarectal anesthetic gel to decrease ultrasound probe discomfort and needle discomfort for periprostatic nerve block. (2) Benzodiazepine for patients with excessive anxiety. (3) Periprostatic nerve block with 5 cc of 1% lidocaine injection at prostate base bilaterally junction with seminal vesicles. The *arrow* on the transverse (*upper*) image points to the marker which indicates the projection of the path that the needle will follow in the sagittal (*lower*) image. Note that this target is exactly at prostate base junction with seminal vesicles

Of other techniques, the data regarding NSAIDs, probe design, and rectal anesthetic gel are unconvincing. Entonox is an effective, simple, and safe form of analgesia, although it is not currently used widely.[47,48] Topical GTN paste (commonly used in the treatment of anal fissures) effectively reduces anal discomfort during probe introduction, but takes 30 min to be effective and a recovery time is necessary.[44,49] Intravenous sedation is useful,[50] but any intravenous administration of sedative has potential problems that may require the attendance of an anesthetist.

Among the various methods, periprostatic nerve block alone or associated with lidocaine gel has been shown to be safe, easy to perform, and highly effective. It can be considered the gold standard at the moment even if the optimal technique remains to be established.

Basic Technique for TRUS-Guided Biopsy

Anatomy

The guiding principle behind prostate biopsy is the anatomical or glandular distribution of prostate cancer. Anatomically, the gland is split into zones as shown in Fig. 6.2. In the young male the peripheral zone (PZ) comprises 75% of the volume of the prostate, the transition zone (TZ) 20%, and the central zone (CZ) 5%, but with age these ratios change. After the age of 40 years, most men develop BPH, which arises from TZ and eventually it may occupy most of the gland. Conversely, the majority (70–80%) of prostate cancers arise from PZ,[51] whatever the gland volume and zonal volume percentages. Whole gland studies have also shown that cancers cluster around the posterolateral margins, apex and base of the gland.[52] This basic knowledge of PCa has been applied to maximize the sampling techniques from areas of high cancer incidence during TRUS-guided prostate biopsy.

Probes

Any biopsy regimen must include sampling from the apical area of the prostate. Endfire probe is suitable for the apical biopsies because the biopsy guide for endfire imaging is placed immediately behind the imaging array (Fig. 6.3a). This ensures the shortest possible biopsy path to the apex. Some of the currently available biplane probes can simultaneously visualize the prostate in both sagittal and transverse planes. A simultaneous biplane view enables more correctly targeted biopsy (Fig. 6.3b).

Imaging of the Prostate

Currently, the most widely used probe is a high-frequency transducer (7 MHz or higher) which can produce precise images of the prostate. Positioning should be left lateral,

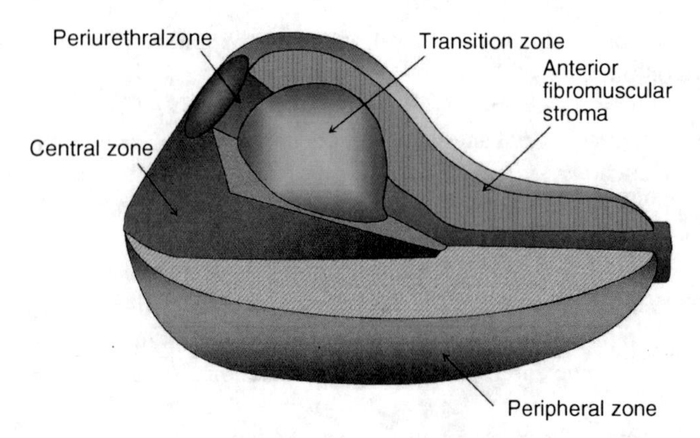

Fig. 6.2. Zonal anatomy of the prostate. Anatomically, the gland is split into five zones: three glandular (*the peripheral zone, the transition zone,* and *the central zone*) and two nonglandular (*the periurethral zone* and *the fibromuscular stroma*). *The peripheral zone*: The peripheral zone constitutes almost 75% of the normal prostate gland. It occupies the distal prostate gland, the area around the urethra distal to the verumontanum. A healthy peripheral zone displays a homogeneous isoechoic ultrasound pattern. The "surgical capsule" that separates the peripheral zone from the transition zone appears as a distinct boundary in ultrasound. *The transition zone*: Approximately 5–10% of the normal prostate gland is transition zone. The transition zone lies superior to the verumontanum, lateral to the proximal urethra, and posterior to the fibromuscular stroma. Enlargement of the transition zone due to BPH may alter the contour of the prostate in older men, compressing the peripheral zone or displacing it laterally. *The central zone*: The central zone makes up 25% of the glandular tissue. The central zone lies posterior to the urethra and superior to the verumontanum. The ejaculatory ducts traverse through the central zone. *The anterior fibromuscular stroma*: The anterior fibromuscular stroma forms the anterior surface of the gland. It may be up to 1-cm thick, but thins out over the distal portion of the gland. The anterior fibromuscular stroma is more prominent sonographically in younger, non-BPH patients. *The periurethral zone*: The periurethral zone is a midline structure of cylindrical, internal smooth muscle sphincter that runs from the base of the verumontanum to the back of the bladder neck. This is the site of origin of the large median lobe of BPH

lithotomy, or knee-elbow. A small amount of urine in the bladder facilitates the examination. When starting scan in the transverse view, from the deepest part, seminal vesicles are identified bilaterally with the ampullae of the vas on either side of the midline (Fig. 6.4a). Next, the base of the prostate is imaged where CZ comprises the posterior part of the gland and often is hypoechoic (Fig. 6.4b). The midgland is the widest portion of the gland (Fig. 6.4c). The echogenicity in PZ is described as isoechoic and closely packed. TZ is the central part of the gland and itself is moderately hypoechoic when compared to PZ. The junction of PZ and TZ is usually distinct and characterized by a hypo- or hyperechoic border (Fig. 6.4d). Scanning at the level of the verumontanum and observing the tower-like appearance help identify the urethra (Fig. 6.4e). The prostate distal to the verumontanum (prostatic apex) is mainly composed of PZ (Fig. 6.4f). The peripro-

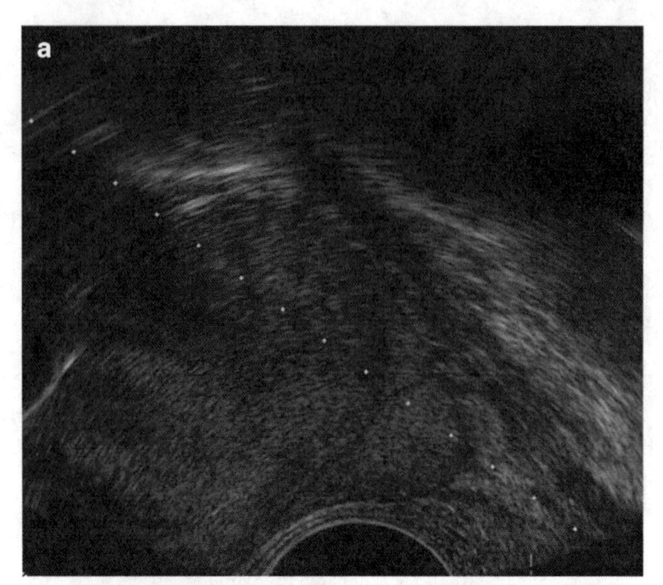

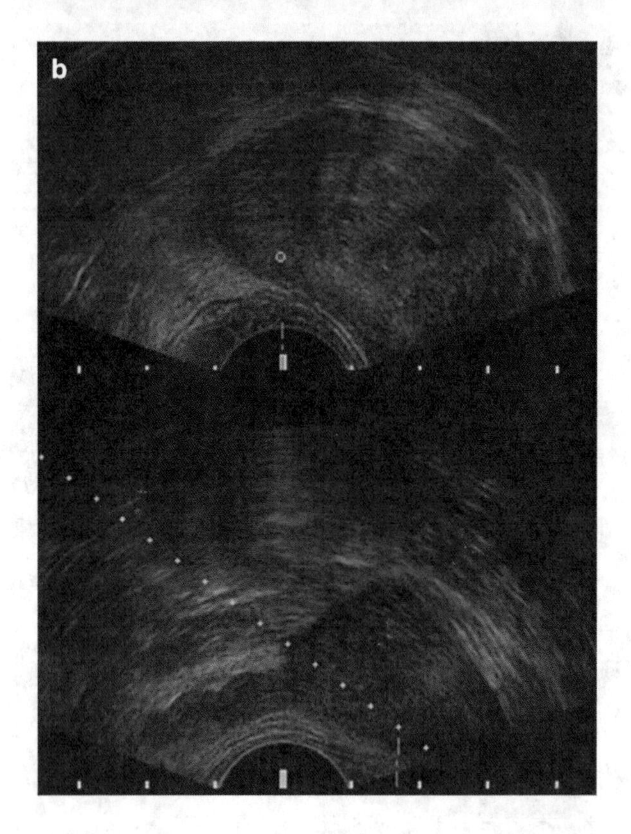

Fig. 6.3. (**a**) Targeting the apical biopsy. The biopsy guide for endfire imaging is placed immediately behind the imaging array. This ensures the shortest possible biopsy path to the apex, thereby helping you avoid accidental piercing of other pelvic floor structures. (**b**) Targeting the right lateral peripheral zone for a biopsy. The *arrow* on the transverse (*upper*) image points to the marker which indicates the projection of the path that the needle will follow in the sagittal (lower) image. Note that this target is exactly in the lateral peripheral zone

static tissue of the prostate is a hyperechoic structure that can be identified all around the gland. Several hypoechoic structures identified anterior to the prostate gland are the

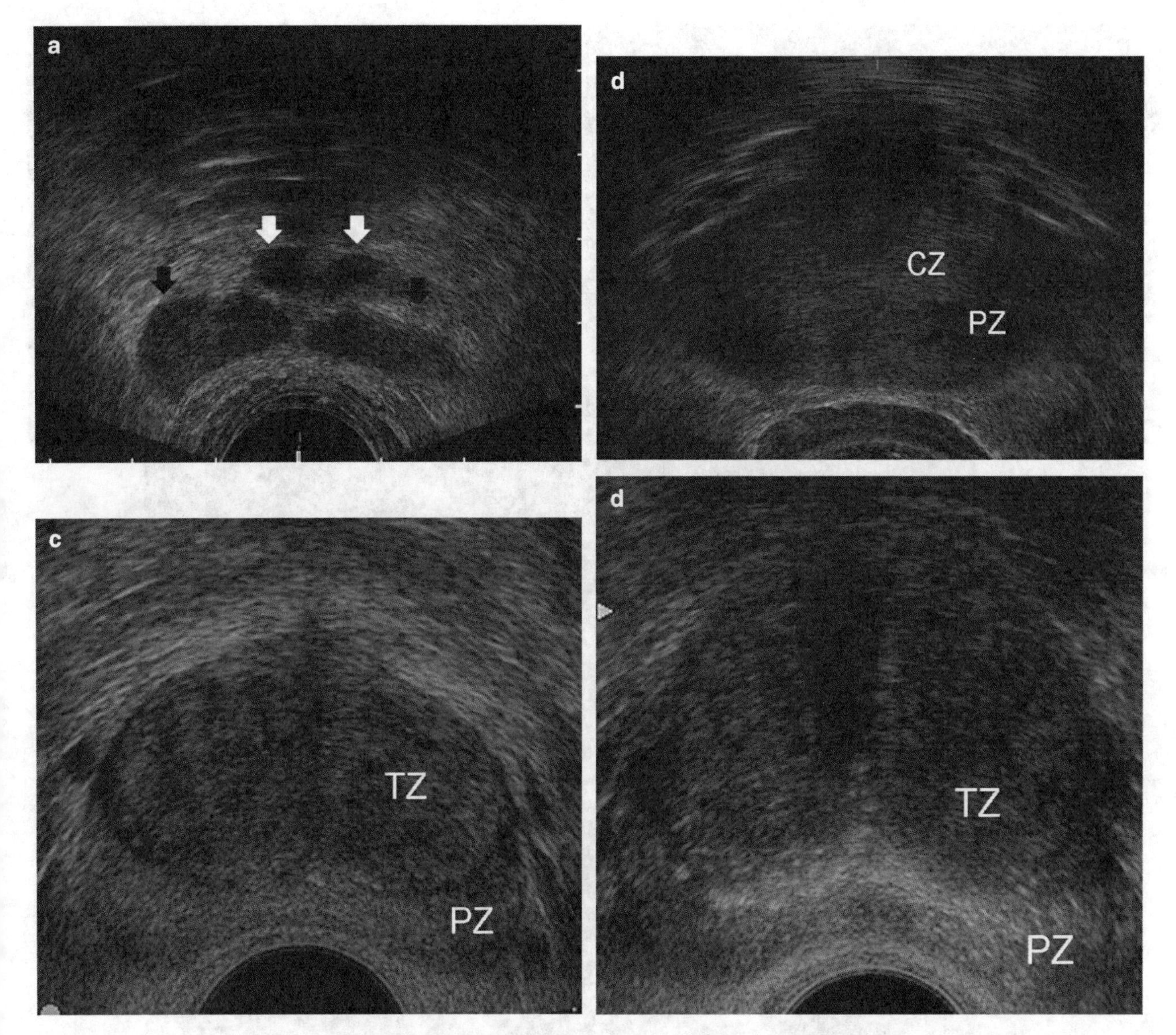

FIG. 6.4. (**a**) The image of seminal vesicles. The seminal vesicles are convoluted cystic structures and are darkly anechoic. The ampullae of the vas are on either side of the midline. (**b**) The base of the prostate. The upper hypoechoic area is composed of the smooth muscle of the internal sphincter and portions of the periurethral tissue. (**c**) The midgland. The junction of the peripheral zone and the transition zone is distinct and hypoechoic. The echogenicity in PZ is described as isoechoic. The transition zone is the central part of the gland and a variety of echogenic areas. (**d**) The midgland. The junction of PZ and TZ may be characterized by a hyperechoic region, which results from prostatic calculi or corpora amylacea. (**e**) The level of the verumontanum. The hypoechoic tower-like appearance helps identify the urethra. (**f**) The apex of the prostate. The periurethral structure is surrounded by the peripheral zone. (**g**) The prostatic venous plexus. Several hypoechoic structures identified anterior to the prostate gland are the prostatic venous plexus. Doppler imaging (*right*) shows blood flow in the venous plexus. (**h**) The neurovascular bundles. The neurovascular bundles can be identified as a hypoechoic bundle located outside posterolateral prostate. Doppler imaging (*right*) shows blood flow in the neurovascular bundle. (**i**) The median lobe of the prostate. The sagittal plane allows visualization of the urethra. The median lobe of the prostate is visualized

prostatic venous plexus (Fig. 6.4g). The neurovascular bundles can be identified as a hypoechoic bundle (mainly by reflection of the relatively large hypoechoic vascular complex surrounded by hyperechoic fat), within which definitive blood flow could be confirmed using Doppler imaging (Fig. 6.4h). Imaging in the sagittal plane allows visualization of the urethra. The median lobes of the prostate are often visualized (Fig. 6.4i).

Diagnostically, TRUS is also used to measure the volume of the prostate gland,[53] an important factor in calculating PSA density, i.e., serum PSA level divided by gland volume. Moreover, the volume as measured with TRUS can be used in predictive nomograms.[54] Several formulas have been used to calculate prostatic volume, but the most common one is the ellipsoid formula, which requires measurement of three prostate dimensions. First, in the transverse view, the width (trans-

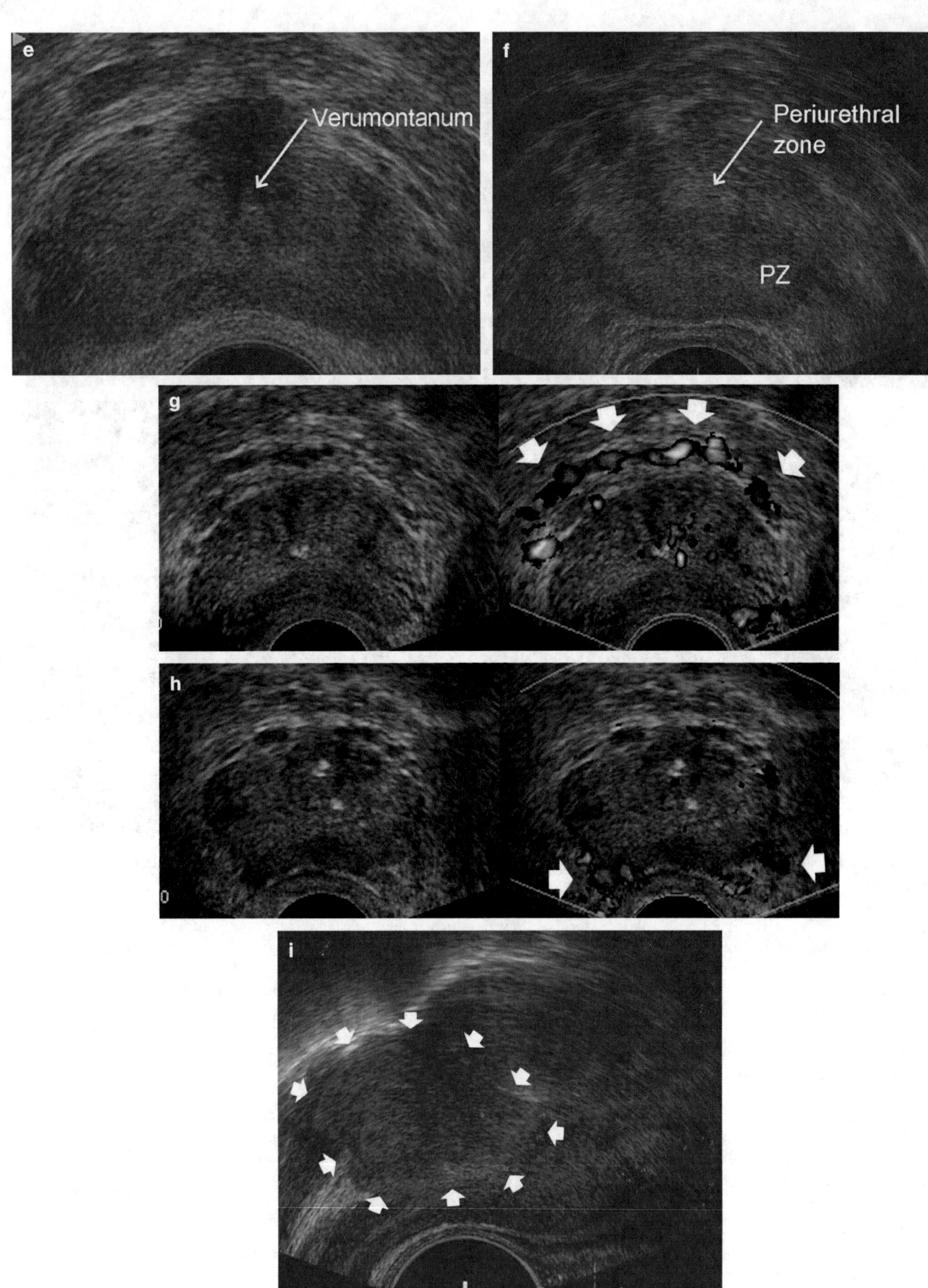

FIG. 6.4. (continued)

verse dimension) and the height (anteroposterior dimension) are measured at its largest diameter (Fig. 6.5a). The length (longitudinal dimension) is measured in the sagittal plane just off the midline because the bladder neck often obscures the cephalad extent of the gland (Fig. 6.5b). The ellipsoid volume formula is then applied as follows:

$$\text{Volume} = \text{height} \times \text{width} \times \text{length} \times 0.52.$$

Basic Biopsy Technique

Biopsies are best performed with a spring-driven needle core biopsy device, which can be passed through the needle guide attached to the ultrasound probe. Most instrumentation provides optimal visualization of the biopsy needle path in the sagittal plane. In general, 18-gauge needles are used, and the tips of the needles are etched with small ridges to increase their echogenicity. Ultrasound images should be superimposed with a ruled puncture line that corresponds to the needle guide of the probe, which allows anticipation of the needle path (Fig. 6.3a,b).

Directed biopsies are obtained from any suggestive (i.e., hypoechoic) area based on ultrasound images or based on palpable abnormalities after DRE. Because the incidence of nonpalpable isoechoic prostate tumors is high, limiting biopsy sites to either sonographically suspicious lesions or to areas of palpable abnormality tends to miss many malignancies.

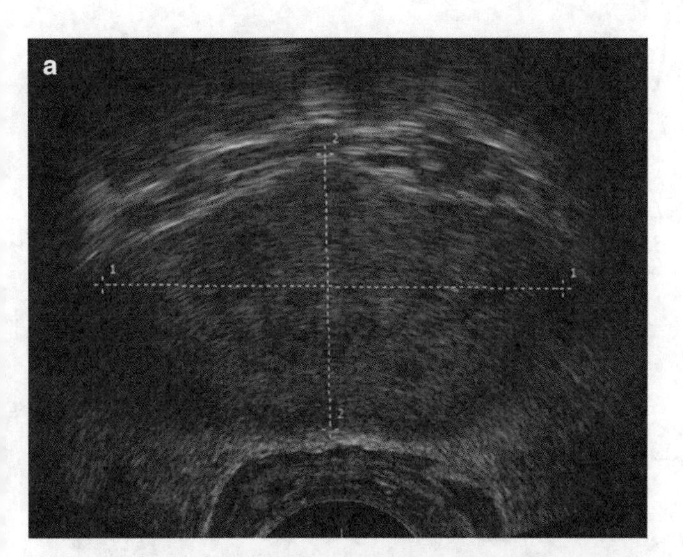

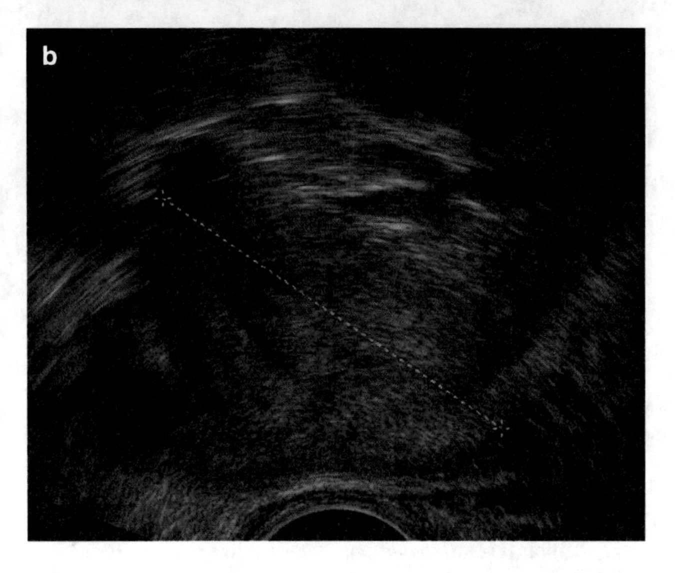

FIG. 6.5. (**a**) A measurement of the prostate in the transverse view. The transverse and anteroposterior dimensions are measured at the estimated point of widest transverse dimension. (**b**) A measurement of the prostate in the sagittal view. The longitudinal dimension is measured in the midline

Cancer Imaging

Cancer, depending on its size, grade, and location, usually appears hypoechoic relative to the normal peripheral zone of the prostate.[55] Modern TRUS probes incorporate wide-band high-frequency transducers capable of detailed multiaxial imaging, but despite greatly improved anatomical representation its diagnostic ability is still disappointing. For cancer diagnosis, TRUS has a positive predictive value of 6% if PSA and DRE are normal.[56] With the shift toward smaller, early-stage cancers, many cancers detected at biopsy are not visible at TRUS (low sensitivity) and many hypoechoic areas do not prove to be malignant at biopsy (low specificity); therefore, TRUS alone, without the addition of biopsy, has limited value in the detection of cancer.

Evolution of Biopsy Technique

Initial Biopsy: Development of the Various Protocols

The first TRUS-guided prostate biopsies (in the early 1980s) were targeted at focal lesions suspicious for cancer. But most of these nodules proved to be histologically benign. Faced with the knowledge that targeted biopsies were inaccurate, various sampling methods were tried. Bilobar or quadrant biopsies were first reported, but the landmark sampling technique was the sextant protocol reported in 1989.[1] As originally described, six biopsies were obtained in a parasagittal line drawn halfway between the lateral border and midline bilaterally, from the base, midgland, and apex (see Fig. 6.6a). This was a major advance, with a 20–25% positive biopsy rate. However, with wider experience, even the sextant technique was found to be inaccurate, principally because it undersamples the PZ. Keetch et al.[2] showed a 20% positive rate on repeat biopsy, and all subsequent studies have confirmed this high false-negative rate of the classical sextant method.[57–59] Modifications of the sextant technique were reported from the mid-1990s onward, based on improved understanding of the origin and location of prostate cancers within the gland. The anteriorly directed trajecto-

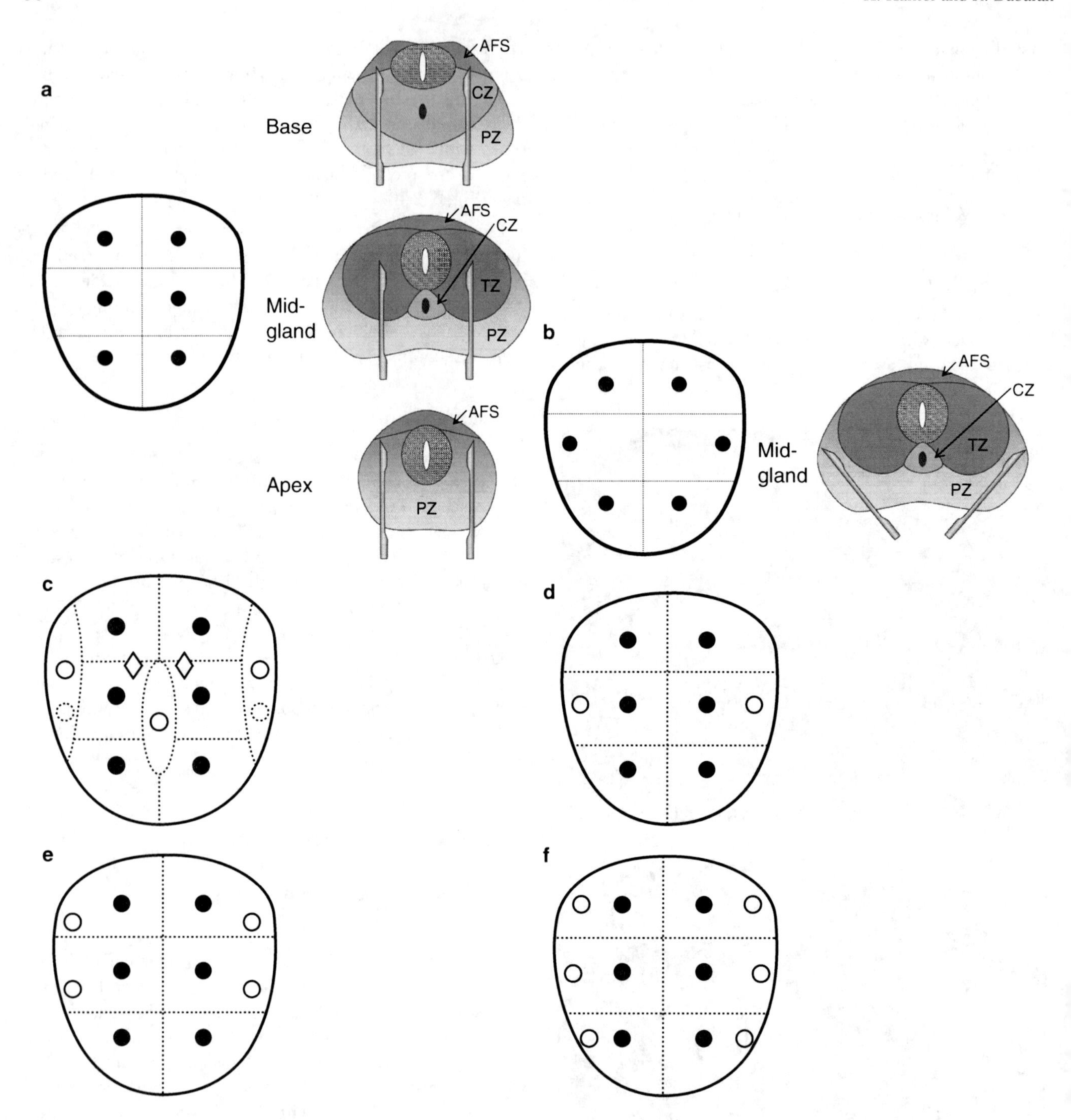

Fig 6.6. Diagrammatic representation of the various sampling patterns. (**a**) This is the original sextant biopsy as described by Hodge et al. The coronal section shows six biopsies (*filled circles*) obtained in the parasagittal line, halfway between the lateral border and midline bilaterally, from the base, midgland, and apex. The corresponding images demonstrate the needle trajectory in the axial plane at points marked on the coronal view. Note the amount of the peripheral zone left unsampled, particularly by the midgland biopsies. (**b**) These coronal and axial figures represent the modified sextant technique. Note, on the corresponding axial image representing the midgland, a larger amount of the PZ is sampled by pointing the needle in an anterolateral direction. (**c**) This coronal figure illustrates 11-core biopsy; sextant (*filled circles*) plus one lateral on each side, one TZ on each side just lateral and anterior to urethra (*open diamond*), and one midline biopsy. (**d**) 13-core biopsy includes one additional lateral biopsy (broken circle) on each side. These coronal representations show the ideal targets for eight PZ biopsies. (**e**) These coronal representations show the ideal targets for 10 PZ biopsies. (**f**) These coronal representations show the ideal targets for 12 PZ biopsies

ries of the traditional sextant model (Fig. 6.6a) undersampled the PZ, particularly around the posterolateral margins. Hence the so-called modified protocol evolved, whereby the middle biopsies of the standard sextant were moved laterally and the biopsy trajectories also angled anterolaterally so that mainly the PZ was sampled (Fig. 6.6b).[60,61]

With time even the modified sextant pattern was shown to miss some tumors,[6,62] and various alternatives were explored. Chen et al.[52] showed that midline, periurethral, and apicolateral PZ tumors were being missed. Therefore extended protocols were introduced to minimize the missing cancers when conventional sextant biopsy was performed. Figure 6.6c illustrates the technique we developed.[7] Other protocols use more cores directed on PZ (Fig. 6.6d–f).[63,64] Although available data show that eight to ten biopsies will improve diagnosis by 20–30% over the traditional sextant protocol, it is still a matter of debate whether extended protocols are substantially better than the modified sextant protocol. A recent survey of US practice showed that 63% obtain eight or more cores per biopsy session, 36% biopsy the lateral and midline locations.[42] Presti[65] reviewed several studies evaluating various biopsy schemes and suggested that a 10–12-core scheme is optimal in most patients having an initial biopsy.

The biopsy protocols described aim to increase PZ sampling. Logically more cores should increase the likelihood of hitting a given tumor volume in the PZ. However, some prostate cancers originate in TZ. It is believed that these tumors may be less aggressive, although they present with higher PSA levels. Studies have varied in the diagnostic yield of TZ biopsies from 3 to 26%.[66–68] Some have advocated routine biopsy of this area, but more contemporary studies suggest that the true yield is around 2%.[69] In reality all biopsy strategies may sample a part of the TZ that immediately adjacent to the PZ and in routine practice deep samples from the TZ are not thought helpful, except in patients requiring repeat biopsies. Indeed at second biopsy, many studies estimate higher diagnostic yields for TZ biopsies.[69]

Naughton et al.[70] have suggested a linear relationship between the number of biopsies required to diagnose prostate cancer and gland volume. The added effects of BPH also need to be considered. An enlarged TZ compresses the PZ into a thin rind and more cores are needed to sufficiently sample a thinned PZ. Two retrospective studies have shown that sextant biopsies in an enlarged gland had a higher false-negative rate compared with the smaller gland.[71,72] Many practitioners use a volume correction method (an example is 8–10 cores for ≤50 ml glands, and 12 cores if the volume is >50 ml). However, the data on the advantages of volume-determined biopsy strategies, over and above an extended policy (eight to ten biopsies), are not yet convincing.[73]

Repeat Biopsies

In some cases clinical suspicion of undisclosed cancer persists after a negative first biopsy. Examples include patients with a high PSA level (a "high" PSA level is also a matter of debate but an example is PSA >10 or 20 ng ml^{-1}, particularly if the gland is of normal size), a rising PSA level, high-grade prostatic intraepithelial neoplasia (HGPIN) or atypical glands suspicious for cancer (AG) on first biopsy.

As a group these patients are few, but repeat biopsy may detect cancer in 19–41% of patients within these subcategories.[2,74,75] Small retrospective studies have looked at methods to stratify patients who require rebiopsy, but this is still an area of debate.[76–78] It is assumed that the first set of biopsies may have missed cancer either because it was of small volume or because it was in the inner gland. Repeat biopsies should therefore include the anterolateral PZ, apex and TZ (inner gland), where cancer may have been missed.[79]

Logically with repeat negative biopsies, the likelihood of missing significant cancer diminishes with each set of biopsies. Djavan et al.[58] studied the value of up to four repeat biopsies. Cancer was found in 10% on the second biopsy (other studies have found a rate between 12–30%[76–78]) but the pick-up rate was low on biopsies 3 and 4 (5 and 4%, respectively). Moreover, the cancers found on biopsies 3 and 4 were of low Gleason grade. They concluded that biopsies 3 and 4 were not mandatory. However the PSA range used in their study was narrow (4–10 ng ml^{-1}) and the sextant technique was used to sample the peripheral zone (with two additional TZ biopsies). The results may therefore not be applicable in patients with higher or rapidly increasing PSA,[2,74] or those who had extended cores at the first biopsy.

HGPIN is said to be a precancerous condition that predates frank cancer by 10 years ("HGPIN in the 40s, cancer in the 50s"). It is characterized by architecturally benign ducts and acini lined by abnormal secretory cells with nucleomegaly and prominent nucleoli visible at ×20.[80] The expected incidence of HGPIN on needle biopsy is between 5 and 8%.[81] Finding HGPIN in a prostate biopsy is associated with a greater risk of cancer being detected in subsequent biopsies. In contemporary studies, the median risk recorded in the literature for cancer following the diagnosis of HGPIN on needle biopsy is 24%.[81] If present, cancer may be at remote sites and repeat biopsies should not focus on the area with HGPIN. Extended cores are thought to be sufficient, but in some, saturation coverage may be appropriate. If repeat biopsies again show HGPIN, then PSA levels may be monitored.

The term AG, or atypical small acinar proliferation, denotes the presence of a small focus of atypical glands suspicious for adenocarcinoma, but with insufficient cytological and/or architectural atypia to establish a definitive diagnosis. The median incidence of AG on prostatic needle biopsies is 4.4% and ranges from 0.7 to 23.4%.[81] The likelihood of finding cancer on repeat biopsy is 40–50%,[82] higher than that with a diagnosis of HGPIN. Unlike the man with a rising PSA or HGPIN, the approach here is site specific. It is assumed that either insufficient diagnostic material was retrieved on the first biopsy because the tumor was too small, or that the biopsy caught the edge of a larger, immediately adjacent tumor (perhaps located in the inner gland).

Saturation Biopsy Protocol

In some men, there remains a continuing suspicion of prostate cancer in spite of repeated negative biopsies. Many centers have reported the value of a saturation biopsy technique in these cases. The assumption here is that the cancer is small and/or located in one of the deeper reaches of the gland. The saturation technique takes the principles of sampling to its logical conclusion – the whole gland is sampled without following any particular zonal pattern. In its simplest form this involves little more than taking 20 or more cores, evenly distributed throughout the gland, including the zone anterior to the urethra. The larger number of evenly distributed samples increases the likelihood of picking up an underlying cancer, regardless of tumor size or location (34% positive rate in one study).[83] A more systematic technique of saturation biopsy uses a transperineal, grid-based method using a brachytherapy template (this method allows better sampling of the area immediately anterior to urethra).[84]

However, given the fact more than 40% of men may develop prostate cancer in their lifetime, no one can be sure that all the tiniest foci of PCa have been detected, despite thorough sampling. Much of this disease may be clinically insignificant.[58,85] Furthermore, although a patient with a negative biopsy can be reassured by saturation biopsy protocol, the concern remains that de novo tumor may develop in his remaining years. Indeed in one study, 11% of patients with a negative biopsy developed cancer over a 7-year follow-up period, and two men died of prostate cancer.[86] The need for future rebiopsy depends on the morbidity and acceptability in each patient.

At our institution, we take 10 cores as an initial biopsy; sextant plus two lateral biopsies on each side at midgland and base (Fig. 6.6e). As a repeat biopsy for men with negative sextant biopsy, we use 11-core biopsy; sextant plus one lateral on each side one TZ on each side just lateral and anterior to urethra one midline biopsy (Fig. 6.6c). When two or more extended biopsies are negative and there remains a high suspicion of cancer we consider systematic 12-core TZ biopsy. If there remains a high suspicion of cancer and systematic 12-core TZ biopsy is negative, saturation biopsy using brachytherapy template is considered.

TRUS-Directed Biopsies

The diagnostic ability of gray-scale TRUS is limited by the intrinsically poor visibility of most contemporary prostate cancers. Described appearances of prostate cancer range from hyperechoic to hypoechoic lesions. Hypoechoic lesions are more common, but the vast majority of contemporary tumors are either isoechoic or distinguished only by a nonspecific echo irregularity.

Color Doppler and power Doppler (looking for neovascularization, a prerequisite for tumor invasion) can improve tumor detection, but not significantly more than extended core sampling.[87] It may have a role in the patient undergoing repeat biopsy. Intravascular microbubble contrast agents can improve the accuracy of prostate cancer detection, missing only low-volume tumors of grade 6 and below.[88] Again its value may be limited to repeat biopsy, but large studies of its routine use are needed. Three-dimensional imaging aids detection of enhancement and morphological asymmetry,[89] but has not been proved additional value. Dynamic enhancement curves may help to distinguish inflammatory change from neovascularization and to assess response to antiandrogen therapy, but its use has not been evaluated for diagnostic purposes. Ultrasound elastography may be used to measure tissue stiffness in order to distinguish hard (malignant) from soft (normal).[90] Trials of its routine use are necessary.

Complications

TRUS-guided prostate biopsy is generally considered safe and is commonly performed in an outpatient setting. Several studies on transrectal prostate biopsy reveal major complication (sepsis, bleeding, or other complication requiring admission) rates of around 1–2%, with the following rates of minor complications: hematuria 1–84%; rectal bleeding 37%; hematospermia 1–28%; vasovagal episodes 0–5%; infective complications 1–4%.[25] Although most subside within 48–72 h, patients should be warned that hematospermia can last for 3–4 weeks. Nevertheless, minor complications occurred frequently with 70% of all patients experiencing at least one complication. Although these complications generally do not need intervention (neither conservative nor surgical), patients need to be informed adequately. Repeat biopsies can be performed 6 weeks later with no significant difference in pain apprehension, infectious or hemorrhagic complications.

Prospective studies report higher percentages of complications, but there may also be a relation with the number of cores taken. Increasing the number of biopsies has been associated with an increase in urinary retention and epididymitis[91,92] and continual monitoring is necessary as we move to an era of more cores per gland. The use of local anesthesia has no bearing on complication rates.[93]

Prostate Cancer Staging

Transrectal US has been used for local staging of prostate cancer in some studies but is generally considered insufficient. The criteria for identifying extracapsular extension (ECE) on transrectal US scans are bulging or irregularity of the capsule adjacent to a hypoechoic lesion (Fig. 6.7). Seminal vesicle invasion (SVI) is heralded by a visible extension of a hypoechoic lesion at the base of the prostate into a seminal vesicle or by echogenic cancer within the normally fluid-filled seminal vesicle.[94] Asymmetry of the seminal vesicles or solid hypoechoic masses within the seminal vesicles are

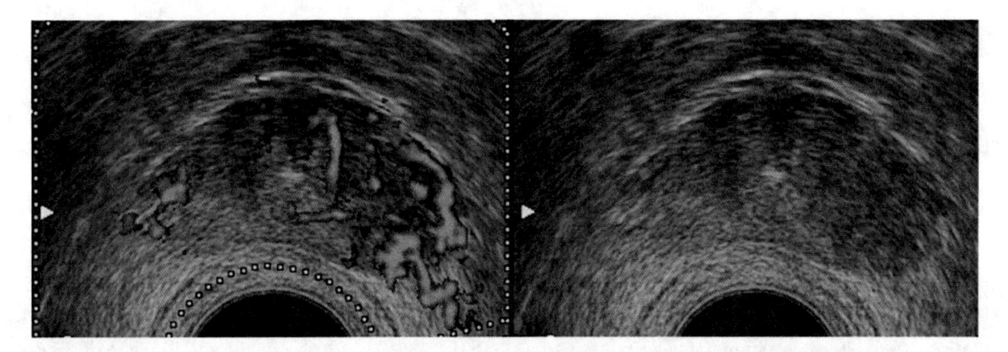

Fig. 6.7. Extracapsular extension of the prostate. The criteria for identifying extracapsular extension on transrectal US scans are bulging or irregularity of the capsule adjacent to a hypoechoic lesion (*right*), and increased vascularity within a region of the gland (*left*)

indirect indicators of disease extension. When extraprostatic extension into the seminal vesicles is suspected, additional transrectal US-guided biopsies of the seminal vesicles can be performed.

The length of the contact of a visible lesion with the capsule is also associated with the probability of ECE. Ukimura et al.[95] reported a monogram predicting the probability of microscopic ECE based on TRUS-determined tumor contact length and preoperative PSA. However, given the substantial stage migration that has occurred, prostate cancer is rarely a systemically detectable disease at presentation. Today, however, tumors are smaller and local extension is uncommon. Modern nomograms more accurately help estimate the probability of ECE, SVI, and lymph node metastases from standard clinical data (stage, grade, and PSA level).[96] Nevertheless, these algorithms provide no information about the location of the cancer or the site of ECE. In most cases management can be decided on biopsy data, supplemented by clinical (age, general health) and biochemical (PSA) data, without the need for any further staging. Therefore, as prostate biopsy lies at the heart of prostate cancer management, it should be carried out with care.

Conclusions

Most prostate cancers are either not visualized on TRUS or indistinguishable from coexisting BPH. Without any fundamental advance in prostate imaging, systematic sampling prostate biopsy will continue to occupy a central management role. However, the diagnostic ultrasound and biopsy of the prostate is a rapidly evolving field with many areas of debate. Looking to the future, ever-younger men are undergoing PSA testing. Less invasive treatments are also under development and some are showing real promise. This will increase the pressure to identify early-stage and small-volume tumors. We can expect further change in our approach to prostate biopsy.

References

1. Hodge KK, McNeal JE, Terris MK, Stamey TA. Random systematic versus directed ultrasound guided transrectal core biopsies of the prostate. J Urol 1989;142:71–4.
2. Keetch DW, Catalona WJ, Smith DS. Serial prostatic biopsies in men with persistently elevated serum prostate specific antigen values. J Urol 1994;151:1571–4.
3. Rabbani F, Stroumbakis N, Kava BR, Cookson MS, Fair WR. Incidence and clinical significance of false-negative sextant prostate biopsies. J Urol 1998;159:1247–50.
4. Stamey TA. Making the most out of six systematic sextant biopsies. Urology 1995;45:2–12.
5. Eskew LA, Bare RL, McCullough DL. Systematic 5 region prostate biopsy is superior to sextant method for diagnosing carcinoma of the prostate. J Urol 1997;157:199–202.
6. Presti JC Jr, Chang JJ, Bhargava V, Shinohara K. The optimal systematic prostate biopsy scheme should include 8 rather than 6 biopsies: results of a prospective clinical trial. J Urol 2000;163:163–6.
7. Babaian RJ, Toi A, Kamoi K, et al. A comparative analysis of sextant and an extended 11-core multisite directed biopsy strategy. J Urol 2000;163:152–7.
8. Naughton CK, Miller DC, Mager DE, Ornstein DK, Catalona WJ. A prospective randomized trial comparing 6 versus 12 prostate biopsy cores: impact on cancer detection. J Urol 2000;164:388–92.
9. Smith RA, Cokkinides V, Eyre HJ. American Cancer Society guidelines for the early detection of cancer, 2006. CA Cancer J Clin. 2006;56:11–25.
10. Aus G, Damber JE, Khatami A, Lilja H, Stranne J, Hugosson J. Individualized screening interval for prostate cancer based on prostate-specific antigen level: results of a prospective, randomized, population-based study. Arch Intern Med 2005;165:1857–61.
11. Carter HB, Landis PR, Metter EJ, Fleisher LA, Pearson JD. Prostate-specific antigen testing of older men. J Natl Cancer Inst 1999;91:1733–7.
12. Thompson IM, Pauler DK, Goodman PJ, et al. Prevalence of prostate cancer among men with a prostate-specific antigen level ≤4.0 ng per milliliter. N Engl J Med 2004;350:2239–46.
13. Catalona W, Smith D, Ornstein D. Prostate cancer detection in men with serum PSA concentrations of 2.6 to 4.0 ng/ml and

benign prostate examination: enhancement of specificity with free PSA measurements. JAMA 1997;277:1452–5.
14. Djavan B, Zlotta A, Kratzik C, et al. PSA, PSA density, PSA density of transition zone, free/total PSA ratio, and PSA velocity for early detection of prostate cancer in men with serum PSA 2.5 to 4.0 ng/ml. Urology 1999;54:517–22.
15. Babaian R, Johnston D, Naccarato W. The incidence of prostate cancer in a screening population with a serum prostate specific antigen between 2.5 and 4.0 ng/ml: relation to biopsy strategy. J Urol 2001;165:757–60.
16 Hugosson J, Aus G, Lilja H, Lodding P, Pihl C. Results of a randomized, population-based study of biennial screening using serum prostate-specific antigen measurement to detect prostate carcinoma. Cancer 2004;100:1397–405.
17. Sokoloff M, Yang X, Fumo M, Mhoon D, Brendler C. Characterizing prostatic adenocarcinomas in men with a serum prostate specific antigen level of <4 ng/ml. BJU Int 2004;93:499–502.
18. Schroeder F, van der Cruijsen-Koeter I, de Koning H, Vis AN, Hoedemaeker RF, Kranse R. Prostate cancer detection at low prostate specific antigen. J Urol 2000;163:806–12.
19. Krumholtz J, Carvalhal G, Ramos C, et al. Prostate specific antigen cutoff of 2.6 ng/ml for prostate cancer screening is associated with favorable pathologic tumor features. Urology 2002;60:469–73.
20. Stamey TA, Caldwell M, McNeal JE, Nolley R, Hemenez M, Downs J. The prostate specific antigen era in the United States is over for prostate cancer: what happened in the last 20 years? J Urol 2004;172:1297–301.
21. Johansson JE, Andren O, Andersson SO, et al. Natural history of early, localized prostate cancer. JAMA 2004;291:2713–9.
22. Carter HB. Prostate cancers in men with low PSA levels – must we find them? N Engl J Med 2004;350:2292–4.
23. Hoffman R, Clanon D, Littenberg B, Frank JJ, Peirce JC. Using the free-to-total prostate-specific antigen ratio to detect prostate cancer in men with nonspecific elevations of prostate-specific antigen levels. J Gen Intern Med 2000;15:739–48.
24. Maan Z, Cutting CW, Patel U, et al. Morbidity of transrectal ultrasonography-guided prostate biopsies in patients after the continued use of low-dose aspirin. BJU Int 2003;91:798–800.
25. Rodriguez LV, Terris MK. Risks and complications of transrectal ultrasound guided prostate needle biopsy: a prospective study and review of the literature. J Urol 1998;160:2115–20.
26. Ihezue CU, Smart J, Dewbury KC, Mehta R, Burgess L. Biopsy of the prostate guided by transrectal ultrasound: relation between warfarin use and incidence of bleeding complications. Clin Radiol 2005;60:459–63.
27. Cochlin DL. Biopsy of the prostate guided by transrectal ultrasound: relation between warfarin use and bleeding complications. Clin Radiol 2005;60:457–8.
28. Ramachandran N, MacKinnon AD, Allen C, Dundas D, Patel U. Re: Biopsy of the prostate guided by transrectal ultrasound: relation between warfarin use and incidence of bleeding complications. Clin Radiol 2005;60:1130.
29. Shandera KC, Thibault GP, Deshon GE. Variability in patient preparation for prostate biopsy among American urologists. Urology 1998;52:644–6.
30. Kapoor DA, Klimberg IW, Malek GH, et al. Single-dose oral ciprofloxacin versus placebo for prophylaxis during transrectal prostate biopsy. Urology 1998;52:552–8.
31. Aron M, Rajeev TP, Gupta NP. Antibiotic prophylaxis for transrectal needle biopsy of the prostate: a randomized controlled study. BJU Int 2000;85:682–5.
32. Puig J, Darnell A, Bermudez P, et al. Transrectal ultrasound-guided prostate biopsy: is antibiotic prophylaxis necessary? Eur Radiol 2006;16:939–43.
33. Shigemura K, Tanaka K, Yasuda M, et al. Efficacy of 1-day prophylaxis medication with Fluoroquinolone for prostate biopsy. World J Urol 2005;23:356–60.
34. Sieber PR, Rommel FM, Agusta VE, Breslin JA, Huffnagle HW, Harpster LE. Antibiotic prophylaxis in ultrasound guided transrectal prostate biopsy. J Urol 1997;157:2199–200.
35. Rees M, Ashby EC, Pocock RD, Dowding CH. Povidone-iodine antisepsis for transrectal prostatic biopsy. BMJ 1980;281:650.
36. Lindert KA, Kabalin JN and Terris MK. Bacteremia and bacteriuria after transrectal ultrasound guided prostate biopsy. J Urol 2000;164:76.
37. Sharpe JR, Sadlowsky RW, Finney RP, Branch WT, Hanna JE. Urinary tract infection after transrectal needle biopsy of the prostate. J Urol 1982;127:255–6.
38. Carey JM, Korman HJ. Transrectal ultrasound guided biopsy of the prostate. Do enemas decrease clinically significant complications? J Urol 2001;166:82–5.
39. Collins GN, Lloyd SN, Hehir M, McKelvie GB. Multiple transrectal ultrasound-guided prostatic biopsies: true morbidity and patient acceptance. Br J Urol 1993;71:460–3.
40. Desmond PM, Clark J, Thompson IM, Zeidman EJ, Mueller EJ. Morbidity with contemporary prostate biopsy. J Urol 1993;150:1425–6.
41. Webb JAW, Shanmuganathan K, McLean A. Complications of ultrasound-guided transperineal prostate biopsy. Br J Urol 1993; 72:775–7.
42. Davis M, Sofer M, Kim SS, Soloway MS. The procedure of transrectal ultrasound guided biopsy of the prostate: a survey of patient preparation and biopsy technique. J Urol 2002;167:566–70.
43. Leibovici D, Zisman A, Siegel YI, Sella A, Kleinmann J, Lindner A. Local anesthesia for prostate biopsy by periprostatic lidocaine injection: a double-blind placebo controlled study. J Urol 2002;167:563–5.
44. Luscombe CJ, Cooke PW. Pain during prostate biopsy. Lancet 2004;363:1840–1.
45. Stirling BN, Shockley KF, Carothers GG, Maatman TJ. Comparison of local anesthesia techniques during transrectal ultrasound-guided biopsies. Urology 2002;60:89–92.
46. Obek C, Onal B, Ozkan B, Onder AU, Yalcin V, Solok V. Is periprostatic local anesthesia for transrectal ultrasound guided prostate biopsy associated with increased infectious or hemorrhagic complications? A prospective randomized trial. J Urol 2002;168:558–61.
47. Manikandan R, Srirangam SJ, Brown SC, O'Reilly PH, Collins GN. Nitrous oxide vs periprostatic nerve block with 1% lidocaine during transrectal ultrasound guided biopsy of the prostate: a prospective, randomized, controlled trial. J Urol 2003;170:1881–3.
48. Masood J, Shah N, Lane T, Andrews H, Simpson P, Barua JM. Nitrous oxide (Entonox) inhalation and tolerance of transrectal ultrasound guided prostate biopsy: a doubleblind randomized controlled study. J Urol 2002;168:116–20.
49. Rochester MA, Le MK, Brewster SF. A double-blind, randomized, controlled trial of topical glyceryl trinitrate for transrectal ultrasound guided prostate biopsy. J Urol 2005;173:418–20.
50. Patel HR, Miller RA. Increased patient satisfaction from transrectal ultrasonography and biopsy under sedation. BJU Int 2002;89:972.

51. McNeal JE, Redwine EA, Freiha FS, Stamey TA. Zonal distribution of prostatic adenocarcinoma. Correlation with histologic pattern and direction of spread. Am J Surg Pathol 1988;12:897–906.
52. Chen ME, Troncoso P, Johnston DA, Tang K, Babaian RJ. Optimization of prostate biopsy strategy using computer based analysis. J Urol 1997;158:2168–75.
53. Terris MK, Stamey TA. Determination of prostate volume by transrectal ultrasound. J Urol 1991;145:984–7.
54. Garzotto M, Hudson RG, Peters L, et al. Predictive modeling for the presence of prostate carcinoma using clinical, laboratory, and ultrasound parameters in patients with prostate specific antigen levels < or =10 ng/mL. Cancer 2003;98:1417–22.
55. Shinohara K, Wheeler TM, Scardino PT. The appearance of prostate cancer on transrectal ultrasonography: correlation of imaging and pathological examinations. J Urol 1989;142:76–82.
56. Coley CM, Barry MJ, Fleming C, Mulley AG. Early detection of prostate cancer. Part I. Prior probability and effectiveness of tests. The American College of Physicians. Ann Intern Med 1997;126:394–406.
57. Djavan B, Zlotta A, Remzi M, et al. Optimal predictors of prostate cancer on repeat prostate biopsy: a prospective study of 1051 men. J Urol 2000;163:1144–8.
58. Djavan B, Ravery V, Zlotta A, et al. Prospective evaluation of prostate cancer detected on biopsies 1, 2, 3 and 4: when should we stop? J Urol 2001;166:1679–83.
59. Fowler Jr JE, Bigler SA, Miles D, Yalkut DA. Predictors of first repeat biopsy cancer detection with suspected local stage prostate cancer. J Urol 2000;163:813–8.
60. Terris MK, Wallen EM, Stamey TA. Comparison of mid-lobe versus lateral systematic sextant biopsies in the detection of prostate cancer. Urol Int 1997;59:239–42.
61. Bauer JJ, Zeng J, Zhang W, et al. Lateral biopsies added to the traditional sextant prostate biopsy pattern increases the detection rate of prostate cancer. Prostate Cancer Prostatic Dis 2000;3:43–6.
62. Borboroglu PG, Comer SW, Riffenburgh RH, Amling CL. Extensive repeat transrectal ultrasound guided prostate bio-psy in patients with previous benign sextant biopsies. J Urol 2000;163:158–62.
63. Durkan GC, Sheikh N, Johnson P, Hildreth AJ, Greene DR. Improving prostate cancer detection with an extended-core transrectal ultrasonography-guided prostate biopsy protocol. BJU Int 2002;89:33–9.
64. Klein EA, Zippe CD. Transrectal ultrasound guided prostate biopsy-defining a new standard. J Urol 2000;163:179–80.
65. Presti JC Jr. Prostate biopsy: how many cores are enough? Urol Oncol 2003;21:135–40.
66. Bazinet M, Karakiewicz PI, Aprikian AG, et al. Value of systematic transition zone biopsies in the early detection of prostate cancer. J Urol 1996;155:605–6.
67. Lui PD, Terris MK, McNeal JE, Stamey TA. Indications for ultrasound guided transition zone biopsies in the detection of prostate cancer. J Urol 1995;153:1000–3.
68. Durkan GC, Sheikh N, Johnson P, Hildreth AJ, Greene DR. Improving prostate cancer detection with an extended-core transrectal ultrasonography-guided prostate biopsy protocol. BJU Int 2002;89:33–9.
69. Liu IJ, Macy M, Lai YH, Terris MK. Critical evaluation of the current indications for transition zone biopsies. Urology 2001;57:1117–20.
70. Naughton CK, Smith DS, Humphrey PA, Catalona WJ, Keetch DW. Clinical and pathologic tumor characteristics of prostate cancer as a function of the number of biopsy cores: a retrospective study. Urology 1998;52:808–13.
71. Karakiewicz PI, Bazinet M, Aprikian AG, et-al. Outcome of sextant biopsy according to gland volume. Urology 1997;49:55–9.
72. Uzzo RG, Wei JT, Waldbaum RS, Perlmutter AP, Byrne JC, Vaughan Jr ED. The influence of prostate size on cancer detection. Urology 1995;46:831–6.
73. Mariappan P, Chong WL, Sundram M, Mohamed SR. Increasing prostate biopsy cores based on volume vs the sextant biopsy: a prospective randomized controlled clinical study on cancer detection rates and morbidity. BJU Int 2004;94:307–10.
74. Ellis WJ, Brawer MK. Repeat prostate needle biopsy: who needs it? J Urol 1995;153:1496–8.
75. Perachino M, di Ciolo L, Barbetti V, et al. Results of rebiopsy for suspected prostate cancer in symptomatic men with elevated PSA levels. Eur Urol 1997;32:155–9.
76. Djavan B, Zlotta AR, Byttebier G, et al. Prostate specific antigen density of the transition zone for early detection of prostate cancer. J Urol 1998;160:411–8.
77. Horninger W, Reissigl A, Klocker H, et al. Improvement of specificity in PSA-based screening by using PSA-transition zone density and percent free PSA in addition to total PSA levels. Prostate 1998;37:133–7.
78. Letran JL, Blase AB, Loberiza FR, Meyer GE, Ransom SD, Brawer MK. Repeat ultrasound guided prostate needle biopsy: use of free-to-total prostate specific antigen ratio in predicting prostatic carcinoma. J Urol 1998;160:426–9.
79. Patel U. Transrectal biopsy of prostate gland: reducing sampling errors. CME Urol 2000;2:35–8.
80. Epstein JI, Grignon DJ, Humphrey PAet-al., Interobserver reproducibility in the diagnosis of prostatic intraepithelial neoplasia. Am J Surg Pathol 1995;19:873–86.
81. Epstein JI, Herawi M. Prostate needle biopsies containing prostatic intraepithelial neoplasia or atypical foci suspicious for carcinoma: implications for patient care. J Urol 2006;175:820–34.
82. Chan TY, Epstein JI. Follow-up of atypical prostate needle biopsies suspicious for cancer. Urology 1999;53:351–5.
83. Stewart CS, Leibovich BC, Weaver AL, Lieber MM. Prostate cancer diagnosis using a saturation needle biopsy technique after previous negative sextant biopsies. J Urol 2001;166:86–91.
84. Bott SR, Henderson A, McLarty E, Langley SE. A brachytherapy template approach to standardize saturation prostatic biopsy. BJU Int 2004;93:629–30.
85. Carter HB. Prostate cancers in men with low PSA levels-must we find them? N Engl J Med 2004;350:2292–4.
86. Boddy JL, Pike DJ, Malone PR. A seven-year follow-up of men following a benign prostate biopsy. Eur Urol 2003;44:17–20.
87. Patel U, Rickards D. The diagnostic value of colour Doppler flow in the peripheral zone of the prostate, with histological correlation. Br J Urol 1994;74:590–5.
88. Halpern EJ, Rosenberg M, Gomella LG. Prostate cancer: contrast-enhanced us for detection. Radiology 2001;219:219–25.
89. Bogers HA, Sedelaar JP, Beerlage HP, et al. Contrast enhanced three-dimensional power Doppler angiography of the human prostate: correlation with biopsy outcome. Urology 1999;54:97–104.
90. Rubens DJ, Hadley MA, Alam SK, Gao L, Mayer RD, Parker KJ. Sonoelasticity imaging of prostate cancer: in vitro results. Radiology 1995;195:379–83.
91. Donzella JG, Merrick GS, Lindert DJ, et al. Epididymitis after transrectal ultrasound-guided needle biopsy of prostate gland. Urology 2004;63:306–8.

92. Ghani KR, Dundas D, Patel U. Bleeding after transrectal ultrasonography-guided prostate biopsy: a study of 7-day morbidity after a six-, eight- and 12-core biopsy protocol. BJU Int 2004;94:1014–20.
93. Soloway MS, Obek C. Periprostatic local anesthesia before ultrasound guided prostate biopsy. J Urol 2000;163:172–3.
94. Ohori M, Shinohara K, Wheeler TM, et al. Ultrasonic detection of non-palpable seminal vesicle invasion: a clinicopathological study. Br J Urol 1993;72:799–808.
95. Ukimura O, Troncoso P, Ramirez EI, Babaian RJ. Prostate cancer staging: correlation between ultrasound determined tumor contact length and pathologically confirmed extraprostatic extension. J Urol 1998;159:1251–9.
96. Partin AW, Mangold LA, Lamm DM, Walsh PC, Epstein JI, Pearson JD. Contemporary update of prostate cancer staging nomograms (Partin Tables) for the new millennium. Urology 2001;58:843–8.

Chapter 7
The Use of High-Intensity Focused Ultrasound in Prostate Cancer

Christian Chaussy and Stefan Thüroff

Introduction

The use of ultrasonic waves for medical purposes was first investigated in the 1950s,[1] and high-intensity focused ultrasound (HIFU) for focal tissue destruction was established in 1955.[2] One of the first clinical applications of HIFU was for the treatment of neurological disorders by the production of small lesions deep inside the cerebral cortex. Routine use of the technique, however, was limited by the need for a large cranial bone flap and by the lack of an appropriate imaging device. Exploration of the use of HIFU for the irradiation of tumors started in 1956,[3] continued during the late 1970s and early 1980s,[4,5] and by the mid-1980s, the technique was being used to treat ocular cancers and glaucoma.[6] The use of HIFU in the treatment of prostate disorders began in the early 1990s with clinical trials of HIFU in the treatment of benign prostatic hyperplasia (BPH)[7,8] and the treatment of organ-confined prostate cancer.[9]

Mechanism of Action

HIFU can be delivered as a pulsed or a continuous beam. Continuous beam processes include solar waves, microwaves, and radar technology, while medical HIFU and extracorporeal shock wave lithotripsy (ESWL) involve pulsed HIFU. HIFU destroys tissues via two mechanisms, acoustic cavitation (similar to bubble formation during boiling) and internal friction; these mechanisms result in the generation of sufficient heat within the tissues to create a necrotic lesion.

In the treatment of prostate cancer with HIFU, ultrasound waves are generated by the high-frequency vibration (0.5–10 MHz) of a piezoelectric or piezoceramic transducer within a probe introduced into the rectum. *The ultrasound waves penetrate the rectal wall with only slight absorption and reflection and therefore, no tissue damage*, but as they are focused (by an acoustic lens or parabolic reflectors) onto a small area (the focal point) in the prostate, the power density increases. At the focal point, bubbles form inside the cells due to the negative pressure of the ultrasound wave. The bubbles increase in size to the point at which resonance is achieved; this triggers their sudden collapse, creating high pressure (20,000–30,000 bars) which damages cells and generates heat (Fig. 7.1). The increase in temperature is determined by the absorption coefficient of the tissue, as well as the size, shape, and thermal response of the heated region. The biological changes that are induced by the rise in temperature depend on the thermal dose, that is, the temperature reached and the length of time that the tissue is exposed to the elevated temperature. A steep temperature gradient exists between the tissue at the focal point and the surrounding tissue; a sharp demarcation between the necrotic lesion and the normal cells can be seen in histological samples (Fig. 7.2). A number of factors affect the extent of the lesion and the process has to be carefully controlled. Treatment parameters important for effective tissue coagulation using HIFU include:

- The power setting (W)
- The piezoelectric frequency (MHz)
- The shot duration
- The delay between shots (this is necessary to avoid accumulation of cavitation bubbles in adjacent lesions)
- The number of shots per prostate volume (dose)

Pros and Cons of Different Commercial Systems

Two commercially available HIFU systems are currently in use: the Ablatherm® (EDAP SA, Lyon, France) and the Sonablate® (Focus Surgery, Inc., Indianapolis, IN, USA). The two systems are similar in TRUS imaging, and treatment is possible with both using a probe encased in a degassed, fluid-filled balloon that cools the rectum. The two systems differ in terms of positioning of the patient, the ultrasound frequencies used during treatment and planning, shoot, and delay times, the treatment mode within the prostate, and the safety measures available to protect the rectal wall.

O. Ukimura and I.S. Gill (eds.), *Contemporary Interventional Ultrasonography in Urology*,
DOI: 10.1007/978-1-84800-217-3_7, © Springer-Verlag London Limited 2009

Fact Sheet

- The use of ultrasound for medical purposes started in the 1950s for the treatment of neurological disorders
- The use of ultrasound for tumor ablation started in 1956, but it was not until the 1990s that ultrasound was used to treat prostate cancer
- Medical HIFU involves a pulsed ultrasound beam
- HIFU destroys tissues by generating heat sufficient to cause necrosis
- When treating prostate cancer, ultrasound waves are generated by a transducer within a probe introduced into the rectum
- The ultrasound waves penetrate the rectal wall with only slight absorption and reflection, but are focused onto a small area (the focal point) in the prostate to generate a lesion
- The HIFU process has to be carefully controlled, and a variety of treatment parameters are important

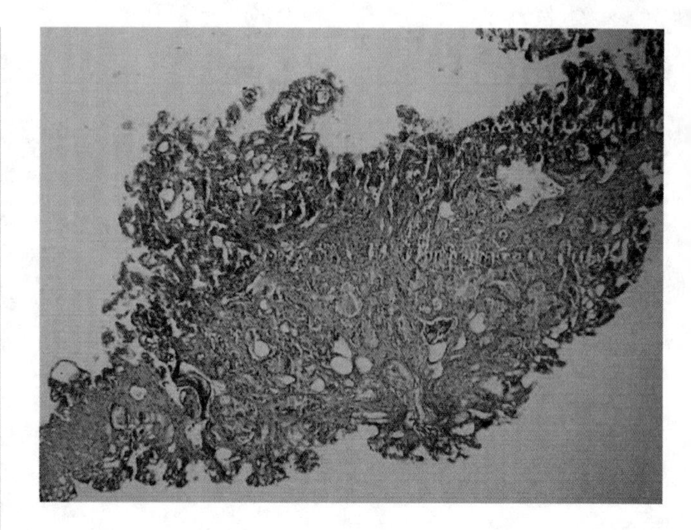

Fig. 7.2. Histological section of the prostate following treatment with high-intensity focused ultrasound

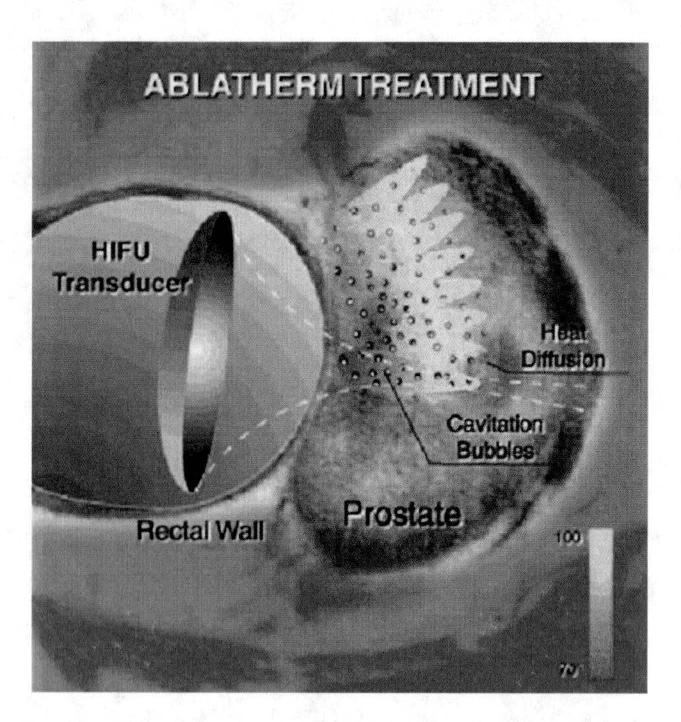

Fig. 7.1. Ultrasound waves generated by the high-intensity focused ultrasound (HIFU) transducer are focused on the tumor lesion within the prostate

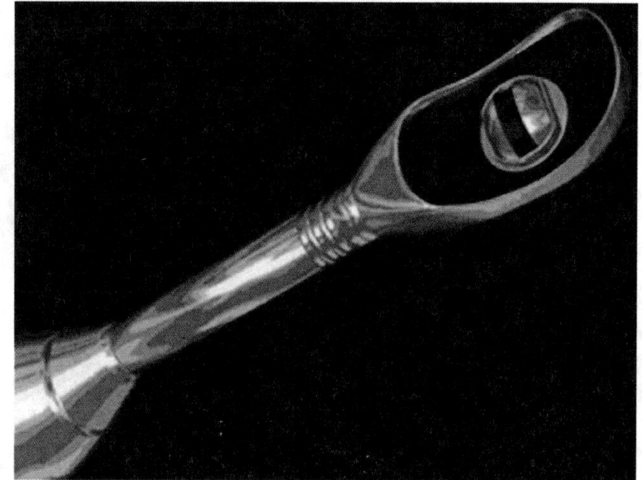

Fig. 7.3. Ablatherm® piezoelectric probe

The Ablatherm® system includes a treatment bed, an endorectal probe, and probe positioning system, an ultrasound power generator, a cooling system for preservation of the rectal wall, and a control module. The endorectal probe (Fig. 7.3) incorporates a two-dimensional imaging probe working at 7.5 MHz and a treatment transducer focused at a maximum of 45 mm and working at 3 MHz. *Thus a single probe fits all prostate sizes and undertakes both imaging and treatment functions*. Variable focusing of the transducer is shown in Fig. 7.4. Real-time rectal wall control is provided by automatic adjustment of the probe toward the rectal wall, and multiple security circuits are in place to prevent accidental focusing on the rectal wall, thereby avoiding rectal injury. In 2005, modifications were made to the Ablatherm® system to allow integrated imaging. The features of the two models (the pre-2005 Ablatherm® Maxis and the post-2005 Ablatherm® device with integrated imaging) are outlined in Table 7.1. *The Ablatherm®system can be used for primary HIFU treatment, HIFU retreatment, and salvage therapy in patients who have previously received radiotherapy*.

The Sonablate® system does not have a dedicated treatment bed; instead, treatment is performed with the patient in the dorsal position under general anesthetic. Furthermore, rather than the single, dual-frequency probe used for gland

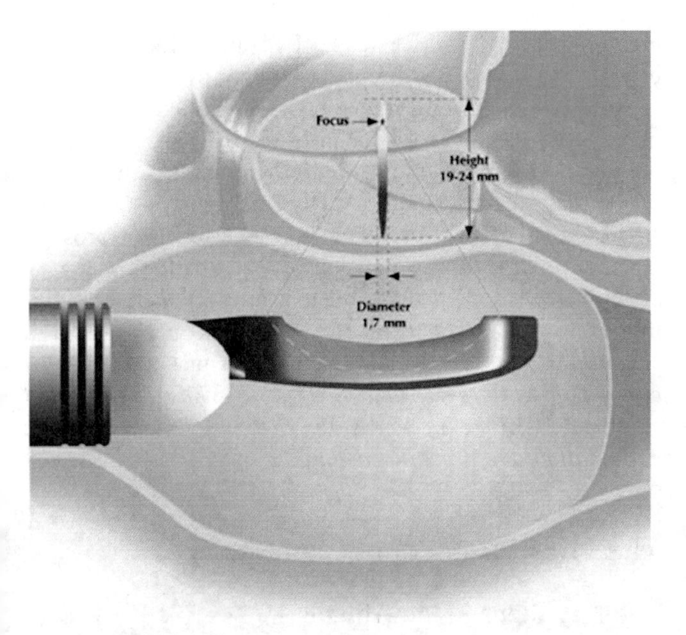

FIG. 7.4. The Ablatherm® transducer demonstrating variable focusing

imaging and treatment used in the Ablatherm® system, *the Sonablate® system uses a range of treatment probes*. Probe selection is determined by the size of the lesion required; a 25- or 45-mm focal length probe results in a lesion that is 10 mm in length and 2 mm in diameter, and a 30-, 35-, or 40-mm focal length probe used with a split beam results in a lesion that is 10 mm in length and 3 mm in diameter. Prostate size also has to be taken into account, and larger glands require probes with a longer focal length. Treatment is usually conducted in three consecutive coronal layers, starting from the anterior prostate and moving from the apex to the base. At least one probe change is required during the treatment process. *No automatic, real-time, rectal wall distance control is present, which means that the operator has to perform manually guided, rectal-wall-orientated HIFU treatment in the peripheral zone (which is the predominant location of a prostate tumor)*. The limitations of the Sonablate® system mean that the indications for this system are restricted to T1–2 prostate cancer; the system cannot be used for salvage or palliative HIFU.

Fact Sheet

- Two commercially available HIFU systems are currently in use – the Ablatherm® system and the Sonablate® system
- Both systems provide simultaneous imaging and treatment using an endorectal probe
- The main differences between the systems are in patient positioning, the ultrasound frequencies used during treatment and planning, shoot and delay times, the treatment mode within the prostate, the measures available to protect the rectal wall, and treatment indications
- Overall, the Sonablate® system has limitations, while the Ablatherm® system provides a number of treatment and safety benefits

Patient Selection: Indications and Contraindications

Indications

HIFU is indicated for patients with localized prostate cancer (stage T1–T2 N0M0 Gleason score [GS] 1–3) who are not candidates for surgery due to their age, general health status or a prohibiting comorbidity, or who would prefer not to undergo a radical prostatectomy. However, the indications have been expanded based on clinical experience to include: partial therapy in unilateral low volume, low GS tumors (T1–2a Nx/0M0, GS1–2, prostate-specific antigen [PSA] < 20 ng ml^{-1}); salvage therapy in recurrent prostate cancer after radical prostatectomy, radiotherapy, or hormone ablation (all T Nx/0M0, all GS/PSA); and advanced prostate cancer as a debulking process (T3–4 Nx/0M0, all GS/PSA). *While other nonsurgical treatment options for localized prostate cancer (e.g., cryotherapy or brachytherapy) cannot generally be repeated in cases of local recurrence, HIFU can be repeated, and can also be used as a salvage therapy.*

TABLE 7.1. Distinguishing features of the two generations of the Ablatherm® high-intensity focused ultrasound device.

Ablatherm® integrated imaging	Ablatherm® maxis
• Electronic applicator with integrated 7.5-MHz real-time TRUS	• Electromechanical applicator with inserted 7-MHz alternating TRUS
• Excellent TRUS resolution by a new diagnostic ultrasound unit	• No real-time control
• Fast and highly precise planning by computerized scanning procedure	• High TRUS resolution with a standard diagnostic ultrasound unit • Manual therapy planning
• Virtual prostate reconstruction	• Real-time TRUS control
• Real-time TRUS control	• Electronic picture and data storage
• Electronic picture and data storage	• Learning curve: 30 treatments
• Ablaview® "blackbox"	
• Treatment time reduced by 25%	
• Learning curve: ten treatments (new users); five treatments (Ablatherm® users)	

TRUS, transrectal ultrasound

Contraindications

Contraindications for the use of HIFU in prostate cancer include a gland size larger than 40 ml (due to the focal length of HIFU). Larger glands can be reduced in size using transurethral resection of the prostate (TURP) and/or hormonal therapy with a luteinizing hormone-releasing agonist (LHRHa) prior to HIFU. Other contraindications include conditions where the rectal wall is damaged or rendered more susceptible to damage (e.g., rectal fistula or conditions when there is a reduced blood supply), following radiotherapy, or when there is active local infection. HIFU is not suitable for patients with rectal stenosis or rectal amputation, as these conditions mean that the probe cannot be placed in the rectum.

Fact Sheet

Ablatherm = A Sonablate = S

- HIFU is indicated:
  - For localized prostate cancer (stages T1–T2 N0M0 Gleason score 1–3) (A + S)
  - For partial therapy in unilateral low-volume, low Gleason score tumors (A + S)
  - For salvage therapy in recurrent prostate cancer after radical prostatectomy, radiotherapy, or hormone ablation (A)
  - For advanced prostate cancer as a debulking process (A)
- HIFU is contraindicated:
  - For gland sizes larger than 40 ml (larger glands can be reduced in size prior to HIFU) (S)
  - In conditions where the rectal wall is damaged or rendered more susceptible to damage (A + S)
  - Following radiotherapy (S)
  - When there is active local infection (A + S)
  - In cases of rectal stenosis or rectal amputation (A + S)

Transurethral Resection of the Prostate Plus HIFU

For prostate gland sizes greater than 40 ml, TURP is conducted 1 month prior to HIFU For prostate sizes less than 40 ml, TURP is carried out at the same time as HIFU. In salvage HIFU, the use of TURP is limited or unnecessary. TURP prior to HIFU can reduce gland size, remove calcification, abscesses, and large adenomas, reduce significantly postoperative side effects, allow more patients to meet the inclusion criteria for HIFU, and help achieve greater efficacy with HIFU. TURP results in the generation of a cavity, which is subsequently compressed by the rectal balloon, increasing the accessibility of the remaining gland to HIFU waves. TURP prior to HIFU should remove the ventral region of the gland, leaving intact a large area of the gland at the bladder neck. This reduces the risk of stenosis of the neck of the bladder as a result of prostate gland shrinkage during HIFU. The rectal balloon that covers the HIFU probe is then able to "squeeze" the gland, fixing it into position. TURP before HIFU has been used as a standard procedure in the Munich clinic since 2000. *TURP carried out at the same time as HIFU also has the benefit of stopping TURP-related prostatic bleeding due to necrotic coagulation and prostate edema.*

Fact Sheet

- TURP before HIFU reduces gland size, improves HIFU efficacy, and expands the indication for the procedure
- TURP carried out at the same time as HIFU reduces TURP-related prostatic bleeding

The HIFU Procedure: Ablatherm®

The Key Steps in the Ablatherm®

HIFU procedure is shown in Table 7.2.

Preoperative Preparation

Approximately 2 h before the procedure, an enema should be given to cleanse the rectum. At the start of treatment, prophylactic antibiotics are administered and a urethral catheter is put into place. Antibiotic prophylaxis is used to avoid urinary tract infections following HIFU, as necrotic tissue provides a good substrate for bacterial growth. Antibiotics should continue for about 1 week or until the catheter is removed. Urethral catheterization is needed during and after treatment to control bladder filling and bleeding, and to avoid patient movement as a result of bladder irritation. Both suprapubic and urethral catheters can be used. Suprapubic catheters tend to be used if TURP and HIFU are performed in the same treatment session. The use of a suprapubic catheter prevents the TURP syndrome and any inflow of cells, and helps continuous bladder washing during the procedure. The urethral catheter can be withdrawn the day following the procedure, and the patient can be discharged with a urine collection bag attached to the suprapubic catheter.

TABLE 7.2. The key steps in the Ablatherm® high-intensity focused ultrasound procedure.

1. *Preoperative preparation*
2. Anesthesia
3. Positioning the patient and keeping him warm
4. Device preparation
5. Introducing the transrectal probe
6. Transrectal ultrasound simulation
7. Treatment planning
8. Robotic treatment
9. The perioperative phase
10. *Follow up*

Anesthesia

While HIFU can be performed using spinal or general anesthesia, spinal anesthesia with analgesic sedation is the preferred anesthetic method in the Munich clinic. *If general anesthesia is used, muscle relaxation should be maintained until the rectal probe has been removed at the end of the procedure, as waking the patient early can lead to spontaneous, uncontrolled movements that can result in rectal perforation by the probe.*

Positioning the Patient and External Warming

It is important that the patient remains perfectly still throughout the procedure. As the treatment time is around 95 min (30–150 min), making sure that the patient is comfortable helps him to stay still, and ensures precise and rapid treatment. The patient is positioned on his right side on the treatment table, with restraints and cushions to support the feet, knees, back and left arm, as appropriate. *Special attention should be paid to the comfortable positioning of the right arm and shoulder, as most disturbances at the end of the HIFU treatment are due to patient movement because of discomfort of the right shoulder.* External warming should be applied to counteract the internal cooling of the rectum that will occur during the procedure. *The patient should be kept warm by keeping the treatment room warm and by draping blankets over him* (Fig. 7.5).

Device Preparation

The endorectal probe containing the transducer is covered with a balloon, which is inserted into the rectum via the anus and then filled with 150 ml degassed transmitter fluid (Ablasonic®) (Fig. 7.6). Device preparation is important; the balloon should be fixed using tape to avoid dilatation of the anus, and inflation of the balloon should be minimal prior to positioning.

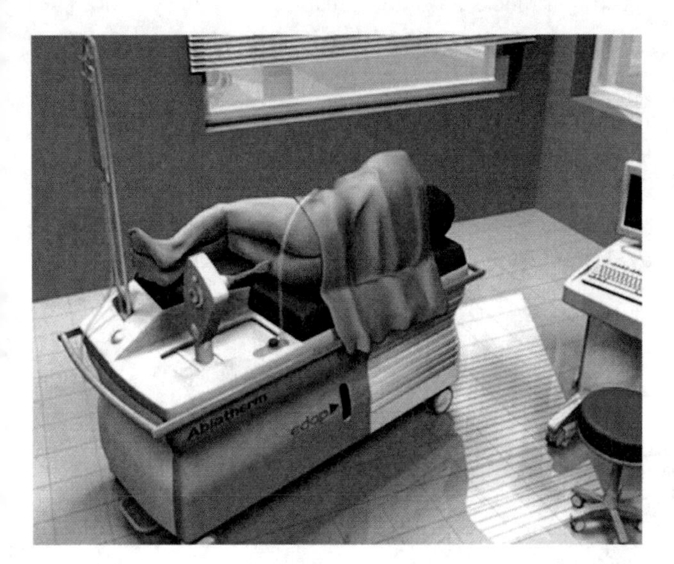

Fig. 7.5. Positioning of the patient in the Ablatherm® table; patient should be kept warm

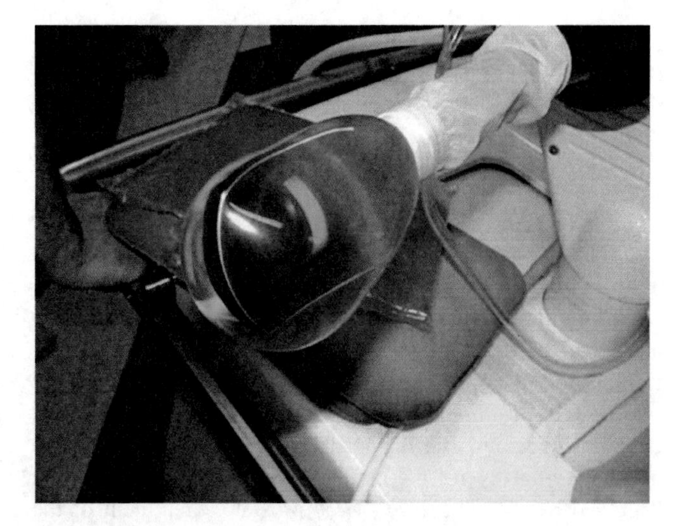

Fig. 7.6. Ablatherm® probe covered with fluid-filled balloon

Introducing the Probe

The balloon-covered probe should be covered with ultrasound gel before it is inserted into the rectum; this is to ensure close, smooth contact between the balloon and the rectal mucosa. Ultrasound gel should not be introduced directly into the rectum. Digital rectal examination using anal dilatation with up to two fingers may be needed to allow smooth introduction of the probe. An absence of feces is important at this point. *Dilatation using more than two fingers can result in the balloon "popping out" during treatment, which can lead to delays.* The presence of hemorrhoids is not a problem – a small amount of bleeding of the anal mucosa due to dilatation is not a cause for concern. *Introduction of the probe is made easier by lifting the patient's left buttock and making small lateral movements with the probe.*

Once the probe is positioned in the rectum, the balloon should be filled with the Ablasonic® liquid. This blue, anti-cavitation coupling and cooling fluid prevents the acoustic cavitation of bubbles within the cooling circuit and in front of the probe. This fluid is cooled to limit the heat damage to the rectal wall by creating a temperature gradient between the rectal mucosa and the prostatic capsule. *It is important that all the liquid supplied is used, as this ensures sufficient dilatation of the rectal ampulla, good contact and compression of the rectal wall, and optimum HIFU treatment and cooling while preventing the passage of feces or air. The rectum cannot be damaged by overfilling the balloon.* A roller pump circulates the liquid slowly through the balloon into a cooling unit and back to the rectum at a temperature of 15°C.

Transrectal Ultrasound Simulation

The prostate is scanned automatically by the integral 7.5 MHz TRUS, from the apex to the base, to generate a high-definition, two-dimensional image of the gland. A three-dimensional

TRUS simulation is generated; this allows accurate treatment planning to be performed, including calculation of the prostate volume and clear definition of the base and apex of the gland (Fig. 7.7).

Treatment Planning

The TRUS image is used to plan a treatment that generates a series of lesions that includes the whole of the prostate, including the seminal vesicles if appropriate. Apex definition is one of the most important aspects of treatment planning; this allows an appropriate balance to be made between the preservation of continence and effective treatment. Planning takes into account starting HIFU treatment 5 mm from the apex, moving toward the bladder, and treating the left lobe followed by the right lobe of the prostate. Treatment of the seminal vesicles is optional and depends on the anatomy of the patient, seminal vesicle length, and location of the tumor. Treatment of the seminal vesicles is desirable if the tumor is located on the base of the prostate, but in small individuals, this can be difficult. Lateral or ventral tissue remaining untreated can be a reason for persistently elevated PSA levels and prostate cancer recurrence.

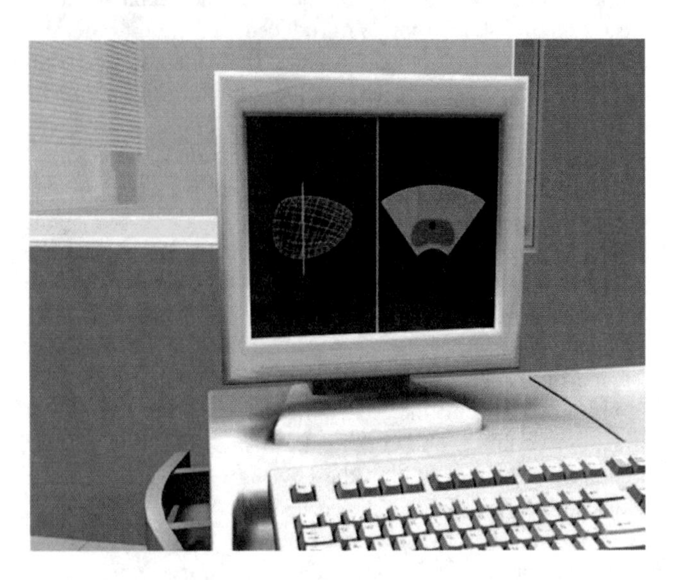

Fig. 7.7. Mapping of the prostate during high-intensity focused ultrasound treatment using transrectal ultrasound simulation

During planning, the prostate is divided ("sliced") into 1.6-mm transverse sections, each representing a single lesion to be generated during active treatment. The length and the diameter of the lesions are defined by the operator on the control screen, tailored to fit the anatomy of the prostate of the individual being treated. Up to 800 lesions may be defined, depending on the size of the prostate.

Tissue type is also taken into consideration, specifically untreated, HIFU pretreated, or irradiated prostate tissue. Three power settings are available, involving the application of different energy levels suited to the three different tissue types. The different power settings used by the Maxis system (pre-2005) and the Integrated imaging system (post-2005) are provided in Table 7.3. Power and shot duration are lower for patients who have received radiotherapy than for those receiving primary HIFU treatment or HIFU retreatment because irradiated prostate tissue has a higher uptake of HIFU energy,[11] so a lower level is used to reduce the risk of rectal wall injury. It is important that the correct software setting is selected from "Standard," "HIFU retreatment," and "Salvage." Failure to select the correct setting can result in side effects such as rectourethral fistula. The actual plan of how the HIFU will be delivered is then generated by the computer software.

Active Treatment

To achieve accurate lesions, it is important that the patient remains perfectly still throughout the procedure. The treatment time is around 95 (30–150) min, and the actual treatment carried out is recorded and can be reviewed after the procedure. For optimal efficacy, the entire prostate is normally treated. Treatment is divided into sequences lasting approximately 30 min; these are referred to as treatment "blocks." The larger the prostate, the more blocks have to be performed. As a rough guide, a standard resection is likely to need four blocks and a local recurrence is likely to need one block. *Before delivering HIFU to the prostate, the urethral catheter should be withdrawn 5 cm into the urethra to prevent the reflection of ultrasound waves.*

Treatment automatically follows the computerized instructions generated during the planning phase. The probe generates a series of pulsed HIFU beams that destroy a small slice of the prostate with intense, localized heat. The zone destroyed by each pulse creates a lesion that is 1.6 mm deep, with a

Table 7.3. Power settings used during high-intensity focused ultrasound (HIFU); standard, re-treatment and radiation failure cases depicted.

	MHz		Power (%)		Shot duration (s)		Delay duration (s)	
	M	ii	M	ii	M	ii	M	ii
Standard	3.0	3.0	100	100	5	6	5	4
HIFU retreatment	3.0	3.0	100	100	4.5	5	5	4
Radiation failure	3.0	3.0	90	95	4	5	7	5

M, maxis; ii, integrated imaging

height and a width that match the anatomy of the prostate at that particular point (Fig. 7.8). The whole gland is treated in this way. In most cases, the only adjustments that the operator needs to make during the procedure are small manual corrections to the inflow or the outflow of fluid to the rectal balloon, or readjustment of the external movement detector. Very rarely, electronic or mechanical disturbances stop treatment and necessitate restarting.

To maximize safety and efficacy, the Ablatherm® system incorporates a number of safety features, including alarm screens, an external movement detector, the Ablaview® function and real-time imaging with post-2005 equipment. Red and yellow alarm screens indicate problems during treatment. If a red alarm occurs, treatment should be stopped; these alarms seldom occur. Yellow alarms indicate the need for small adjustments by the operator. An external movement detector provides an additional warning if the patient moves. *Changing the position of the probe to treat the right prostate almost always triggers this alarm due to movement of the pelvis as the probe is adjusted.*

The Ablaview® function registers and retains all planning and treatment sequences. This enables previously untreated areas to be easily distinguished if treatment is restarted or if there has to be a change of operators for any reason. This function also provides the ability to check whether all areas of a prostate have been treated correctly. The endorectal probe is held away from the rectal wall by means of the balloon filled with Ablasonic® fluid. This anticavitation coupling and cooling fluid prevents the formation of acoustic cavitation bubbles within the cooling circuit and in front of the probe. This fluid is cooled to limit the heat damage to the rectal wall by creating a temperature gradient between the rectal mucosa and the prostatic capsule.

The Ablatherm® Integrated Imaging system has real-time imaging as a result of improvements to the piezoelectric probe. Less local movement has also been achieved through fixation of the HIFU probe (Fig. 7.9) allowing greater accuracy in the delivery of HIFU. The device also has inbuilt controls which detect when the probe is too close to the rectal wall and allows the device to "fire" with an accuracy of ±1 mm.

The Perioperative Phase

Following HIFU treatment, the prostate swells immediately due to inflammation and edema. This effect can compress the urethra, hence the need for a urethral catheter. The inflammation and the edema usually resolve over the following 3–8 days. TURP carried out at the same time as HIFU often reduces the level of urethral compression and the need for a urinary catheter. Perioperative morbidity is low following HIFU; significant bleeding is unusual, the need for blood transfusions or intensive care, and the occurrence of thrombo-

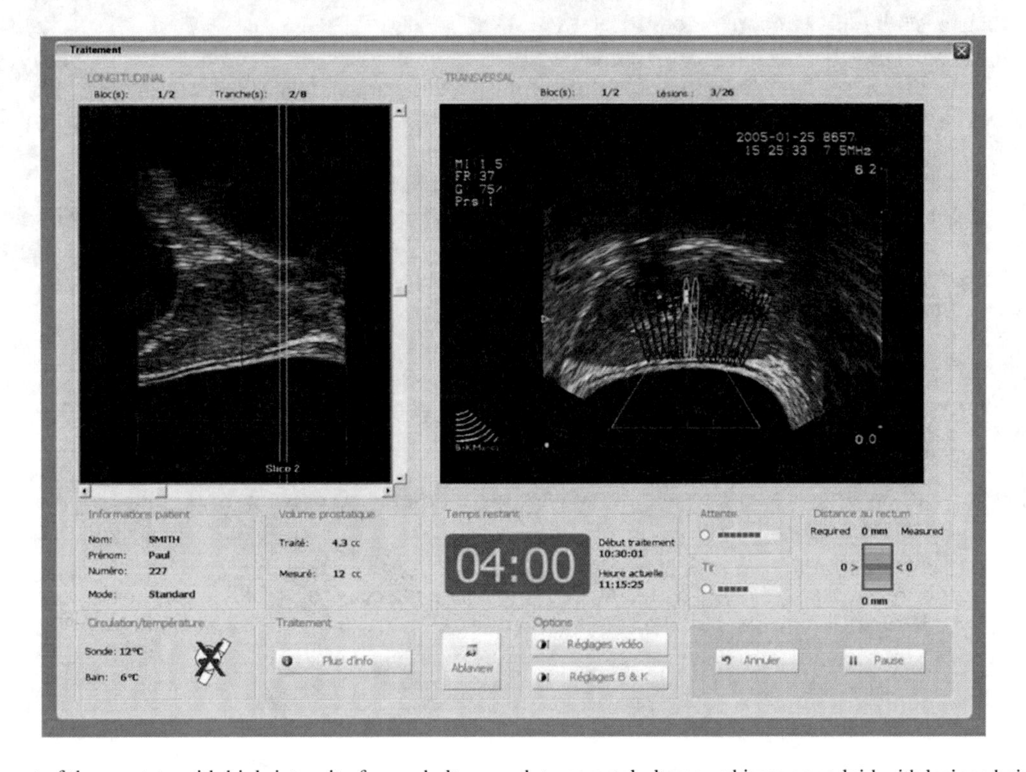

FIG. 7.8. Treatment of the prostate with high-intensity focused ultrasound; transrectal ultrasound image overlaid with lesions being generated

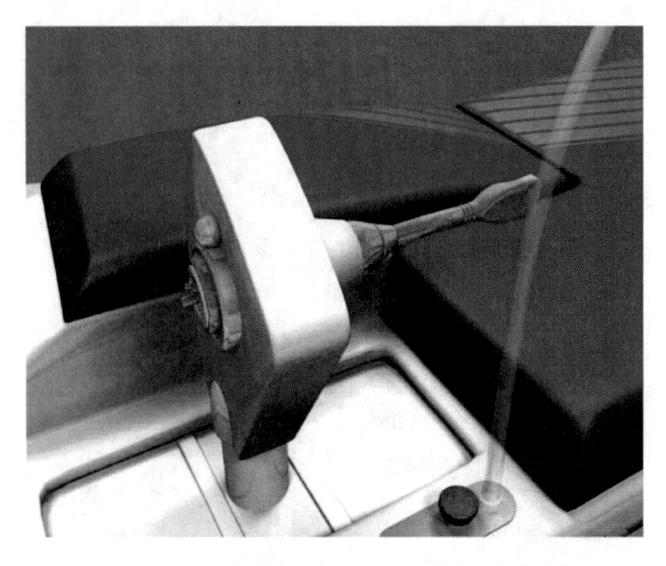

FIG. 7.9. Fixation of the high-intensity focused ultrasound probe

sis or pulmonary embolism is uncommon. Usually there is minimal postoperative pain for the patient making analgesic medication unnecessary. *Should pain occur following spinal anesthesia, it is likely to be in the lower left abdomen; this can be managed using intravenous analgesics.* Antibiotic prophylaxis is usually continued until removal of the suprapubic catheter at about 1 week following the procedure.

Follow up

PSA levels should be measured every 3 months for all patients. Other follow-up activities depend on whether the goal of treatment is curative or palliative. In cases where HIFU constitutes curative treatment, biopsies are necessary if the PSA velocity increases above a rate of 0.5 ng $ml^{-1}yr^{-1}$; such biopsies will identify small residual tumor volumes that may require retreatment with HIFU. Complete remission is indicated by negative biopsies, low PSA levels, and a PSA velocity that

Fact Sheet

1. *Preoperative preparation*: Preoperative preparation for HIFU includes the administration of an enema, prophylactic antibiotics, and catheter placement
2. *Anesthesia*: Spinal or general anesthesia can be used for HIFU; spinal anesthesia with sedation is recommended
3. *Positioning the patient and keeping him warm*: It is important to position the patient carefully in a comfortable position and to keep him warm
4. *Device preparation*: Correct preparation of the endorectal probe and its balloon cover is essential for speed, safety, and efficacy
5. *Introducing the probe*: A number of things can be done to make introduction of the endorectal probe easier; using all the supplied Ablasonic® liquid is important for efficacy and safety
6. *Transrectal ultrasound (TRUS) simulation*: Automatic TRUS simulation allows accurate treatment planning, including calculation of the prostate volume and clear definition of the base and apex of the gland
7. *Treatment planning*: Based on the TRUS simulation, treatment is planned to generate a series of lesions tailored to fit the anatomy of the prostate being treated and to include the whole gland
8. *Treatment*: Treatment automatically follows the computerized instructions generated during the planning phase to generate a series of pulsed HIFU beams that produce lesions that are 1.6 mm deep, with a height and a width that match the anatomy of the gland (robotic treatment)
   - Treatment is divided into sequences lasting approximately 30 min; these are referred to as treatment "blocks"; the larger the prostate, the more blocks have to be performed
   - Safety and efficacy are maximized by a number of safety features, including alarm screens, an external movement detector, the Ablaview® function, and real-time imaging with post-2005 equipment
9. *The perioperative phase*: In the perioperative phase, the prostate immediately swells due to inflammation and edema, necessitating the use of a urethral catheter; these symptoms tend to resolve over 3–8 days
   - Other perioperative morbidity is low following HIFU; it is unusual for there to be significant pain, bleeding, the need for blood transfusions or intensive care, and the occurrence of thrombosis or pulmonary embolism is uncommon
10. *Follow up*: Follow up should include measurement of PSA levels every 3 months for all patients; other follow-up activities depend on whether the goal of treatment is curative or palliative
    - In cases where HIFU constitutes curative treatment, biopsies are necessary if the PSA velocity increases above a rate of 0.5 ng ml−1 yr−1; such biopsies will identify small residual tumor volumes that may require HIFU retreatment
    - In cases where HIFU constitutes palliative therapy, biopsies should be done only if a local treatment could provide a benefit

remains stable below 0.2 ng $ml^{-1}yr^{-1}$. In cases where HIFU constitutes adjuvant palliative therapy, biopsies should be done only if a local treatment could provide a benefit.

Specific Measures to Avoid and Manage Complications

Clinically significant complications that can occur with HIFU include incontinence and erectile dysfunction (ED). Specific measures can be taken to avoid ED, while the incidence of incontinence is rare.

Incontinence

HIFU can result in urinary obstruction, and fibrosis or tissue shrinkage of the urethra, although incontinence is often due to TURP or the combination of TURP and HIFU. Grade 1 and 2 incontinence after primary HIFU is rare and can be managed using pelvic floor training. Grade 3 incontinence is very rare and can only be managed by invasive treatment (Table 7.4).

ED

ED following HIFU is caused by heat-induced nerve damage. Potency protection relies on preservation of neurovascular bundles within the prostate. *If the tumor is unilateral, low grade, and low volume, sparing the nerves by leaving a 5-mm margin of subcapsular tissue is possible and can protect potency in 80% of cases.* If ED does occur, patients can be advised that this often decreases over time following the procedure. Oral pharmacological therapy (e.g., sildenafil) can be helpful in the management of ED following HIFU.

Fact Sheet

- Clinically significant complications that can occur with HIFU include incontinence and ED
- In the rare cases where incontinence occurs, it is due to TURP or the combination of TURP and HIFU; little can be done to avoid the occurrence of this complication
- Specific measures can be taken to avoid ED; if the tumor is unilateral, low grade, and low volume, it is possible to spare the nerves by leaving a 5-mm margin of subcapsular tissue and protect potency in 80% of cases

Outcome: Munich Database

HIFU has been in use in the Munich Clinic for over 10 years, and during this time much research has gone into the optimization of the procedure.[12–14] A registration of all patients treated in the Munich Clinic was started in 1996, and this database records all relevant information on each patient, including treatment parameters, outcome, and side effects. Up to 2007 there were over 1,350 patients registered on the database.[15–19] Patients were categorized into the following risk groups: low risk: T1–T2a, PSA ≤10 ng ml^{-1}, GS < 7; intermediate risk: T2b or PSA 10 ng ml^{-1} to ≤ 20 ng ml^{-1} or GS 7; high risk: T2c or PSA > 20 ng ml^{-1} or GS > 7. *Outcome in 1,000 patients treated between 1996 and 2004* with a median follow-up time of 2.5 years (max: 6.5 years) is shown in Table 7.4. *As can be observed, a high negative biopsy rate of 93.7% at a mean of 9 months and a zero PSA nadir at 3 months have been achieved in patients with localized cancer who have low- or medium-risk disease.* PSA velocity was also very low in this group and PSA stability, defined according to the ASTRO criteria, was recorded in 81%. *At the other end of the spectrum, in the metastatic patient, a negative biopsy rate of 60–66% was achieved, which is very high for this group of patients.* Considering that this patient group comprised patients with GS 9

TABLE 7.4. The Munich database of patients treated with high-intensity focused ultrasound.

Prostate cancer risk group	Negative biopsy (%)	Median PSA nadir (ng ml^{-1})	PSA velocity (ng yr^{-1})	PSA stability (%)	Additional PCa therapy (%)	Stress incontinence Grades II-III (%)	Potency preservation (%)
Localized Low + medium risk (n = 400)	93.7	0	0.11	81	4.9	1.6	36
Localized high risk (n = 332)	87.6	0	0.15	73	14.7	2.7	27
Locally advanced (n = 209)	79.4	0.1	0.78	23	28.2	2.3	20
Metastatic N + (n = 26)	60	0.1	0.62	NR	42.9	3.6	0
Metastatic M + (n = 33)	66	0.15	16.9	NR	100	2.9	0

PSA, prostate-specific antigen; PCa, prostate cancer; NR, not recorded

Fact Sheet

- A total of 1,350 patients have been entered into a database of patients treated with HIFU at the Munich center between 1996 and 2007; low-, intermediate-, and high-risk patients have been treated
- Outcome in 1,000 patients indicates a 93.7% negative biopsy rate at a mean of 9 months and a zero PSA nadir at 3 months in patients with localized, low/medium-risk prostate cancer. In patients with metastatic disease, the equivalent negative biopsy rate was 60–66%
- The incidence of severe complications was low in this patient series, and preservation of potency was high, particularly in patients with localized cancer at low and medium risk

and 10, the PSA nadir values recorded were very promising. The objective of treating these patients was not to obtain cure but to reduce local morbidity and increase survival time by delaying metastasis from the primary tumor. *The incidence of severe complications was low in this patient series* and preservation of potency was high, particularly in patients with localized cancer at low and medium risk.

Future Directions

Promising advances in HIFU include the formulation of new treatment strategies for specific patient groups, and improvements in the visualization and assessment of HIFU lesions.

New Treatment Strategies

In the case of a unilateral tumor and where potency is an important issue for the patient, rather than treating the entire prostate, the contralateral lobe/capsule and neurovascular bundle could be excluded. This would be achieved by excluding 5 mm of tissue on the contralateral lobe and treating only 90% of the prostate. This approach might be appropriate in young patients, with small, low GS, unilateral tumors. Patients requesting this approach would need to be advised of the risk of tumor recurrence in the untreated area and the requirement for good compliance with follow up.

Improvements in the Visualization and Assessment of HIFU Lesions

The application and the continued development of a variety of imaging techniques are likely to provide improvements in the visualization and assessment of HIFU lesions in the near future. Magnetic resonance imaging (MRI) is the gold-standard technique used for assessing the efficacy of HIFU treatment, and the extent of necrosis can be clearly visualized on gadolinium-enhanced T1-weighted images.[20] MRI has also been used to guide HIFU treatment by monitoring temperature changes within the tissues.[20,21] Magnetic resonance elastography (MRE) may also provide a means of assessing the effects of thermal tissue ablation by measuring the mechanical properties of the lesion.[22] HIFU-induced lesions are visible using standard ultrasound,[23] although there are limitations to the accuracy of this approach. Other ultrasound-based techniques that might prove useful for assessing the extent of HIFU-induced lesions include MRE,24 contrast-enhanced power Doppler,[25] and other techniques that characterize the acoustic properties of tissues.

Fact Sheet

Promising advances in HIFU include the formulation of new treatment strategies for specific patient groups, and improvements in the visualization and assessment of HIFU lesions

- New treatment strategies include partial treatment of the prostate gland in selected patients; this approach does carry an increased risk of tumor recurrence
- A variety of imaging techniques are likely to provide improvements in the visualization and assessment of HIFU lesions in the near future

Conclusions

HIFU is an effective standard treatment for prostate cancer, with a broad range of indications in all tumor stages. Specifically, HIFU is indicated for localized prostate cancer (stage T1–T2 N0M0 Gleason score 1–3), partial therapy in unilateral low-volume, low Gleason score tumors, salvage therapy in recurrent prostate cancer after radical prostatectomy, radiotherapy, or hormone ablation, and as a debulking approach in advanced prostate cancer. HIFU destroys carefully selected tissue by generating heat sufficient to cause necrosis, while leaving surrounding tissue unharmed. Of the two commercially available HIFU systems, the Ablatherm® system provides well-defined, computer-controlled treatment planning and execution, supported by a variety of safety measures to maximize efficacy and safety. While other nonsurgical treatment options for localized prostate cancer (e.g., cryotherapy or brachytherapy) cannot generally be repeated in cases of local recurrence, HIFU can be repeated and can also be used as a salvage therapy. Postoperative morbidity is low. Clinically significant complications that can occur with HIFU include incontinence and ED, and specific measures can be taken to avoid the latter. HIFU is a highly effective treatment of patients with localized prostate cancer and can also be considered for patients with metastatic disease. Promising advances in HIFU include the formulation of new treatment strategies for specific patient groups, and improvements in the visualization and assessment of HIFU lesions

Overview

HIFU is an effective standard treatment for prostate cancer, with a broad range of indications in all tumor stages, including:

- Localized prostate cancer (stage T1–T2 N0M0 Gleason score 1–3)
- Partial therapy in unilateral low-volume, low Gleason score tumors
- Salvage therapy in recurrent prostate cancer after radical prostatectomy, radiotherapy, or hormone ablation
- For advanced prostate cancer as a debulking process

The contraindications for HIFU are well defined and include:

- Gland sizes larger than 40 ml (larger glands can be reduced in size prior to HIFU by TURP)
- Conditions where the rectal wall is damaged or rendered more susceptible to damage (e.g., following radiotherapy or when there is active local infection)
- In cases of rectal stenosis or rectal amputation

When treating prostate cancer using HIFU, ultrasound waves are generated by a transducer within a probe introduced into the rectum. The ultrasound waves penetrate the rectal wall with only slight absorption and reflection, but are focused onto a small area (the focal point) in the prostate to generate a lesion by generating heat sufficient to cause necrosis.

Two commercially available HIFU systems are currently in use – the Ablatherm® system and the Sonablate® system. Both systems provide TRUS imaging and treatment using an endorectal probe. The main differences between the systems are in the indications that can be treated, patient positioning, the ultrasound frequencies used during treatment and planning, shoot and delay times, the treatment mode within the prostate, and the range of safety measures available. Overall, the Sonablate® system has a number of limitations, while the Ablatherm® system provides features that maximize treatment efficacy and safety.

While other nonsurgical treatment options for localized prostate cancer (e.g., cryotherapy or brachytherapy) cannot generally be repeated in cases of local recurrence, HIFU can be repeated and can also be used as a salvage therapy. HIFU utilizes information available from prostate biopsies and TURP and can be combined with TURP for large volume tumors.

The steps in the Ablatherm® HIFU procedure are well defined and can be thought of as follows:

1. Preoperative preparation
2. Anesthesia
3. Patient positioning and external warming
4. Device preparation
5. Introducing the probe
6. TRUS simulation
7. Treatment planning
8. Robotic treatment
9. The perioperative phase
10. Follow up

Practical tips and tricks refine the procedure further and improve the speed and ease with which the treatment can be conducted.

Apart from immediate swelling of the prostate which tends to resolve over 3–8 days, perioperative morbidity is low following HIFU; significant pain, bleeding, the need for blood transfusions, or intensive care are unusual, and the occurrence of thrombosis or pulmonary embolism is uncommon. Clinically significant complications that can occur with HIFU include incontinence and ED. Specific measures can be taken to avoid ED, such as leaving a 5-mm margin of subcapsular tissue to spare the nerves if the tumor is unilateral, low grade and low volume; this approach protects potency in 80% of cases.

A total of 1,350 patients have been entered into a database of patients treated with HIFU at the Munich center between 1996 and 2007. Patients treated include those with low-, intermediate-, and high-risk disease. Outcome in 1,000 patients treated up until 2004 with a median follow-up of 2.5 years has been analyzed. Data indicate a 93.7% negative biopsy rate at a mean of 9 months and a zero PSA nadir at 3 months in patients with localized, low/medium-risk prostate cancer. In patients with metastatic disease, the equivalent negative biopsy rate was 60–66%. The incidence of severe complications was low in this patient series and preservation of potency was high, particularly in patients with localized disease at low and medium risk.

Advances promising to improve HIFU further in the near future include:

- New treatment strategies such as partial treatment of the prostate gland in selected patients (although this approach does carry an increased risk of tumor recurrence).
- The application and the continued development of a variety of imaging techniques are likely to provide improvements in the visualization and assessment of HIFU lesions in the near future.

References

1. Fry WJ, Mosberg WH, Barnard JW, et al. Production of focal tissue destructive lesions in the central nervous system with ultrasound. J Neurosurg 1954;11:471–8.
2. Fry WJ, Barnard JW, Fry FV, et al. Ultrasonic lesions in mammalian central nervous system. Science 1955;122:517–8.
3. Burov AK. High-intensity ultrasonic vibrations for action on animal and human malignant tumours. Dokl Akad Nauk SSSR 1956;106:239–41.
4. Fry FJ, Johnson LK. Tumor irradiation with intense ultrasound. Ultrasound Med Biol 1978;4:337–41.
5. Goss SA, Fry FJ. The effects of high-intensity ultrasonic irradiation on tumour growth. IEEE Trans Sonics Ultrason 1984;SU-31:491–6.
6. Lizzi FL, Coleman DJ, Driller J, et al. A therapeutic ultrasound system incorporating real time ultrasonics scanning. In: *Proceedings of the 1986 Ultrasonics Symposium Institute of Electrical and Electronic Engineers.* MacAvoy BR (ed), (New York, 1987), pp. 981–4.

7. Bihrle R, Foster RS, Sanghvi NT, et al. High intensity focused ultrasound for the treatment of benign prostatic hyperplasia: early United States clinical experience. J Urol 1994;151:1271–5.
8. Vallancien G, Chartier-Kastler E, Chopin D, et al. Focused extracorporeal pyrotherapy: experimental results. Eur Urol 1991;20:211–9.
9. Gelet A, Chapelon JY, Bouvier R, et al. Treatment of prostate cancer with transrectal focused ultrasound: early clinical experience. Eur Urol 1996;29:174–83.
10. Uchida T, Sanghvi NT, Gardner TA, et al. Transrectal high-intensity focused ultrasound for treatment of patients with stage T1b-2N0M localized prostate cancer: a preliminary report. Urology 2002;59:394–8.
11. Gelet A, Chapelon JY, Poissonnier L, et al. Local recurrence of prostate cancer after external beam radiotherapy: early experience of salvage therapy using high-intensity focused ultrasonography. Urology 2004;63:625–9.
12. Thuroff S, Chaussy C. Status of high intensity focused ultrasound (HIFU) in Urology in 2005. In Chaussy C et al. (eds): Therapeutic Energy Applications in Urology. Thieme Vlg. 2005, pp. 92–102.
13. Chaussy C, Thüroff S. High Intensity focused ultrasound for the treatment of prostate cancer. In Moore RG, Bishoff JT (eds): Minimally Invasive Uro-oncologic Surgery. London: Taylor and Francis, 2005, pp. 327–35.
14. Chaussy C, Thüroff S, Rebillard X, Gelet A. 2005Technology insight: high intensity focused ultrasound for urologic cancers. Nat Clin Pract Urol ;2:191–8.
15. Chaussy C, Thuroff S. High-intensity focused ultrasound in prostate cancer: results after 3 years. 2000Mol Urol ;4(3):179–82.
16. Thuroff S, Chaussy C, Vallancien G, et-al. 2003High-intensity focused ultrasound and localized prostate cancer: efficacy results from the European multicentric study. J Endourol ;17(8):673–7.
17. Chaussy C, Thuroff S. 2003The status of high-intensity focused ultrasound in the treatment of localized prostate cancer and the impact of a combined resection. Curr Urol Rep ;4(3):248–52.
18. Chaussy C, Thuroff S: 2001Results and side effects of high-intensity focused ultrasound in localized prostate cancer. J Endourol ;15(4):437–40.
19. Thüroff S, Chaussy C, Gelet A. Focused ultrasound (HIFU) in the treatment of prostate cancer: energy/efficacy correlation. WCE Congress, November 2001, J Endourol 2001;15(Suppl 1):Abstract A3-P10, p. A32
20. Hynynen K, Freund WR, Cline HE, et al. A clinical, noninvasive, MR imaging-monitored ultrasound surgery method. Radiographics 1996;16:185–95.
21. Damianou C, Pavlou M, Velev O, et al. High intensity focused ultrasound ablation of kidney guided by MRI. Ultrasound Med Biol 2004;30:397–404.
22. Wu T, Felmlee JP, Greenleaf JF, et al. Assessment of thermal tissue ablation with MR elastography. Magn Reson Med 2001;45:80–7.
23. Vaezy S, Shi X, Martin RW, et al. Real-time visualization of high-intensity focused ultrasound treatment using ultrasound imaging. Ultrasound Med Biol 2001;27:33–42.
24. Souchon R, Rouviere O, Gelet A, et al. Visualisation of HIFU lesions using elastography of the human prostate in vivo: preliminary results. Ultrasound Med Biol 2003;29:1007–15.
25. Sedelaar JP, Aarnink RG, van Leenders GJ, et al. The application of three-dimensional contrast-enhanced ultrasound to measure volume of affected tissue after HIFU treatment for localized prostate cancer. Eur Urol 2000;37:559–68.

Chapter 8
Harmonic Scalpel

David D. Thiel and Howard N. Winfield

Few surgeons will argue against the benefit of a bloodless operative field and the ability to achieve this in a safe and timely manner. Since the first electrosurgical unit was put into surgical practice in the 1920s, there has been a quest to discover safer and more efficient hemostatic surgical instruments. The ideal intraoperative hemostatic energy source would accurately coagulate, cut like a knife without charring or sticking to tissue, have minimal smoke production, and keep the patient out of the electrical circuit. Ultrasonic coagulating shears or the Harmonic Scalpel (Ethicon Endo-Surgery, Cincinnati, OH) was developed as an alternative to electrical energy for surgical use. The instrument became commercially available in 1993. Few instruments developed in the past 20 years have facilitated a surgeon's ability to perform complex open and minimally invasive procedures like the Harmonic Scalpel.[1] The instrument's efficacy combined with stellar safety profile has led to the gradual replacement of older monopolar and bipolar electrocautery in many instances.

Hemostatic Principles in Relation to Active Surgical Temperatures

Regardless of the mechanism, generation of heat inside a cell will increase intracellular temperature. The cell can tolerate temperatures up to approximately 40°C without significant cell damage. At temperatures up to 50°C, cellular processes terminate and enzymatic activity ceases in a reversible fashion dependent on the duration of heating. Above 50°C there is irreversible cell damage (denaturation). The tissue will blanch and proteins disorganize to form a coagulum that seals vessels. As temperatures approach 100°C the internal water reaches its boiling point, water changes from the liquid to vapor phase, the cell wall ruptures, and tissue is dessicated. Above 200°C the tissue will carbonize (turn black) from dehydration and no further current can go through it. An eschar forms as the tissue burns.[1–3]

Electrosurgery and laser energy denature protein to form a hemostatic coagulum that tamponades and seals vessels. Electric current (electrocautery) or light (laser) is used to transfer electrons or photons to tissue that results in excitation of the electron orbitals of molecules. When the electrons return to their resting state, heat is generated which denatures protein to form the coagulum.[4]

The Harmonic Scalpel

The Harmonic Scalpel cuts and coagulates tissue without the use of electrosurgical or laser energy. The device itself is composed of a generator, a hand piece, and a blade (Figs. 8.1 and 8.2). Electrical energy is transferred from a microprocessor-controlled generator to a transducer in the hand piece. The generator pulses the transducer with AC electrical current at its natural frequency of 55,500 Hz. The transducer consists of piezoelectric ceramic disks in a stack that are compressed between two metal cylinders (Fig. 8.3). The disks convert the electrical energy from the generator into mechanical energy in the form of vibrating "harmonic" ultrasonic waves at the same frequency (55,500 Hz). The energy is transferred to an active blade at the tip of the instrument that will vibrate longitudinally over a distance of 50–100 μm. The microprocessor in the generator will sense changes in the acoustic system and alter the power delivered.[1,4,5]

Hemostatic Mechanism of the Harmonic Scalpel

The conversion of electrical current into mechanical vibrations at 55,500 times per second will couple with tissue and transfer mechanical vibrational energy that breaks hydrogen bonds in proteins. As the proteins denature, they change conformation and form a sticky coagulum that welds tissue around bleeding vessels. Larger vessels are sealed with coaptation followed by "welding."[5] Heat is generated in the tissue from friction and stress, but much less than that of electrocautery or laser. This will lead to less smoke production and decreases thermal energy spread to surrounding tissues. The lower temperatures

O. Ukimura and I.S. Gill (eds.), *Contemporary Interventional Ultrasonography in Urology*,
DOI: 10.1007/978-1-84800-217-3_8,

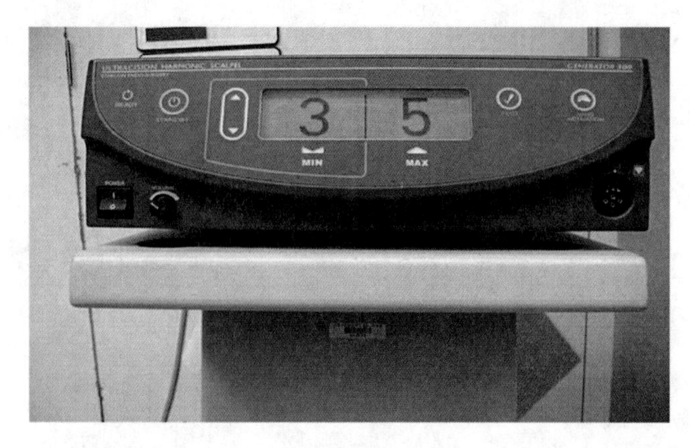

FIG. 8.1. Harmonic Scalpel Generator. The microprocessor-controlled generator utilizes AC current to pulse the transducer (Fig. 8.2) with electrical energy. The generator alters the power delivered based on microprocessors in the device. Note the LED screen demonstrating power settings (level 1–5)

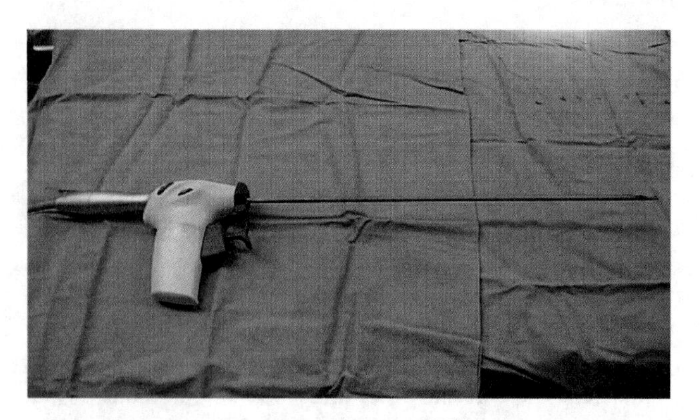

FIG. 8.2. Hand Piece and Blade. Gross photos of the hand piece containing a transducer that converts electrical energy to mechanical energy and transfers this energy to the distal blade

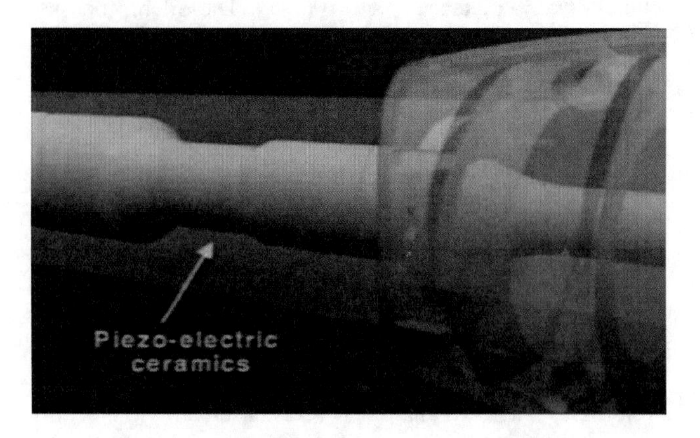

FIG. 8.3. Transducer Schematic. The transducer consists of piezoelectric ceramic disks in a stack that are compressed between two metal cylinders. The disks convert the electrical energy from the generator into mechanical energy in the form of vibrating "harmonic" ultrasonic waves at a frequency of 55,500 Hz

used to coagulate tissue avoid the charring of tissues seen with higher temperature modalities such as electrocautery and laser. This allows for more precise dissection due to absence of tissue plane alteration.

Cutting Mechanism of the Harmonic Scalpel

In addition to the aforementioned coaptive coagulation, the Harmonic Scalpel simultaneously cuts or dissects tissue via two mechanisms. Tissue layers are separated by fluid vapors produced when the instrument is activated. This "cavitational fragmentation" occurs when cells are fragmented into cellular debris and water, and is especially prominent in avascular tissue planes. The Harmonic Scalpel also acts as a "scalpel" cutting high protein collagen containing tissue by vibrating a sharp blade at 55,500 Hz. It should be noted that the vibrational action of the blade will "self-clean" the instrument and avoids tissue or coagulum sticking to the blade.[1,4,5]

Use of the Harmonic Scalpel

The generator has settings to alter cutting and coagulation capabilities. This is done mainly by altering the blade excursion from 50 to 100 μm. There is an inverse relationship between cutting and coagulation. A power setting of five (blade excursion of 100 μm) will increase the cutting speed at the expense of coagulation. A power setting of 1 (blade excursion 50 μm) will slow the cutting speed in favor of improved hemostasis. A power setting of three (blade excursion 70 μm) is the most versatile and most commonly used setting.

There are numerous types of blades and shears available to deliver the ultrasonic energy to the tissue (Fig. 8.4). The blades range from sharp blades for maximal cutting power to flat blades with blunt edges for maximal coagulation. A sharper blade will increase cutting power, precision, and speed at the expense of more reliable hemostasis.[1] Increasing the tension on the tissue or a firmer grip on the tissue being coagulated will give faster cutting with less coagulation. The time of instrument activation is important as well. The less time the instrument is activated on the tissue, the lower the hemostasis potential.

Newer technology has allowed the Harmonic Scalpel to be either foot or hand activated. Ergonomic hand controls have eliminated the need for a foot pedal and seem easier to use (Fig. 8.5). The newer generators allow for more efficient power use in generating the ultrasonic energy. A variety of hand grips now exist to provide easier alteration of tissue tension.

Safety

The Harmonic Scalpel is approved by the United States Food and Drug Administration (FDA) for division of tissue and coagulation of vessels up to 3 mm in diameter. Some animal

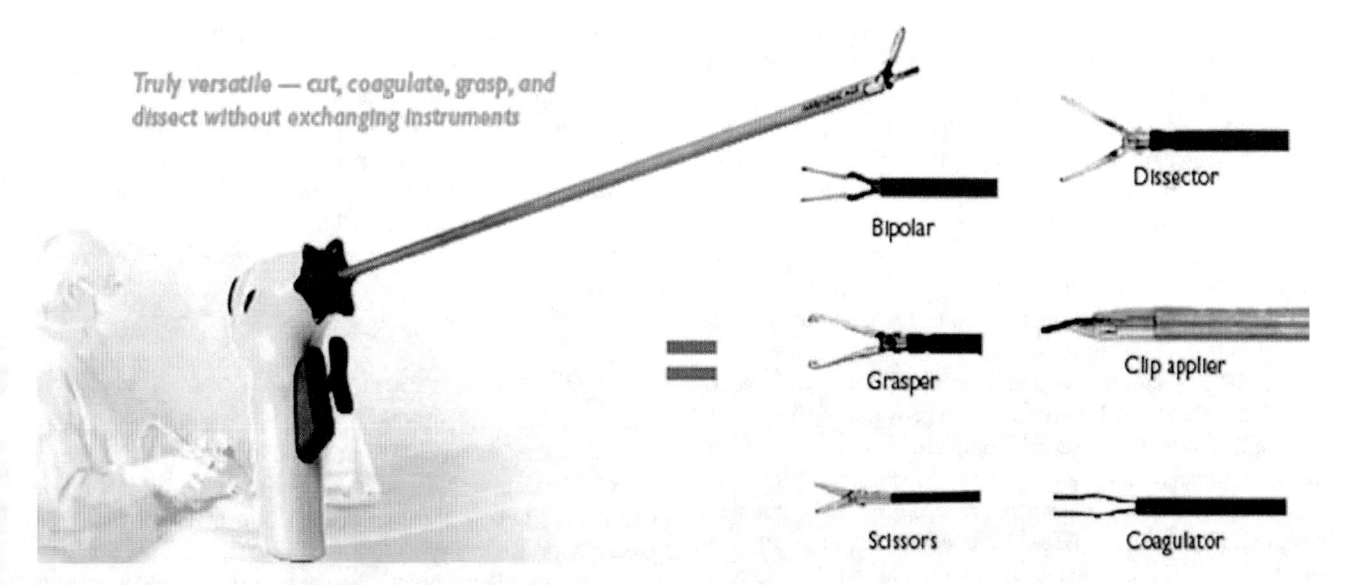

FIG. 8.4. Blade and Shears. Picture demonstrating the multitude of contemporary blades and shears available for use

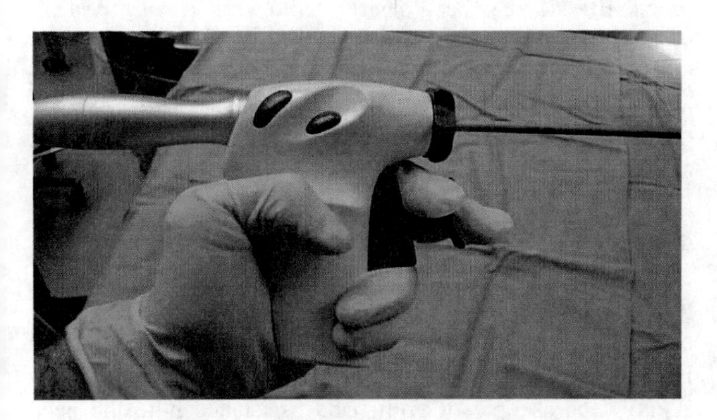

FIG. 8.5. Hand Controls. Ergonomic hand controls like that shown have made Harmonic Scalpel use easier and eliminated the necessity of a foot pedal in many instances

studies suggest that the Harmonic Scalpel can reliably seal vessels up to 5 mm and withstand bursting pressures up to at least 250 mmHg.[6] The product insert lists the indications for the Harmonic Scalpel as "soft tissue incisions when bleeding control and minimal thermal injury are desired. The instrument can be used as an adjunct or substitute for electrocautery, lasers, and steel scalpels." The only two contraindications listed in the product insert are that the Harmonic Scalpel should not be used for incision into bone and it is not indicated for contraception tubal ligation.

Collateral thermal tissue damage is a risk with any method of coagulation. The optimal surgical instrument would be one that coagulates without dispersal of thermal energy outside the area it has been focally applied. Since the functional temperatures of the Harmonic Scalpel are lower than traditional electrocautery, the risk of thermal energy spread to peripheral tissues should be lower. Histologic studies comparing lateral thermal spread of the Harmonic Scalpel to other energy-producing hemostatic modalities (monopolar electrocautery, bipolar electrocautery, and advanced bipolar tissue sealing devices) demonstrate the Harmonic Scalpel to have the least histologic evidence of peripheral energy spread (0–2.18 mm).[6,7] A histologic study completed in rabbits comparing ligation of the short gastric vessels (diameter under 1 mm) with these modalities demonstrated ultrasonic shears to have the least amount of thermal damage to the adjacent stomach tissue. Histologic evidence of thermal tissue effect was confined to the subserosal and muscular layers of the stomach compared to deeper submucosal and mucosal injuries created by monopolar and bipolar electrocautery.[8] Intraoperative thermal mapping of ultrasonic shears demonstrates temperatures 1 cm away from the instrument secondary to heat dissipation to vary depending on power setting and time in use.[9] Mean peak temperatures were noted to be directly proportional to the activation time and the power setting. Significant thermal spread can be noted up to 25 mm away from the instrument with maximal power settings and activation times over 10 s.

Despite the minimization of peripheral thermal spread and the lower functional temperatures of the Harmonic Scalpel, the functioning blade is hot and will remain so seconds after an application. Contact with bowel or other surrounding vital structures with the functioning blade should be avoided at all times.[1] Contact with the functional blade can cause thermal injury or pain to the operating surgeon during hand-assisted laparoscopy and should be avoided as well.

Any energy-producing hemostatic device will result in smoke and aerosol emission. The lower functioning temperatures of the Harmonic Scalpel and lack of tissue carbonization lead to less surgical smoke production. This will greatly improve visibility especially in the laparoscopic setting. The amount of cellular debris found in the plume created by the Harmonic Scalpel (>1 × 10^7 particles ml^{-1}) is about one-fourth that produced by electrocautery.[10] The low temperature vaporization of tissue by the Harmonic Scalpel is concerning to some authors due to the fact that cool aerosols have a higher chance of carrying infection and viable cells than higher temperature aerosols.[11] Conflicting studies exist as to exactly how many viable cancer and blood cells are present in the aerosols produced by the Harmonic Scalpel.[9,12] However, the aerosols have not been completely studied, and there is no consensus regarding its composition or its potential effect on operating room personnel.

The FDA Manufacturer and User Facility Device Experience Database (MAUDE) lists reported adverse events involving medical devices. A search completed since 1993 relating the Harmonic Scalpel and mortality lists ten occurrences. There is one case of inadvertent enterotomy not recognized intraoperatively and two cases of delayed bleeding following splenectomy. There is one death reported from a laparoscopic nephrectomy although Harmonic Scalpel malfunction played no role in the death. In the same time period there are 230 reported intraoperative injuries involving the Harmonic Scalpel, with the most common being inadvertent injury to adjacent small intestine or large bowel. The most commonly reported adverse events of the Harmonic Scalpel involve failure of the device to test properly before activation at the beginning of the case. This does not add to patient morbidity and seems only to increase operative time. There are a few reported instances of the blades becoming overheated and melting trocars during certain laparoscopic procedures. There are also occasional reported events of the distal tip of the instrument falling off during surgery requiring retrieval. Again there appears to be no added morbidity with this occurrence except for an increase in operative time.

Since no electrical current is passed into or through the patient with the Harmonic Scalpel, there is no risk of direct coupling or capacitive coupling injuries. The entire device is internally grounded eliminating electrical risk to the surgeon. There is also no risk of neuromuscular stimulation causing inadvertent patient movement. This is especially important in patients with pacemakers or implanted defibrillators. Electrocautery (monopolar and bipolar) can cause faulty pacemaker sensing or reset the pacemaker device. Ultrasonic energy is the safest alternative for surgical coagulation in this patient population.[1] Despite the proven safety of the Harmonic Scalpel, proper training and experience with the device is necessary to prevent inadvertent damage to surrounding structures.

Clinical Applications of the Harmonic Scalpel

Harmonic scalpel technology has been utilized in several fields of surgery including otorhinolaryngologic, gastrointestinal, vascular, and obstetric and gynecologic surgery in addition to urology.[13] In open surgery and especially laparoscopic surgery, the Harmonic Scalpel has demonstrated advantages over conventional hemostatic techniques with regard to decreased operative time and intraoperative bleeding. The instrument is disposable and its cost must be figured in to any surgical treatment plan. However, many surgeons will argue the cost effectiveness of the extra expense by factoring reduced operative time and decreased blood loss.[14] In urology, there are numerous published reports of the benefits of Harmonic Scalpel use.

Renal Surgery

The Harmonic Scalpel plays a large role in modern-day laparoscopic renal surgery. We utilize the Harmonic Scalpel in every laparoscopic renal surgery completed at our institution. The scalpel will fit through ports 5 mm or larger making it versatile for use in any abdominal port at any angle. Since the first laparoscopic nephrectomy was reported in 1991, multiple modifications in technique have been proposed for improving hemostasis without compromising visualization and operative time.[15] Efficacy has been clearly demonstrated with the Harmonic Scalpel for reflection of the colon medially and freeing the kidney from all its attachments during laparoscopic nephrectomy without switching instruments.[16] The Harmonic Scalpel allows this to be completed in a bloodless field without need for suction of blood or smoke.

Laparoscopic partial nephrectomy remains a difficult procedure for most urologists secondary to the requirement of intracorporeal knot tying to control renal parenchymal bleeding following mass excision. The Harmonic Scalpel has been proposed for wedge resections of smaller exophytic renal tumors. However, all series commenting on this technique either by a pure laparoscopic or with hand assistance note the need for use of adjuvant hemostatic agents (argon beam, holmium laser, TissueLink radiofreqency device, fibrin based products, etc.).[17] When using the Harmonic Scalpel for mass resection during laparoscopic partial nephrectomy, it is recommended that the generator be set at power level 2 or 3 for slower cutting and increased hemostasis.[18] Pig studies have confirmed that the Harmonic Scalpel will attain complete hemostasis of the renal parenchyma in most cases of peripheral renal wedge resections or biopsies, whereas larger resections (polar nephrectomies or heminephrectomies) will require supplemental coagulation.[19,20] Small interlobular vessels are controlled sufficiently with the Harmonic Scalpel, but larger interlobar and arcuate parenchymal vessels will require adjuvant hemostatic control. The same studies have demonstrated the mean depth of acute cellular injury demonstrated histologically is approximately 1.3 mm. However, studies completed on various canine organs demonstrate that the Harmonic Scalpel will not compromise microscopic examination of the tissue by the pathologists, and in most tissues there is no alteration in specimen quality when compared to standard sharp resection.[21] We have not found pathologic examination of renal masses to be compromised by any hemostatic method we employ on the renal parenchyma for partial nephrectomy including the Harmonic Scalpel.

We find the Harmonic Scalpel to be very useful in controlling tributaries to the renal vein. This is especially imperative in left-sided laparoscopic donor nephrectomies. The use of endovascular staplers to control the renal vein prohibits clip placement near the vein that could potentially interfere with placement or deployment of the vascular stapler. We find the tributaries of the renal vein (gonadal, adrenal, and lumbar veins) to be well controlled with bipolar cautery followed by Harmonic Scalpel division. We utilize a power level of 3 for this step. Caution must be used with the Harmonic Scalpel during laparoscopic donor nephrectomies during periureteral dissection. Pig studies utilizing the Harmonic Scalpel parallel to the ureter have noted no visible evidence of injury, but marked transmural coagulation microscopically. This transmural coagulation was more pronounced than that seen with standard electrocautery.[22] We do not utilize the Harmonic Scalpel to dissect out periureteral tissue in laparoscopic donor nephrectomies.

Laparoscopic cyst decortication has been proven to provide prolonged relief of flank discomfort in patients with large renal cysts. Significant cyst fluid in the operative field may render standard electrocautery ineffective during laparoscopic cyst decortication. Published reports document the efficacy of the Harmonic Scalpel in laparoscopic renal cyst decortication for removal of the cyst wall and hemostasis. One series with eight procedures noted significant postoperative bleeding requiring transfusion in two patients. However, both patients had heparin flushes in their dialysis catheters postoperatively.[23] The authors of this manuscript note that caution should be used when utilizing the Harmonic Scalpel alone for hemostasis of the renal parenchyma in patients with prolonged bleeding times. The Harmonic Scalpel has been utilized to divide the isthmus of horseshoe kidneys laparoscopically. The renal isthmus of horseshoe kidneys is often too thick for laparoscopic staplers, and the Harmonic Scalpel has been published as an efficacious safe method for isthmus division.[24,25]

Adrenal Surgery

Laparoscopic adrenal surgery is now the gold standard for surgical management of incidentally discovered adrenal masses. Many authors believe that the Harmonic Scalpel has been the one technological innovation to improve cost, safety, learning curve, and operating room time of laparoscopic adrenalectomy. The Harmonic Scalpel has demonstrated cost saving compared to conventional instruments by dramatically reducing the number of clips used to control vasculature in proximity to the adrenal gland.[26,27] For a right-side adrenalectomy, all vessels can usually be controlled with the Harmonic Scalpel including the main adrenal vein, although use of clips is certainly reasonable and safe. On the left side all vessels can be managed with the Harmonic Scalpel, but larger veins branching toward the left renal vein may require clipping or stapling.

Pediatric Urologic Surgery

Use of the Harmonic Scalpel has been published in pediatric urologic literature as well. Partial nephrectomies are often performed in the pediatric population for entities such as nonfunctioning renal units, ectopic ureteroceles, and severe reflux nephropathy. Laparoscopic partial nephrectomy has proven benefit of improved cosmesis and shorter hospital stay compared to open partial nephrectomy. The Harmonic Scalpel is used to transect the renal moiety in a bloodless fashion. There have been no published complications of the Harmonic Scalpel in pediatric renal surgery.[28,29] The Harmonic Scalpel has been published to be a critical tool in pediatric laparoscopic adrenalectomy for children as young as 3 years of age.[30]

Laparoscopic varicocelectomy has become a viable treatment option in adolescents with large or symptomatic varicoceles. Harmonic Scalpel use has allowed this procedure to be performed via two 5-mm port sites. One port is used for a 5-mm camera and another port is used for dissection and sacrifice of the spermatic cord with the Harmonic Scalpel.[31] In most cases no attempt is made to separate the artery and vein before division of the cord cephalad to the divergence of the vas deferens.

Prostate and Bladder Surgery

Prevention of neurovascular bundle injury during radical prostatectomy is imperative to preserve sexual function. Athermal dissection of the neurovascular bundles during open radical prostatectomy appears to be the best method to preserve cavernosal nerve function. The rapid increase of laparoscopic and robotic prostatectomies being performed has led to a rise in the use of hemostatic energy sources to control intraoperative bleeding. The Harmonic Scalpel has been utilized in laparoscopic radical prostatectomy for hemostatis. Canine studies show that the Harmonic Scalpel may provide less damage to surrounding neurovascular bundles than other energy sources (bipolar or monopolar electrocautery) but provide statistically more damage and less postoperative nerve function that conventional athermal neurovascular bundle dissection.[32] Surgeons performing other procedures in close proximity of nerve bundles have noted the Harmonic Scalpel to cause nerve impairment secondary to thermal energy spread. Recurrent laryngeal nerve injuries have been noted following Harmonic Scalpel use during endoscopic parathyroid surgery.[33]

Simple prostatectomy or adenomectomy is performed on patients with benign obstructing prostates that are too large for standard transurethral resection of the prostate. While traditionally performed with an open incision, there are recent reports of this procedure being performed laparoscopically. The Harmonic Scalpel is used in two recent publications to resect the adenoma from the prostatic capsule in a relatively bloodless field. The mean blood loss in these reports is less than that traditionally seen with open simple adenomectomies.[34,35]

The Harmonic Scalpel has proven beneficial in laparoscopic cystoprostatectomy as well. The lateral and posterior vascular pedicles of the prostate can be controlled with the Harmonic Scalpel in conjunction with bipolar electrocautery as needed. Many authors have found the Harmonic Scalpel to be more beneficial and cost effective than sequential firings of Endo-GIA staplers.[36]

References

1. Harrell AG, Kercher KW, Heniford BT. Energy sources in laparosopy. Semin Laparosc Surg. 2004; 11(3):201–209.
2. Shimi SM. Dissection techniques in laparoscopic surgery: A review. J R Coll Surg Edinb. 1995; 40:249–259.
3. Elashry OM, Wolf JS, Rayala HJ, McDougall EM, Clayman RV. Recent advances in laparoscopic partial nephrectomy: Comparative study of electrosurgical snare electrode and ultrasonic dissection. J Endourol. 1997; 11(1):15–22.
4. Amaral JF. Laparoscopic application of an ultrasonically activated scalpel. Gastrointest Endosc Clin North Am. 1993; 3(2):381–391.
5. Amaral JF. The experimental development of an ultrasonically activated scalpel for laparoscopic use. Surg Laparosc Endosc. 1994; 4(2):92–99.
6. Landman J, Kerbel K, Rehman J, Andreoni C, Humphery PA, Collyer W, Olweny E, Sundaram C, Clayman RV. Evaluation of a vessel sealing system, bipolar electrocautery, harmonic scalpel, titanium clips, endoscopic gastrointestinal anastomosis vascular staples and sutures for arterial and venous ligation in a porcine model. J Urol. 2003; 169:697–700.
7. Harold KL, Pollinger H, Matthews BD, Kercher KW, Sing RF, Heniford BT. Comparison of ultrasonic energy, bipolar thermal energy, and vascular clips for the hemostasis of small-, medium-, and large-sized arteries. Surg Endosc. 2003; 17:1228–1230.
8. Diamantis T, Kontos M, Arvelakis A, Syroukis S, Koronarchis D, Papalois A, Agapitos E, Bastounis E, Lazaris AC. Comparison of monopolar electrocoagulation, bipolar electrocoagulation, ultracision, and Ligasure. Surg Today. 2006; 36:908–913.
9. Emam TA, Cuscheri A. . How safe is high-power ultrasonic dissection? Ann Surg. 2003; 2:186–191.
10. Ott DE, Moss E, Martinez K. Aerosol exposure from an ultrasonically activated (harmonic) device. J Am Assoc Gyn Laparoscopists. 1998; 5:29–32.
11. Barrett WL, Garber SM. Surgical smoke – a review of the literature. Surg Endosc. 2003; 17:979–987.
12. Nduka CC, Poland N, Kennedy M, Dye J, Darzi A.. Does the ultrasonically activated scalpel release airborne cancer cells? Surg Endosc. 1998; 12:1031–1034.
13. Miccoli P, Berti P, Dionigi GL, D'Agostino J, Orlandini C, Donatini G. Randomized controlled trial of harmonic scalpel use during thyroidectomy. Arch Otolaryngol Head Neck Surg. 2006; 132:1069–1073.
14. Ortega J, Sala C, Flor B, Liedo S. Efficacy and cost-effectiveness of the UltraCision harmonic scalpel in thyroid surgery: an analysis of 200 cases in a randomized trial. J Laparoendosc Adv Surg Tech A. 2004; 14:9–12.
15. Clayman RV, Kavoussi LR, Soper NJ, et-al.. Laparoscopic nephrectomy: initial case report. J Urol. 1991; 146:278–282.
16. Helal M, Albertini J, Lockhart J, Albrink M. Laparoscopic nephrectomy using the harmonic scalpel. J Endourol. 1997; 11(4):267–268.
17. Simon SD, Ferrigni RG, Novicki DE, Lamm DL, Swanson SS, Andrews PE. Mayo clinic scottsdale experience with laparoscopic nephron sparing surgery for renal tumors. J Urol. 2003; 169:2059–2062.
18. Zhang XU, Li HZ, Ma X, Zheng T, Li LC, Ye ZQ. Retroperitoneal laparoscopic nephron-sparing surgery for renal tumors: Report of 32 cases. Urology. 2005; 65:1080–1085.
19. Jackman SV, Cadeddu JA, Chen RN, Micali S, Bishoff JT, Lee BR, Moore RG, Kavoussi LR. Utility of the harmonic scalpel for laparoscopic partial nephrectomy. J Endourol. 1998; 12(5):441–444.
20. Elashry OM, Wolf JS, Rayala HJ, McDougall EM, Clayman RV. Recent advances in laparoscopic partial nephrectomy: Comparative study of electrosurgical snare electrode and ultrasonic dissection. J Endourol. 1997; 11(1):15–22.
21. Barnes RF, Greenfield CL, Schaeffer DJ, Landolfi J, Andrews J. Comparison of biopsy samples obtained using standard endoscopic instruments and the Harmonic Scalpel during laparoscopic and laparoscopic-assisted surgery in normal dogs. Vet Surg. 2006; 35:243–251.
22. Kadesky KM, Schopf B, Magee JF, Blair GK. Proximity injury by the ultrasonically activated scalpel during dissection. J Pediatr Surg. 1997; 32(6):878–879.
23. Mcnally ML, Erturk E, Oleyourryk G, Schoeniger L. Laparoscopic cyst decortication using the Harmonic Scalpel for symptomatic autosomal dominant polycystic kidney disease. J Endourol. 2001; 15(6):5597–599.
24. Lapointe SP, Houle AM, Barrieras D. Retroperitoneoscopic left nephrectomy in a horseshoe kidney with the use of the harmonic scalpel. Can J Urol. 2002; 9(5):1651–1652.
25. Nadler RB, Thaxton CS, Kim SC. Hand-assisted laparoscopic pyeloplasty and isthmectomy in a patient with a horseshoe kidney. J Endourol. 2003; 17(10):909–910.
26. Valeri A, Borrelli A, Presenti L, Lucchese M, Manca G, Tonelli P, Bergamini C, Borrelli D, Palli M, Saieva C. The influence of new technologies on laparoscopic adrenalectomy. Surg Endosc. 2002; 16:1274–1279.
27. Tazaki H, Baba S, Murai M. technical improvements in laparoscopic adrenalectomy. Tech Urol. 1995; 1(4):222–226.
28. Horowitz M, Shah SM, Ferzli G, Syad PI, Glassberg KI. Laparoscopic partial upper pole nephrectomy in infants and children. BJU Int. 2001; 87:514–516.
29. Sydorak RM, Shaul DB. Laparoscopic partial nephrectomy in infants and toddlers. J Pediatr Surg. 2005; 40:1945–1947.
30. Pampaloni E, valeri A, Mattei R, Presenti L, Centonze N, Neri AS, Salti R, Noccioli B, Messineo A. Initial experience with laparoscopic adrenal surgery in children: is endoscopy surgery recommended and safe for the treatment of adrenocortical neoplasms? Pediatr Med Chir. 2004; 26(6):450–459.
31. Link BA, Kruska JD, Wong C, Kropp BP. Two trocar laparoscopic varicocelectomy: Approach and outcomes. JSLS. 2006; 10:151–154.
32. Ong AM, Su LM, Varkarakis I, Inagaki T, Link RE, Bhayani SB, Patriciu A, Crain B, Walsh PC. Nerve sparing radical prostatectomy: effects of hemostatic energy sources on the recovery

of cavernous nerve function in a canine model. J Urol. 2004; 172:1318–1322.

33. Owaki T, Nakano S, Arimura K, Aikou T. The ultrasonic coagulating and cutting system injures nerve function. Endoscopy. 2002; 34:575–579.
34. Rehman J, khan SA, Sukkarieh T, Chughtai B, Waltzer WC. Extraperitoneal laparoscopic prostatectomy (adenomectomy) for obstructing benign prostatic hyperplasia: transvesical and transcapsular (Millin) techniques. J Endourol. 2005; 19(4):491–496.
35. van Velthoven R, Peltier A, Laguna MP, Piechaud T. Laparoscopic extraperitoneal adenomectomy (Millim): Pilot study on feasibility. Eur Urol. 2004; 45:103–109.
36. Simonato A, gregori A, Lissiani A, Bozzola A, Galli S, Gaboardi F. Laparoscopic radical cystoprostatectomy: A technique illustrated step by step. Eur Urol. 2003; 44:132–138.

Chapter 9
Intravascular Ultrasound

Srinivasa Kalidindi, Stephen J. Nicholls, and Steven E. Nissen

Introduction

In the half century since it was initially performed, coronary angiography has become the preferred imaging modality for the diagnosis of atherosclerotic coronary artery disease (CAD). Angiography has been employed to triage patients to a range of medical and revascularization therapies. At the same time, it has become apparent that conventional angiographic techniques are limited in their ability to evaluate atherosclerotic plaque. This has prompted the search to develop new imaging modalities to more extensively visualize atherosclerosis in order to gain further insight into the mechanisms driving the disease process and to facilitate the therapeutic approach to the patient with CAD. Intravascular ultrasound (IVUS) has emerged as a sensitive tool for the evaluation of the natural history of atherosclerosis.

Role of Angiography in the Evaluation of Atherosclerosis

A number of important observations suggest that angiography is limited in its ability to characterize atherosclerosis. While early studies demonstrated a relationship between the number of vessels diseased on angiography and clinical outcome, more recent data suggest that the angiographic severity of a lesion is a poor predictor of its propensity to cause clinical events.[1–3] Several groups have reported that culprit lesions are often mild-to-moderately stenotic in patients undergoing angiography during hospitalization for an acute myocardial infarction.[12] These observations have stimulated the concept of the importance of plaque composition, rather than its extent, in determining the likelihood of acute ischemic syndromes. In addition, while studies employing serial quantitative coronary angiography have demonstrated a beneficial impact of medical therapies on the rate of progression of obstructive disease, the degree of benefit appeared to be of a much smaller magnitude than the effect of these therapies on clinical events. These observations highlight the potential discord between studying the luminal stenoses and making conclusions about atherosclerosis.

Angiography provides a two-dimensional silhouette of the arterial lumen. It does not visualize the vessel wall, in which plaque accumulates. As a result, angiography does not image atherosclerotic plaque. This has important implications for the precise quantitation of the extent of atherosclerosis within the coronary arteries. Quantitative angiography compares the lumen diameter at the site of a lesion with a segment of artery that is presumed to be free of disease. Given that atherosclerosis is a diffuse process, this approach is limited by the likelihood that the "reference" segment is not normal. This is supported by the finding of necropsy studies that angiography underestimates the extent of atherosclerosis.[4–6]

Angiographic analysis is confounded by arterial remodeling. In the presence of early plaque accumulation, the external elastic membrane (EEM) typically expands, with relative preservation of the luminal diameter.[7] Contraction of the lumen does not typically occur until later stages of atherosclerosis. As a result, angiographic abnormalities may not appear until a substantial amount of atheroma is present within the artery wall. This is supported by the observation from imaging modalities that visualize the entire vessel that substantial plaque is often present in segments that appear normal or minimally diseased on angiography.[8] As a result, there is a need to develop imaging modalities that visualize the artery wall to gain a greater insight into the natural history of atherosclerosis and its regulation.

Intravascular Ultrasound

Technological advances in ultrasound technology permit the placement of transducers within the coronary arteries. The ability to place high-frequency ultrasound transducers (20–50 MHz) in close proximity to the endothelial surface generates high-resolution (axially 80 mm, laterally 200 mm) tomographic cross-sectional images of the entire artery wall (Fig. 9.1). Transducer

O. Ukimura and I.S. Gill (eds.), *Contemporary Interventional Ultrasonography in Urology,*
DOI: 10.1007/978-1-84800-217-3_9,

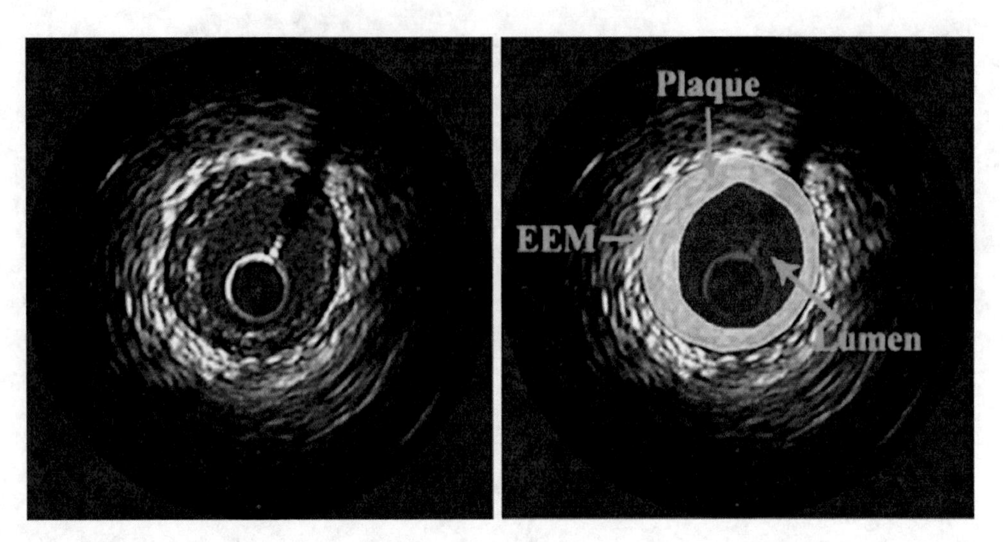

FIG. 9.1. IVUS Image: An intravascular ultrasound image demonstrating the external elastic membrane (EEM), plaque, and lumen areas

systems incorporate mechanically rotated devices or electronically switched multielement electronic arrays. Mechanical systems employ a single piezoelectric transducer, rotated at 1,800 rpm, generating 30 images per second. Electronic systems employ up to 64 transducer elements, organized in an annular array, which are sequentially activated to generate images. Mechanical rotation systems are preferred due to superior image quality.

Ultrasonic imaging is performed following anticoagulation and administration of nitroglycerin. For adjunctive use during percutaneous coronary interventions, the catheter tip is advanced beyond the segment of interest. In the setting of clinical trials that assess the natural history of atherosclerosis, the catheter is typically placed as distally as possible in the longest and least angulated epicardial artery. The catheter is subsequently withdrawn through the coronary artery either manually or at a constant speed (0.5 mm s^{-1}) using a motorized pullback device.

The requirement for invasive cardiac catheterization limits the application of IVUS to the setting of percutaneous coronary interventions or evaluation of the patient undergoing a clinically indicated angiogram. Despite this, several studies have documented that IVUS can be performed safely, with reported complications varying from 1 to 3%.[9–11] The most commonly cited adverse reaction is transient, focal coronary spasm, which responds rapidly to administration of intracoronary nitroglycerin. Serious complications, including dissection and vessel closure, are rare (less than 0.5%), typically occurring during coronary intervention rather than diagnostic imaging. Sequential IVUS imaging has not been shown to accelerate vasculopathy in both transplant and nontransplant patients.[11,12]

Evaluation of Atherosclerosis by Intravascular Ultrasound

The ability to visualize the entire vessel wall permits the opportunity to detect the full extent of atherosclerosis within an imaged arterial segment. Invasive ultrasonic imaging has provided a number of important insights into the natural history of coronary atherosclerosis. Coronary ultrasound reveals more extensive and diffuse atherosclerosis than suggested by angiography. It also highlights that atherosclerosis is typically present much earlier than previously thought. In a study of 262 heart transplant recipients, shortly following their operation, macroscopic atheroma was detected in the coronary arteries of one in six teenage, apparently healthy, donors.[13] The prevalence of coronary plaque rises exponentially with age. This dispels the myth that atherosclerosis is a disease which commences in middle age.

IVUS has been extensively employed to characterize the in vivo remodeling response of the arterial wall in response to plaque accumulation. The typical expansive pattern of remodeling in early atherosclerosis, initially described on the basis of necropsy specimens, has been confirmed by ultrasonic imaging.[14] Further studies provided important insights into the interaction between atherosclerosis, remodeling, and the clinical expression of disease.[15] In particular, culprit lesions in the setting of acute ischemic syndromes are more likely to be associated with expansive remodeling. In contrast, patients with more stable, exercise-related symptoms are more likely to have culprit lesions with constrictive remodeling, promoting lumen contraction and obstruction. These findings are consistent with the observation that expansive remodeling is associated with higher systemic levels of matrix metalloproteinases, factors involved in fibrous cap rupture, the pathological stimulus of acute ischemic syndromes.[16]

IVUS has been employed to characterize the morphology of culprit lesions in the setting of acute coronary syndromes. Echolucent, lipid-rich plaques with evidence of rupture (Fig. 9.2) and luminal thrombus can be identified in the setting of unstable clinical syndromes.[17] Investigations in patients with unstable angina reveal the presence of multiple ruptured plaques, throughout the coronary tree.[18] This is consistent with the concept that acute ischemic syndromes are triggered by systemic inflammatory factors.

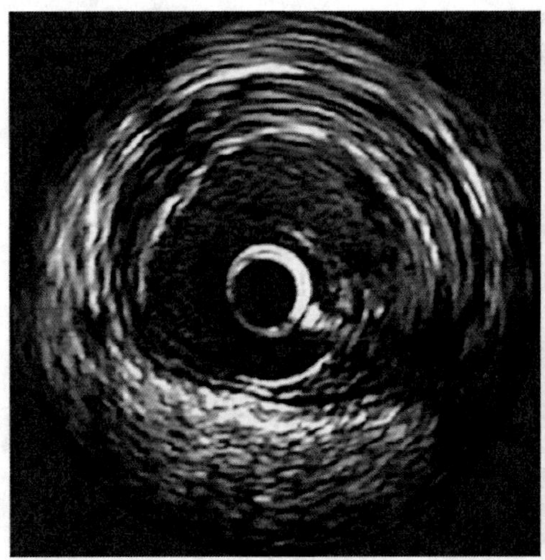

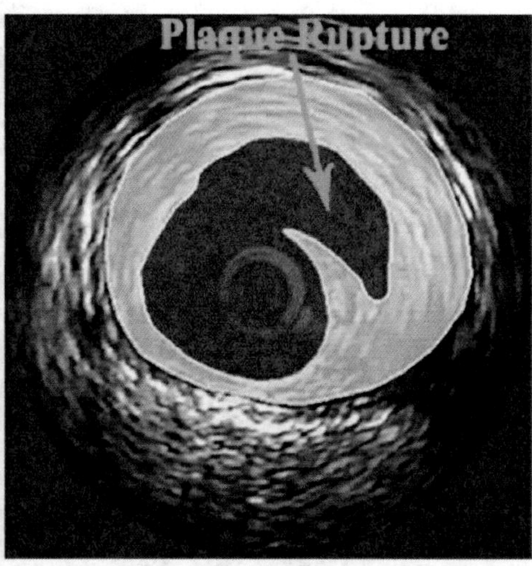

Fig. 9.2. Plaque Rupture: The site of plaque rupture can be identified in an IVUS image as a blood-filled recess in the plaque beginning at the luminal-intimal border

IVUS provides an important role in the diagnostic assessment of lesions which cannot be accurately evaluated by angiography.[8] Overlapping contrast-filled structures on angiography may obscure ostial and bifurcation lesions. IVUS has been employed in the catheterization laboratory to characterize these segments and other indistinct lesions, including those at sites of aneurysms, focal spasm, and angiographic haziness.[8,19] The left main coronary artery can be a challenge to accurately assess angiographically, as a result of its short length, aortic cusp opacification obscuring the ostium, and concealment of the distal part by bifurcation or trifurcation branches.[20] Slow withdrawal of the ultrasound catheter into the aorta, with the guiding catheter disengaged from the left main ostium, facilitates accurate characterization of the left main coronary artery.[21,22]

IVUS has also been employed to investigate the natural history of other pathological processes within the coronary arteries. The development of vasculopathy as result of neointimal hyperplasia is the leading cause of poor clinical outcome following heart transplantation. Given that the transplanted heart is denervated and patients tend to be asymptomatic until late stages, surveillance for development of vasculopathy in recipients is imperative. IVUS is the most sensitive modality for the detection and quantitation of the extent of vasculopathy in transplant patients.[23] As a result, IVUS has been incorporated into clinical surveillance strategies of heart transplant recipients in many large centers.

Utility of Intravascular Ultrasound in Interventional Cardiology

IVUS has been used extensively in the setting of percutaneous coronary interventions. Ultrasonic imaging has characterized that restenosis following interventions results from a combination of arterial recoil, remodeling, and neointimal hyperplasia.[8] IVUS has provided an important tool for the guidance of coronary interventions and to evaluate the efficacy of new devices. Lesions of intermediate stenosis are often difficult to evaluate using angiography. Assessment is also difficult in the setting of atypical symptoms, vessel tortuosity, plaque eccentricity, and severe calcification. IVUS facilitates the decision whether to proceed with revascularization in such patients. Correlation with functional studies, such as fractional flow reserve, has provided guidelines from IVUS measurements, to identify hemodynamically significant lesions.[24] The presence of a minimum lumen cross-sectional area of at least 4.0 mm^2 typically suggests that the lesion can be medically managed.[25,26] Additional criteria, including the presence of a percent cross-sectional area stenosis greater than 70%, provide increasing support for the need for intervention in the setting of a minimum lumen area between 3.0 and 4.0 mm^2.[24,25]

Adjunctive imaging with IVUS guides the appropriate choice of intervention required for management of a specific lesion. The choice of intervention is often dependent on the extent and distribution of plaque, extent of calcification, and the presence of thrombi or dissections. Ultrasonic imaging provides valuable information for the treatment of ostial lesions and coronary artery dissections, which are not sufficiently discernable on angiography. Accurate imaging of the full longitudinal extent of a lesion reduces the requirement to deploy multiple stents to achieve adequate lesion coverage.

Directional coronary atherectomy (DCA) employs a mechanically driven cutter to shave off plaque. IVUS identifies specific lesions, which are suitable for this approach. As calcification impedes tissue removal by DCA, and its detection by ultrasonic imaging minimizes the chance of procedural failure. Calcified lesions are more amenable to high-speed rotational atherectomy, in which a rotating burr debulks plaque. IVUS imaging has demonstrated that rotablation selectively removes less compliant plaque material.[27]

Advances in stent technology have revolutionized the interventional approach to coronary lesions. Early stents were complicated by significant rates of acute thrombosis, requiring the use of

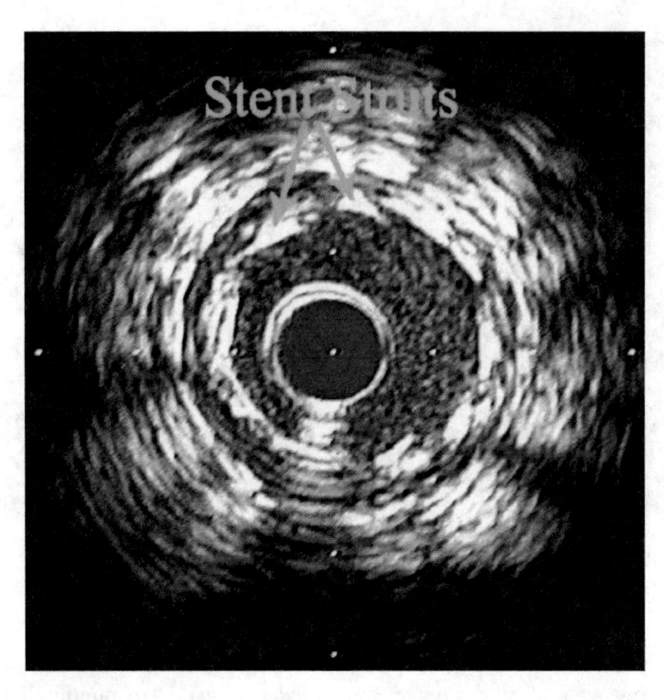

FIG. 9.3. Stent: An IVUS image demonstrating an implanted stent

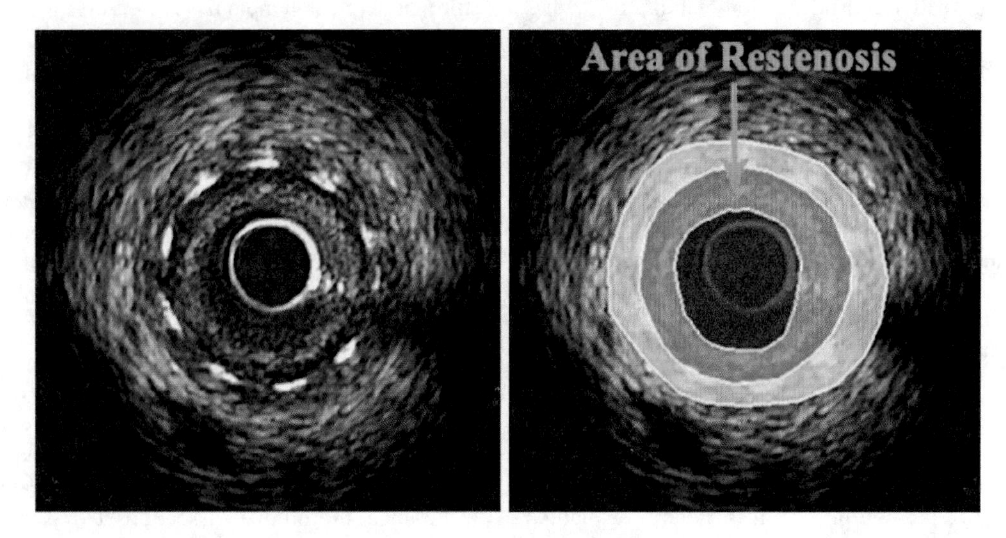

FIG. 9.4. Restenosis: In-stent restenosis is characterized by the proliferation of neointimal tissue inside the stent struts, as demonstrated in this IVUS image

intensive anticoagulation. Seminal IVUS observations demonstrated that low-pressure stent deployment resulted in inadequate stent expansion and apposition of the struts to the vessel wall, both factors increasing the risk of acute thrombosis.[28] Subsequent studies revealed that high inflation pressures could be applied in a safe manner without the use of ultrasound, promoting acceptable stent expansion and strut apposition[29,30] (Fig. 9.3). This practice was associated with lowering the risk of thrombosis and the need for intense anticoagulation, improving clinical outcomes. As IVUS demonstrated that high inflation pressures could be safely employed for stent deployment, the routine use of ultrasonic guidance in the majority of interventional procedures was no longer required.

Neointimal proliferation within stents promotes late lumen loss and restenosis (Fig. 9.4). The detection of inadequate stent expansion on ultrasound has been reported to predict subsequent restenosis.[31] IVUS imaging has provided important insights into the development of neointimal proliferation within stents and has guided the development of strategies to prevent its formation. Coronary ultrasound demonstrated that application of intracoronary radiation had a profound inhibitory effect on the development of neointimal proliferation.[8] IVUS studies assisted in the definition of optimal radiation dose and location of delivery to result in the most effective prevention of restenosis.

The development of drug-eluting stents, coated with antiproliferative and immunosuppressive agents, has had a substantial impact on restenosis rates. Their widespread use has limited the role of radiation therapy to a small number of resistant cases. Clinical trials comparing the efficacy of various drug-eluting stents have employed IVUS to monitor for the incidence and extent of structural change within the stented region.[32] However, increasing use has highlighted a significant association between stent underexpansion and subsequent thrombosis within these devices.[33] The ability of guidance with IVUS has the potential to enable the use of larger diameter stents and higher inflation pressures. In fact, achieving a postprocedure minimum lumen area of 5.0 mm^2 is the most significant predictor of a decreased prospective incidence of developing angiographic restenosis, in patients receiving sirolimus-coated stents.[34] While IVUS helped define the optimal use of a series of interventional approaches, it is likely that with ongoing problems of restenosis and thrombosis within stents that they are likely to be used in an increasing manner, in order to achieve more effective management of symptomatic lesions.

Evaluating the Impact of Medical Therapies on Plaque Progression

Visualization of the entire artery wall thickness permits accurate quantitation of atheroma burden. The leading edges of the lumen and EEM can be defined by manual planimetry or automatic edge detection software packages (Fig. 9.1), in accordance with consensus guidelines for acquisition and analysis of IVUS images by the American College of Cardiology and European Society of Cardiology.[35] Given that the medial layer of the artery wall has a negligible thickness (less than 500 μm) the area between these leading edges is conventionally regarded to be atherosclerotic plaque.

$$\text{Plaque area} = \text{EEM area} - \text{Lumen area}$$

The ability to continuously acquire images during catheter withdrawal generates a series of consecutive cross-sectional images. A pullback rate of 0.5 mm s^{-1} results in a spatial separation of 1 mm between every 60th. Summation of plaque areas in images spaced 1-mm apart permits calculation of the total atheroma volume (Fig. 9.5).

$$\text{Total Atheroma Volume}\,(mm^3) = \sum(\text{EEM}_{\text{area}} - \text{Lumen}_{\text{area}})$$

The ability to evaluate the same arterial segment at different time points provides an important opportunity to evaluate factors that influence the natural history of plaque progression. Given that atherosclerosis is a systemic and not focal process, determination of atheroma volume provides a significant advantage compared with investigations at a single site. This is further supported by the difficulty in precisely matching a single site at two different time points. In contrast, segments that are defined by the fixed, anatomic location of arterial side branches can be precisely matched, allowing for accurate comparisons (Figs. 9.6 and 9.7).

Differences in the length of segment evaluated in subjects participating in clinical trials will have a profound impact on

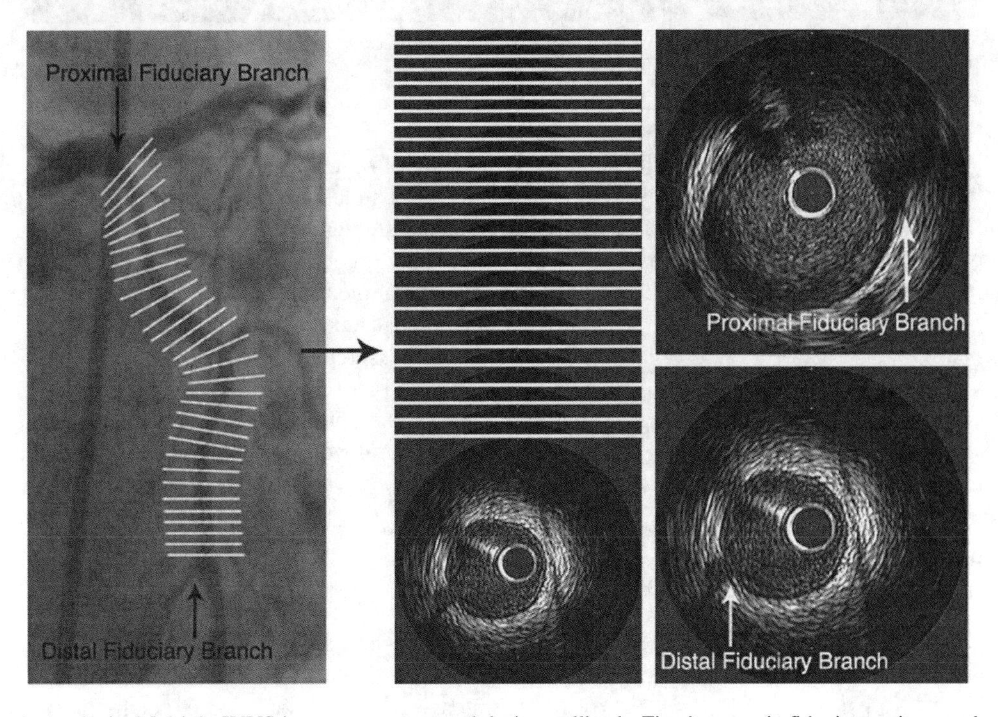

FIG. 9.5. Volumetric Analysis: Multiple IVUS images are generated during pullback. Fixed anatomic fiduciary points, such as side branches, define the segment of interest. Volumetric extent of atheroma (and other measures) can then be calculated by summating plaque areas in equally spaced individual images within the segment of interest. The fiduciary points, as seen in the IVUS pullback images, are shown on the right

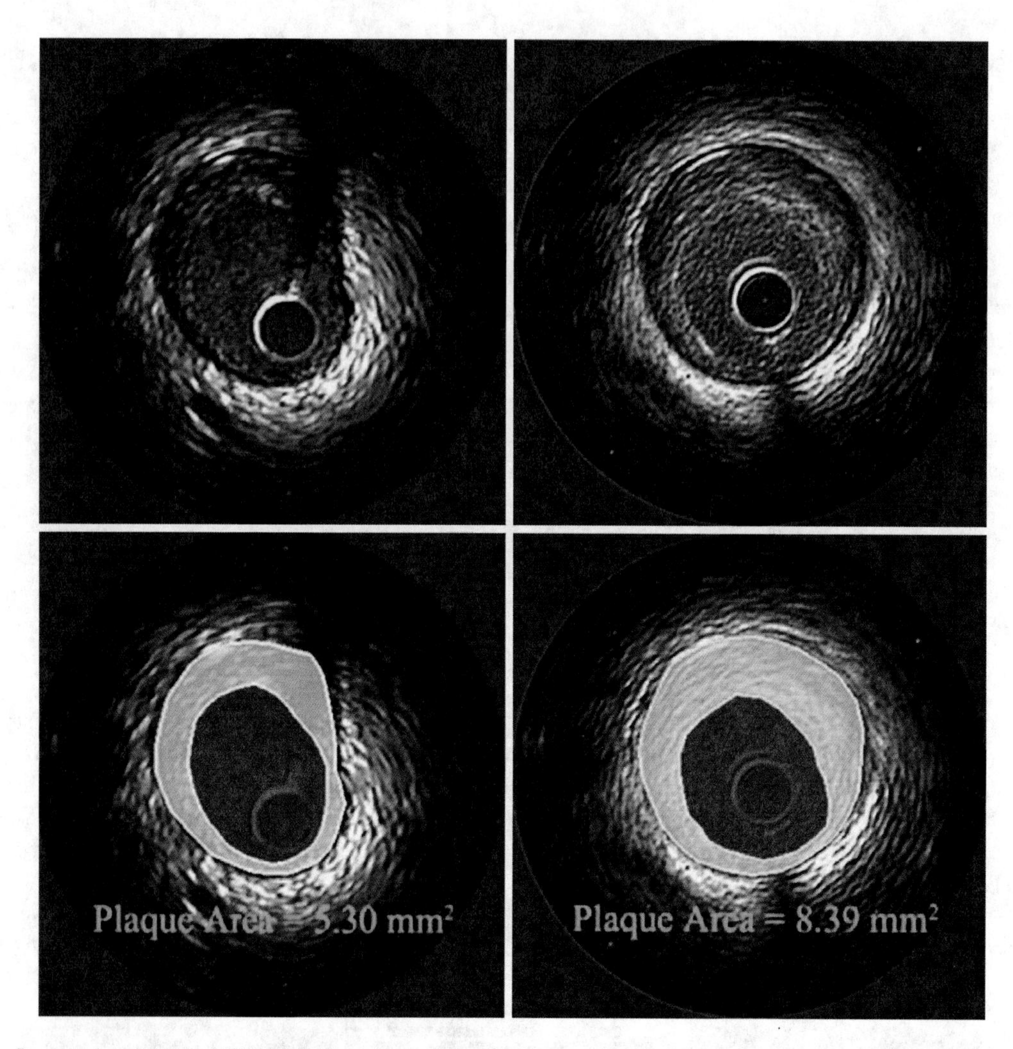

FIG. 9.6. Plaque Progression: Matched IVUS images demonstrating an increase in plaque area from baseline (*left*) to follow-up (*right*)

the calculated atheroma volume. To control for the heterogeneity in segment length, atheroma volume is adjusted, or normalized, by multiplication of the mean plaque area within a segment by the median number of evaluable images for the entire study cohort.

$$\text{Normalized TAV}(\text{mm}^3) = \frac{\sum(\text{EEM}_{\text{area}} - \text{Lumen}_{\text{area}})}{\text{Number of Frames per Patient}} \times \text{Median Number Frames for all Patients}$$

The extent of atherosclerosis can also be calculated as the percent atheroma volume (PAV), which defines the amount of atheroma as a proportion of the volume occupied by the entire arterial wall.

$$\text{Percent Atheroma Volume} = \frac{\sum(\text{EEM}_{\text{area}} - \text{Lumen}_{\text{area}})}{\sum \text{EEM}_{\text{area}}} \times 100$$

The lower variability in PAV measurements permits the use of smaller sample sizes and has become the primary end point in many studies that assess the impact of medical therapies on plaque progression. A number of additional measures are obtained at the time of analysis. These include maximum and minimum plaque thickness and the degree of plaque calcification. Serial measurements of each of these parameters have been performed in a number of studies that evaluate the impact of medical therapies that target established atherosclerotic risk factors and novel pathologic targets within the artery wall.

Lowering Low-Density Lipoprotein Cholesterol

While lowering levels of low-density lipoprotein cholesterol (LDL-C) with statins reduces event rates in placebo-controlled trials,[36–38] their optimal use in clinical practice remains uncertain. In particular, considerable debate has focused on whether intensive lowering of LDL-C results in incremental benefit. The Reversal of Atherosclerosis with Aggressive Lipid Lowering (REVERSAL)[39] trial compared the effects of a

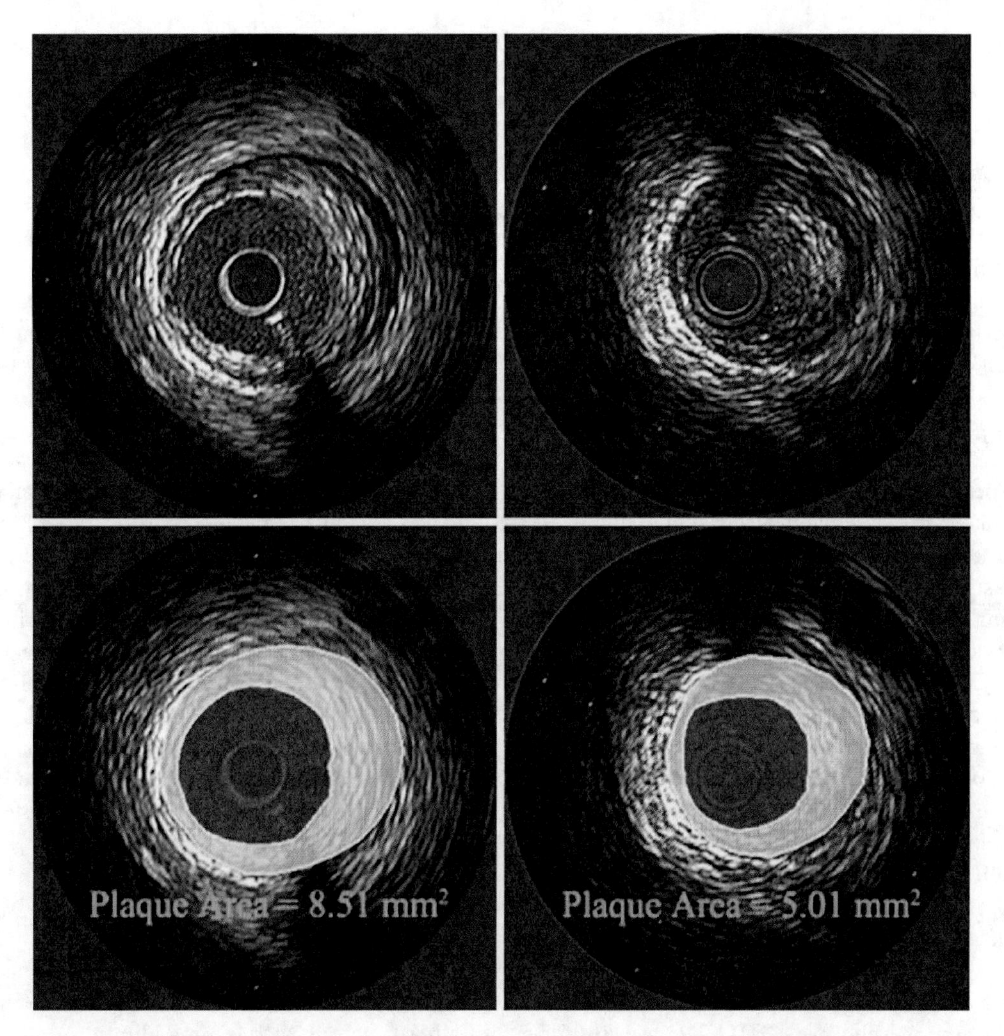

FIG. 9.7. Regression: Matched IVUS images demonstrating a decrease in plaque area from baseline (*left*) to follow-up (*right*)

moderate (pravastatin 40 mg) and intensive lipid-lowering (atorvastatin 80 mg) strategy in 502 patients with angiographic CAD and LDL-C between 125 and 210 mg dL^{-1}. The mean LDL-C levels were reduced to 110 and 79 mg dL^{-1} in the pravastatin- and atorvastatin-treated groups, respectively. After 18 months of therapy, serial IVUS measurements demonstrated no significant change in atheroma volume (−0.4%) compared with baseline in atorvastatin-treated patients, while there was evidence of disease progression in the pravastatin group (+2.7% change in total atheroma volume). The direct relationship between LDL-C lowering and rate of plaque progression suggested that intensively lowering levels of LDL-C could halt the natural history of atheroma progression.

Subsequent analysis revealed that pravastatin-treated patients required an additional 30 mg dL^{-1} lowering of LDL-C to achieve the same impact on plaque progression. This suggested that factors, in addition to differences in LDL-C lowering, contributed to the observed benefit of high-dose atorvastatin. The finding of greater reductions in levels of the inflammatory marker C-reactive protein (CRP) with atorvastatin and a direct relationship between changes in CRP and atheroma volume suggest that anti-inflammatory properties of statins may contribute to their benefit.[40] These findings correlate well with the results of the Pravastatin or Atorvastatin Evaluation and Infection Therapy-Thrombolysis in Myocardial Infarction 22 (PROVE-IT) study,[41] which demonstrated a beneficial impact of atorvastatin 80 mg compared to pravastatin 40 mg on clinical events in patients with acute coronary syndromes. Furthermore, it was reported that patients who achieved the greatest lowering of both LDL-C and CRP demonstrated the lowest number of clinical events and rate of plaque progression. The National Cholesterol Education Program subsequently included an optional treatment goal of 70 mg dL^{-1} for management of high-risk patients.

A Study to Evaluate the Effect of Rosuvastatin on Intravascular Ultrasound-Derived Coronary Atheroma Burden (ASTEROID)[42] investigated the impact of lowering LDL-C to very low levels. 349 patients with angiographic CAD were treated with rosuvastatin 40 mg for 24 months, resulting in lowering of LDL-C by 53.2% to 60.8 mg dL^{-1} and raising high-density lipoprotein cholesterol (HDL-C) levels by 14.7% to 49 mg dL^{-1}. These changes were associated with significant reductions in all measures of atheroma burden, consistent with regression. Statistically significant reductions in atheroma burden were only observed in patients who achieved LDL-C levels less than 70 mg dL^{-1}. This result supported the concept that lowering LDL-C levels to very low levels with statin monotherapy could reverse plaque accumulation within the coronary arteries. These findings also support early reports of regression in response to statin therapy in small cohorts of subjects.

Promoting the Biological Activity of HDL

The protective role of HDL in atherosclerosis has been consistently demonstrated in epidemiological and animal studies.[43–45] The finding that current therapies raise HDL-C levels by modest degrees has stimulated the search to develop new strategies to promote HDL function. IVUS has recently been employed in clinical trials that have evaluated the potential efficacy of experimental agents that can be administered either by intravenous infusion or chronic oral therapy.

Carriers of the mutant apolipoprotein A-I Milano (AIM) have low levels of HDL-C, but are protected from atherosclerotic cardiovascular disease. Administration of AIM in animal models has a substantial impact on atherosclerotic lesion formation. A small clinical trial was subsequently performed to assess the impact of infusing AIM in humans.[46] 47 patients, within 2 weeks of an acute coronary syndrome, received weekly intravenous infusions of saline or low (15 mg kg^{-1}) or high (45 mg kg^{-1}) doses of reconstituted HDL particles containing AIM and phospholipids (ETC-216) weekly for 5 weeks. IVUS performed within 2 weeks of the final infusion revealed regression of coronary atherosclerosis in patients receiving either dose of ETC-216. The rapid regression observed is consistent with the observation that lipid-depleted forms of HDL are efficient promoters of cholesterol efflux. The recent report from the Effect of rHDL on Atherosclerosis – Safety and Efficacy (ERASE) study[47] that infusing reconstituted HDL particles containing wild-type apoA-I promotes plaque regression provides further support for the concept that infusing HDL may be of clinical utility in the management of patients with acute ischemic syndromes. The impact of these therapies on clinical outcome remains to be defined in large-scale clinical trials.

While current therapies raise HDL-C levels to a modest degree, emerging evidence suggests that this can have a substantial impact on clinical outcome. In a recent pooled analysis of clinical trials that employed serial assessments by IVUS, the modest elevation of HDL-C levels was found to be an independent predictor of the impact of statin therapy on atheroma progression.[48] In fact, raising HDL-C levels by as little as 7.5%, in addition to intensive lowering of LDL-C, resulted in the greatest degree of plaque regression. This observation further supported the concept that improvements in the functional quality of HDL may be the most important target for new therapies.

Inhibiting cholesteryl ester transfer protein (CETP) has been proposed as a therapeutic strategy to raise HDL-C levels. CETP facilitates the transfer of esterified cholesterol from HDL to LDL particles. Pharmacological inhibitors of CETP have been demonstrated to inhibit lesion formation in animal models and to raise HDL-C levels by greater than 50% in humans.[49] Serial IVUS recently evaluated the impact of CETP inhibition in humans. The Investigation of Lipid Level Management Using Coronary Ultrasound to Assess Reduction of Atherosclerosis by CETP Inhibition and HDL Elevation (ILLUSTRATE) study[50] randomized 910 patients with CAD to treatment with either atorvastatin as monotherapy or in combination with 60 mg of torcetrapib daily for 24 months. Atorvastatin was administered at a dose to achieve a LDL-C level less than 100 mg dL^{-1}. Addition of torcetrapib resulted in a 61% increase in HDL-C and 20% decrease in LDL-C. Despite the remarkable effect on plasma lipids, torcetrapib had no effect on the change in PAV. It remains to be determined whether the lack of benefit was due to the formation of dysfunctional forms of HDL, the ability of torcetrapib to raise blood pressure, or some unknown vascular toxicity of the compound. The finding that torcetrapib does not slow progression of coronary atherosclerosis or carotid intimal-medial thickness is consistent with its lack of efficacy in a large clinical trial.[50]

Inhibition of Cholesterol Esterification

Uptake of cholesterol ester by macrophages is the pivotal event in the formation of foam cells, the cellular hallmark of atherosclerotic plaque. In addition to lowering systemic levels of LDL-C, it has been proposed that inhibition of cholesterol esterification may be a therapeutic strategy of potential utility in cardiovascular prevention. Serial IVUS has demonstrated that two pharmacological inhibitors of acyl-coenzyme A:cholesterol acyltransferase (ACAT), a pivotal factor in promoting cholesterol esterification, do not have a beneficial impact on atheroma progression. The Avasimibe and Progression of Lesions on Ultrasound (A-PLUS) study[51] evaluated the impact of the ACAT inhibitor avasimibe compared to placebo on the rate of plaque progression. No significant difference was observed between the treatment groups with regard to the change in atheroma volume. LDL-C levels were higher in avasimibe-treated patients, consistent with its ability to induce cytochrome P450 3A4 and statin metabolism.

The ACAT Intravascular Atherosclerosis Treatment Evaluation (ACTIVATE)[52] study compared the effect of pactimibe, an ACAT inhibitor with no influence on statin metabolism, and placebo on the serial change in atheroma burden after 18 months of treatment. The groups did not differ with regard to the primary end point, the change in PAV. However, greater reductions in atheroma volume throughout the entire segment evaluated and the most diseased 10-mm segment were observed in placebo-treated patients. This suggested that pactimibe may have a detrimental influence on plaque progression. Accumulation of cytotoxic, intracellular-free cholesterol has been proposed as a potential mechanism that may contribute to the detrimental effects of pactimibe on plaque accumulation.[53,54]

Blood Pressure-Lowering Therapies

While the role of hypertension in promoting cardiovascular disease is well established, the optimal management of blood pressure in patients with CAD is controversial. Epidemiological observations suggest that cardiovascular risk begins to increase at levels of systolic blood pressure considered to be within the normal range.[55,56] In the Comparison of Amlodipine versus Enalapril to Limit Occurrences of Thrombosis (CAMELOT)[57] trial, 1991 patients with angiographically documented CAD and diastolic blood pressure less than 100 mm Hg were treated with amlodipine 10 mg daily, enalapril 20 mg daily, or placebo for 24 months. Treatment with amlodipine significantly reduced a combination of cardiovascular clinical events. In a unique study design, 274 patients also underwent serial evaluation of atheroma burden by IVUS. This revealed progression in placebo-treated patients, a trend toward progression with enalapril and no change in atheroma volume with amlodipine. In particular, the findings on imaging complemented the impact of therapy on clinical events. A direct relationship was observed between blood pressure reduction and change in atheroma volume. These findings suggest that blood pressure should be more intensively lowered in patients with CAD.

Monitoring the Impact of Therapies on Transplant Vasculopathy

The use of ultrasonic imaging within the coronary arteries has been employed to evaluate the impact of medical therapies aimed at preventing formation and propagation of transplant vasculopathy. Emerging evidence of the inflammatory events promoting formation of neointimal hyperplasia in the coronary arteries following heart transplantation has stimulated the search to develop immunomodulatory therapies. Serial IVUS monitored the impact of the immunomodulatory and antiproliferative agent, everolimus, in heart transplant recipients.[58] Treatment with everolimus reduced the incidence and progression of vasculopathy compared with standard medical therapy with azathioprine. This beneficial impact on the coronary arterial wall was associated with a reduction in the incidence of clinical events including death, rejection and retransplantation.

Limitations of Intravascular Ultrasound

The invasive nature of IVUS limits its application to patients who require a coronary angiogram for clinical indications. It precludes the opportunity to study the natural history of atherosclerosis in patients without clinical symptoms and to directly translate the impact of medical therapies to the setting of primary prevention. The emerging ability of computed tomography and magnetic resonance imaging to image the artery wall may provide a potential option to study the natural history of atherosclerosis in a noninvasive fashion. As imaging is typically performed within one coronary artery, it is uncertain whether the impact of medical therapies in regression-progression studies is homogenous throughout the coronary arterial tree.

The quality of information obtained is critically dependent on the ability to generate high-resolution images of the vessel wall. Limitations in catheter size preclude ultrasonic imaging in small vessels and at sites of severe luminal stenosis. A number of imaging artifacts impair the ability to directly visualize the entire artery wall. Imaging artifacts are commonly due to the presence of the guidewire, arterial side branches, calcium, bright haloes surrounding the imaging catheter, geometric distortion due to imaging in an oblique plane, and nonuniform rotational distortion due to uneven drag on the catheter resulting in cyclical oscillations and image distortion. Technological advances in catheter profile and ultrasound frequency have made substantial improvements in the ability to consistently acquire high-resolution imaging within the coronary arteries.

IVUS provides a suboptimal characterization of plaque composition to evaluate the natural history of atherosclerosis. The broad distinction between lipidic, fibrotic, and calficic plaque lacks the precision required to assess serial changes in plaque components in response to use of medical therapies. Technological developments permit analysis of the radiofrequency backscatter, providing a tissue map with good correlation with plaque composition on histology. Preliminary studies using this approach have suggested that lowering levels of LDL-C with statins reduces the lipidic and increases the fibrotic components of atherosclerotic plaque.[59]

Another major challenge for clinical trials that employ imaging modalities as surrogate markers of atherosclerosis is to define the relationship between the impact of therapies on the artery wall and clinical outcome. A number of observations suggest complementary effects of interventions on clinical events and the rate of atheroma progression. However, further evidence is required to directly associate atheroma burden and its change with clinical outcome.

Overview

The evolution of IVUS provides the opportunity to directly visualize the arterial wall with high-resolution imaging. This has permitted a greater understanding of the factors influencing the natural history of atherosclerosis and other vasculopathies within the coronary arteries. Its use has played a pivotal role in the development and validation of new medical and interventional approaches to the management of patients with CAD.

References

1. Falk E, Fuster V. Angina pectoris and disease progression. Circulation 1995;92(8):2033–5.
2. Falk E, Shah PK, Fuster V. Coronary plaque disruption. Circulation 1995;92(3):657–71.
3. Topol EJ, Nissen SE. Our preoccupation with coronary luminology. The dissociation between clinical and angiographic findings in ischemic heart disease. Circulation 1995;92(8):2333–42.
4. Grondin CM, Dyrda I, Pasternac A, Campeau L, Bourassa MG, Lesperance J. Discrepancies between cineangiographic and postmortem findings in patients with coronary artery disease and recent myocardial revascularization. Circulation 1974;49(4):703–8.
5. Vlodaver Z, Frech R, Van Tassel RA, Edwards JE. Correlation of the antemortem coronary arteriogram and the postmortem specimen. Circulation 1973;47(1):162–9.
6. Roberts WC, Jones AA. Quantitation of coronary arterial narrowing at necropsy in sudden coronary death: analysis of 31 patients and comparison with 25 control subjects. Am J Cardiol 1979;44(1):39–45.
7. Glagov S, Weisenberg E, Zarins CK, Stankunavicius R, Kolettis GJ. Compensatory enlargement of human atherosclerotic coronary arteries. N Engl J Med 1987;316(22):1371–5.
8. Nissen SE, Yock P. Intravascular ultrasound: novel pathophysiological insights and current clinical applications. Circulation 2001;103(4):604–16.
9. Hausmann D, Erbel R, Alibelli-Chemarin MJ, et al. The safety of intracoronary ultrasound. A multicenter survey of 2207 examinations. Circulation 1995;91(3):623–30.
10. Batkoff BW, Linker DT. Safety of intracoronary ultrasound: data from a Multicenter European Registry. Cathet Cardiovasc Diagn 1996;38(3):238–41.
11. Guedes A, Keller PF, L'Allier PL, Lesperance J, Gregoire J, Tardif JC. Long-term safety of intravascular ultrasound in nontransplant, nonintervened, atherosclerotic coronary arteries. J Am Coll Cardiol 2005;45(4):559–64.
12. Ramasubbu K, Schoenhagen P, Balghith MA, et al. Repeated intravascular ultrasound imaging in cardiac transplant recipients does not accelerate transplant coronary artery disease. J Am Coll Cardiol 2003;41(10):1739–43.
13. Tuzcu EM, Kapadia SR, Tutar E, et al. High prevalence of coronary atherosclerosis in asymptomatic teenagers and young adults: evidence from intravascular ultrasound. Circulation 2001;103(22):2705–10.
14. Hermiller JB, Tenaglia AN, Kisslo KB, et al. In vivo validation of compensatory enlargement of atherosclerotic coronary arteries. Am J Cardiol 1993;71(8):665–8.
15. Schoenhagen P, Ziada KM, Kapadia SR, Crowe TD, Nissen SE, Tuzcu EM. Extent and direction of arterial remodeling in stable versus unstable coronary syndromes: an intravascular ultrasound study. Circulation 2000;101(6):598–603.
16. Schoenhagen P, Vince DG, Ziada KM, et al. Relation of matrix-metalloproteinase 3 found in coronary lesion samples retrieved by directional coronary atherectomy to intravascular ultrasound observations on coronary remodeling. Am J Cardiol 2002;89(12):1354–9.
17. Hodgson JM, Reddy KG, Suneja R, Nair RN, Lesnefsky EJ, Sheehan HM. Intracoronary ultrasound imaging: correlation of plaque morphology with angiography, clinical syndrome and procedural results in patients undergoing coronary angioplasty. J Am Coll Cardiol 1993;21(1):35–44.
18. Schoenhagen P, Stone GW, Nissen SE, et al. Coronary plaque morphology and frequency of ulceration distant from culprit lesions in patients with unstable and stable presentation. Arterioscler Thromb Vasc Biol 2003;23(10):1895–900.
19. Ziada KM, Tuzcu EM, De Franco AC, et al. Intravascular ultrasound assessment of the prevalence and causes of angiographic "haziness" following high-pressure coronary stenting. Am J Cardiol 1997;80(2):116–21.
20. Isner JM, Kishel J, Kent KM, Ronan JA, Jr., Ross AM, Roberts WC. Accuracy of angiographic determination of left main coronary arterial narrowing. Angiographic – histologic correlative analysis in 28 patients. Circulation 1981;63(5):1056–64.
21. Hermiller JB, Buller CE, Tenaglia AN, et al. Unrecognized left main coronary artery disease in patients undergoing interventional procedures. Am J Cardiol 1993;71(2):173–6.
22. Iyisoy A, Ziada K, Schoenhagen P, et al. Intravascular ultrasound evidence of ostial narrowing in nonatherosclerotic left main coronary arteries. Am J Cardiol 2002;90(7):773–5.
23. Pinto FJ, Chenzbraun A, Botas J, et al. Feasibility of serial intracoronary ultrasound imaging for assessment of progression of intimal proliferation in cardiac transplant recipients. Circulation 1994;90(5):2348–55.
24. Takagi A, Tsurumi Y, Ishii Y, Suzuki K, Kawana M, Kasanuki H. Clinical potential of intravascular ultrasound for physiological assessment of coronary stenosis: relationship between quantitative ultrasound tomography and pressure-derived fractional flow reserve. Circulation 1999;100(3):250–5.
25. Briguori C, Anzuini A, Airoldi F, et al. Intravascular ultrasound criteria for the assessment of the functional significance of intermediate coronary artery stenoses and comparison with fractional flow reserve. Am J Cardiol 2001;87(2):136–41.
26. Abizaid AS, Mintz GS, Mehran R, et al. Long-term follow-up after percutaneous transluminal coronary angioplasty was not performed based on intravascular ultrasound findings: importance of lumen dimensions. Circulation 1999;100(3):256–61.
27. Kovach JA, Mintz GS, Pichard AD, et al. Sequential intravascular ultrasound characterization of the mechanisms of rotational atherectomy and adjunct balloon angioplasty. J Am Coll Cardiol 1993;22(4):1024–32.
28. Colombo A, Hall P, Nakamura S, et al. Intracoronary stenting without anticoagulation accomplished with intravascular ultrasound guidance. Circulation 1995;91(6):1676–88.
29. Goods CM, Al-Shaibi KF, Yadav SS, et al. Utilization of the coronary balloon-expandable coil stent without anticoagulation or intravascular ultrasound. Circulation 1996;93(10):1803–8.
30. Karrillon GJ, Morice MC, Benveniste E, et al. Intracoronary stent implantation without ultrasound guidance and with replacement of conventional anticoagulation by antiplatelet therapy. 30-day clinical outcome of the French Multicenter Registry. Circulation 1996;94(7):1519–27.
31. Nakamura S, Colombo A, Gaglione A, et al. Intracoronary ultrasound observations during stent implantation. Circulation 1994;89(5):2026–34.
32. Moses JW, Leon MB, Popma JJ, et al. Sirolimus-eluting stents versus standard stents in patients with stenosis in a native coronary artery. N Engl J Med 2003;349(14):1315–23.
33. Fujii K, Carlier SG, Mintz GS, et al. Stent underexpansion and residual reference segment stenosis are related to stent thrombosis after sirolimus-eluting stent implantation: an intravascular ultrasound study. J Am Coll Cardiol 2005;45(7):995–8.

34. Sonoda S, Morino Y, Ako J, et al. Impact of final stent dimensions on long-term results following sirolimus-eluting stent implantation: serial intravascular ultrasound analysis from the sirius trial. J Am Coll Cardiol 2004;43(11):1959–63.
35. Mintz GS, Nissen SE, Anderson WD, et al. American College of Cardiology Clinical Expert Consensus Document on Standards for Acquisition, Measurement and Reporting of Intravascular Ultrasound Studies (IVUS). A report of the American College of Cardiology Task Force on Clinical Expert Consensus Documents. J Am Coll Cardiol 2001;37(5):1478–92.
36. Scandinavian Simvastatin Survival Study Group.Randomised trial of cholesterol lowering in 4444 patients with coronary heart disease: the Scandinavian Simvastatin Survival Study (4S). Lancet 1994;344(8934):1383–9.
37. Prevention of cardiovascular events and death with pravastatin in patients with coronary heart disease and a broad range of initial cholesterol levels. The long-term intervention with Pravastatin in Ischaemic Disease (LIPID) Study Group. N Engl J Med 1998;339(19):1349–57.
38. MRC/BHF Heart Protection Study of cholesterol lowering with simvastatin in 20,536 high-risk individuals: a randomised placebo-controlled trial. Lancet 2002;360(9326):7–22.
39. Nissen SE, Tuzcu EM, Schoenhagen P, et al. Effect of intensive compared with moderate lipid-lowering therapy on progression of coronary atherosclerosis: a randomized controlled trial. JAMA 2004;291(9):1071–80.
40. Nissen SE, Tuzcu EM, Schoenhagen P, et al. Statin therapy, LDL cholesterol, C-reactive protein, and coronary artery disease. N Engl J Med 2005;352(1):29–38.
41. Cannon CP, Braunwald E, McCabe CH, et al. Intensive versus moderate lipid lowering with statins after acute coronary syndromes. N Engl J Med 2004;350(15):1495–504.
42. Nissen SE, Nicholls SJ, Sipahi I, et al. Effect of very high-intensity statin therapy on regression of coronary atherosclerosis: the ASTEROID trial. JAMA 2006;295(13):1556–65.
43. Gordon T, Castelli WP, Hjortland MC, Kannel WB, Dawber TR. High density lipoprotein as a protective factor against coronary heart disease. The Framingham Study. Am J Med 1977;62(5):707–14.
44. Badimon JJ, Badimon L, Fuster V. Regression of atherosclerotic lesions by high density lipoprotein plasma fraction in the cholesterol-fed rabbit. J Clin Invest 1990;85(4):1234–41.
45. Duverger N, Kruth H, Emmanuel F, et al. Inhibition of atherosclerosis development in cholesterol-fed human apolipoprotein A-I-transgenic rabbits. Circulation 1996;94(4):713–7.
46. Nissen SE, Tsunoda T, Tuzcu EM, et al. Effect of recombinant ApoA-I Milano on coronary atherosclerosis in patients with acute coronary syndromes: a randomized controlled trial. JAMA 2003;290(17):2292–300.
47. Tardif JC, Gregoire J, L'Allier PL, et al. Effects of reconstituted high-density lipoprotein infusions on coronary atherosclerosis: a randomized controlled trial. JAMA 2007;297(15):1675–82.
48. Nicholls SJ, Tuzcu EM, Sipahi I, et al. Statins, high-density lipoprotein cholesterol, and regression of coronary atherosclerosis. JAMA 2007;297(5):499–508.
49. Brousseau ME, Schaefer EJ, Wolfe ML, et al. Effects of an inhibitor of cholesteryl ester transfer protein on HDL cholesterol. N Engl J Med 2004;350(15):1505–15.
50. Nissen SE, Tardif JC, Nicholls SJ, et al. Effect of torcetrapib on the progression of coronary atherosclerosis. N Engl J Med 2007;356(13):1304–16.
51. Tardif JC, Gregoire J, L'Allier PL, et al. Effects of the acyl coenzyme A:cholesterol acyltransferase inhibitor avasimibe on human atherosclerotic lesions. Circulation 2004;110(21):3372–7.
52. Nissen SE, Tuzcu EM, Brewer HB, et al. Effect of ACAT inhibition on the progression of coronary atherosclerosis. N Engl J Med 2006;354(12):1253–63.
53. Warner GJ, Stoudt G, Bamberger M, Johnson WJ, Rothblat GH. Cell toxicity induced by inhibition of acyl coenzyme A:cholesterol acyltransferase and accumulation of unesterified cholesterol. J Biol Chem 1995;270(11):5772–8.
54. Kellner-Weibel G, Jerome WG, Small DM, et al. Effects of intracellular free cholesterol accumulation on macrophage viability: a model for foam cell death. Arterioscler Thromb Vasc Biol 1998;18(3):423–31.
55. Vasan RS, Larson MG, Leip EP, et al. Impact of high-normal blood pressure on the risk of cardiovascular disease. N Engl J Med 2001;345(18):1291–7.
56. Borghi C, Dormi A, L'Italien G, et al. The relationship between systolic blood pressure and cardiovascular risk – results of the Brisighella Heart Study. J Clin Hypertens (Greenwich) 2003;5(1):47–52.
57. Nissen SE, Tuzcu EM, Libby P, et al. Effect of antihypertensive agents on cardiovascular events in patients with coronary disease and normal blood pressure: the CAMELOT study: a randomized controlled trial. JAMA 2004;292(18):2217–25.
58. Eisen HJ, Tuzcu EM, Dorent R, et al. Everolimus for the prevention of allograft rejection and vasculopathy in cardiac-transplant recipients. N Engl J Med 2003;349(9):847–58.
59. Kawasaki M, Sano K, Okubo M, et al. Volumetric quantitative analysis of tissue characteristics of coronary plaques after statin therapy using three-dimensional integrated backscatter intravascular ultrasound. J Am Coll Cardiol 2005;45(12):1946–53.

Chapter 10
Ultrasound Application for Penile Disorders: Color Doppler Ultrasound Hemodynamic Evaluation for Erectile Dysfunction and Priapism

Rei K. Chiou, Christopher R. Chiou, and Fleur L. Broughton

Keywords: Color Doppler sonography, Erectile dysfunction, Impotence, Priapism

Color Doppler Ultrasound Hemodynamic Study for Erectile Dysfunction

Erection is achieved through hemodynamic mechanisms that involve the increase of cavernosal arterial flow, relaxation of corporal smooth muscle, and veno-occlusive function. Hemodynamic studies are important in the evaluation of patients with impotence. Among the methods of hemodynamic study, color Doppler sonography is currently the best.

In 1985, Lue et al. described Duplex ultrasonography as a noninvasive tool to study penile hemodynamics of patients with erectile dysfunction.[1] The advent of color Doppler imaging and continuous improvements in ultrasound technology have greatly enhanced the capacity of ultrasound to assess hemodynamics. Modern ultrasound equipment is also able to analyze blood flow parameters to measure velocity more quickly and more accurately. These characteristics allow the changes in various blood flow parameters be assessed in a dynamic fashion.[2]

The reported methods of performing color Doppler sonography for erectile dysfunction (or impotence) vary. The methods of early reports mostly consist of measuring peak systolic velocity (PSV) and end diastolic velocity (EDV) at 5- or 10-min intervals. The "highest PSV" is commonly used to diagnose arterial insufficiency, and an EDV-based criterion (such as resistive index or RI) is used to diagnose venous leak. However, in our early experience we noted a number of pitfalls associated with these methods. Various diagnostic criteria have also been used; early reports recommended the degree of cavernosal artery dilatation to be a key criterion, while more recent reports commonly use "highest PSV" for arterial insufficiency and resistive index for venous leak.[1–4] Meuleman and associates studied normal volunteers and found that they had a mean PSV of 41–44 cm s^{-1} during the erectile phases.[4] A "highest PSV" of 35 cm s^{-1} was subsequently accepted as normal. In addition to these criteria, we believe that a dynamic observation and interpretation of the study is desirable. The pathophysiology of erectile dysfunction is no less complicated than that of urinary dysfunction. The hemodynamic evaluation for erectile dysfunction should be performed with the same attention to detail as urodynamic studies. We believe that a dynamic study with continuous observation and frequent recording of hemodynamic parameters is preferable.[2,5,6]

Indications

Our current indications for color Doppler ultrasound hemodynamic study in patients with erectile dysfunction are as follows:

1. Primary impotence
2. Erectile dysfunction following penile, perineal, or pelvic injuries
3. Medical legal case
4. Peyronie's disease
5. Young patients (< 50 years old) suspicious for vascular cause of impotence
6. Young patients suspicious for psychogenic cause of impotence
7. Patients or their spouse desire investigation for cause of impotence

Procedure

Our current procedure for color Doppler ultrasound hemodynamic study is as follows:

1. Studies are performed in a "do not disturb" environment with only essential personnel involved.
2. We perform an intracorporeal injection using a 0.2 c.c. Papaverine/phentolamine/PGE1 (30 mg/1 mg/20 μg) mixture (Tri-Mix) or 0.3 ml of the standard Tri-Mix for most patients. We may administer a second injection in the

O. Ukimura and I.S. Gill (eds.), *Contemporary Interventional Ultrasonography in Urology*,
DOI: 10.1007/978-1-84800-217-3_10,

opposite corpora 15–20 min later for patients with an inadequate erectile response and abnormal arterial flow of the opposite side cavernosal artery.

3. We use an ATL HDI ultrasound machine for color Doppler ultrasound studies at our Urology clinic. With the penis gently retracted toward the abdomen, the transducer is placed ventrally at the base of penis to measure blood flow parameters at a consistent proximal location. The cavernosal artery blood flow is traced continuously (switching from one side to another). The hemodynamic parameters including PSV, EDV, and RI are recorded frequently (usually every 1–3 min, depends on the change of hemodynamic parameters observed) for about 30 min. The measurement of cavernosal artery diameter before and after injection is optional.
4. The status of erection is observed and rigidity manually evaluated periodically during the study. Self-stimulation is performed if the patient does not achieve a rigid erection.

Phases of Erection and Hemodynamic Events

Cavernosal arteries at a flaccid state prior to penile injection usually have a low and intermittent flow (Fig. 10.1). After injection of pharmacologic agent, we typically observe the following five phases of hemodynamic events:

In Phase I, both systolic and diastolic flows increase and become continuous. Patients begin to have penile engorgement (Fig. 10.2).

In Phase II, with an increase in intracorporeal pressure, a progressive decrease in EDV occurs. The PSV remains high. In this phase, partial erection is achieved (Fig. 10.3).

In Phase III, when the intracorporeal pressure increases to near systemic diastolic blood pressure, the EDV reaches 0 and the PSV remains high. Patients usually have a full erection with modest rigidity at this phase (Fig. 10.4).

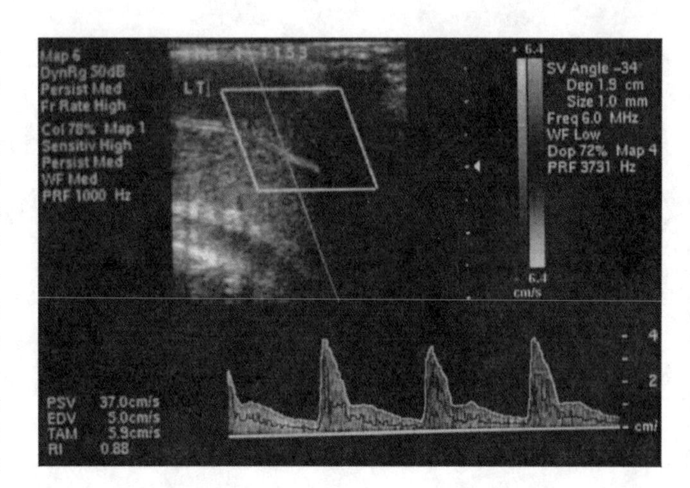

Fig. 10.2. In Phase I of pharmacologic erection, both systolic and diastolic flows increase and become a continuous flow

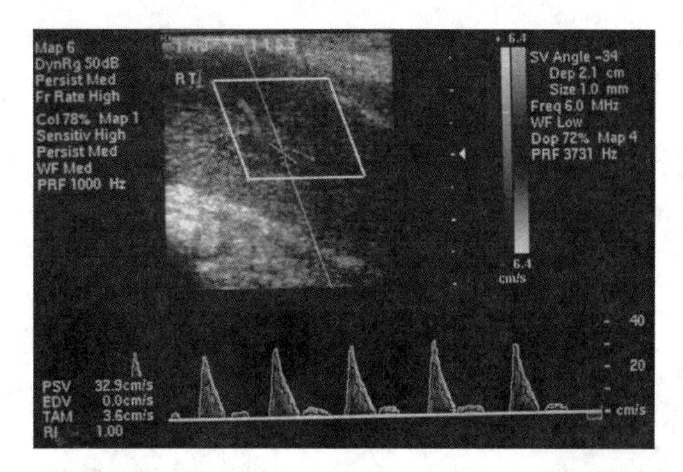

Fig. 10.3. In Phase II of pharmacologic erection, with increase in intracorporeal pressure, a progressive decrease in EDV occurs. The PSV remains high. In this picture, some diastolic flow remains, but the EDV has become zero (phase III)

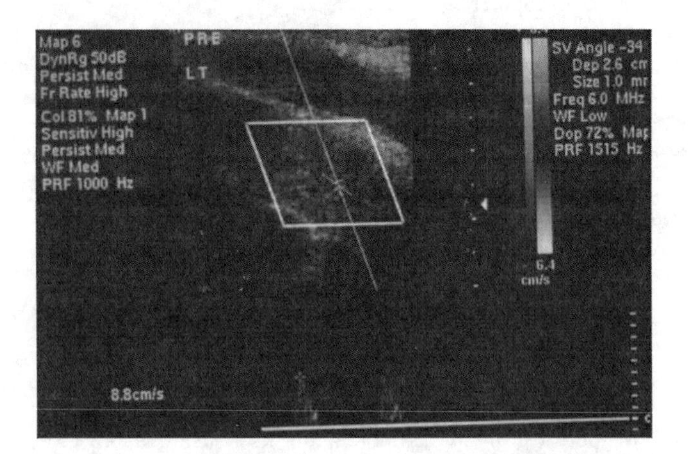

Fig. 10.1. Cavernosal arteries at a flaccid state prior to penile injection usually have a low and intermittent flow with zero end diastolic velocity

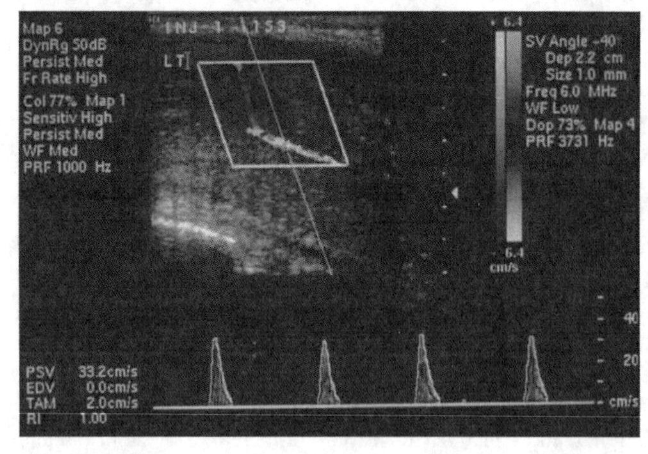

Fig. 10.4. In Phase III of pharmacologic erection, when the intracorporeal pressure increases to near systemic diastolic blood pressure, the EDV reaches 0. PSV remains high

In Phase IV, EDV becomes negative and PSV remains high. The penis further increases in its rigidity (Fig. 10.5).

In Phase V, with further increases in intracorporeal pressure and rigidity, PSV also decreases. EDV remains negative.

Hemodynamic Patterns

The hemodynamic events vary among individual patients. We stratify the color Doppler hemodynamic findings into the following eight patterns[1,2]:

I. Normal maximal PSV ($\geq$35 cm s^{-1}), sustained ($\geq$5 min)
Ia. EDV $\leq$0 with complete erectile response
Ib. EDV >0 or incomplete erectile response
II. Normal maximal PSV ($\geq$ 35 cm s^{-1}), transient (<5 min)
IIa. EDV $\leq$0 with complete erectile response
IIb. EDV > 0 or incomplete erectile response
III. Borderline maximal PSV (30–35 cm s^{-1})
IIIa. EDV $\leq$0 with complete erectile response
IIIb. EDV > 0 or incomplete erectile response
IV. Low maximal PSV (<30 cm s^{-1})
IVa. EDV $\leq$0 with complete erectile response
IVb. EDV > 0 or incomplete erectile response

Interpretation of Color Doppler Ultrasound Hemodynamic Studies

We interpret the entire dynamic study and consider the maximum PSV, erectile response, and injection dose required. The dosage of pharmacologic agents used in color Doppler ultrasound studies varies among investigators. We used a modest dose (as described in procedure) for the first injection since most normal individuals respond to such dose with a complete erection. Patients responding only to higher doses are likely to have abnormal hemodynamics, and their hemodynamic abnormalities may be masked if a high dose is used from the beginning. A smaller dose also decreases the possibility of priapism. Using a modest dose priapism can still occur. All patients were informed of this possibility before the study and we emphasized the prompt and appropriate treatment for priapism. Patients were asked to call our emergency contact number if an erection lasted longer than 3 h. The option of giving a second injection to the opposite side helps avoid misdiagnosing a low PSV in the contralateral cavernosal artery.

Patients with a normal maximum PSV and a rigid erection (patterns Ia, IIa) with one injection are considered *normal.* Patients with a sustained normal maximum PSV but an incomplete erection (patterns Ib) are diagnosed as having *veno-occlusive dysfunction.* Patients with a transient normal maximum PSV but an incomplete erection (patterns IIb) may have *arterial insufficiency* and/or *veno-occlusive dysfunction.* Patients with a borderline or low maximal PSV yet complete erectile response (patterns IIIa, IVa) probably have arterial insufficiency that is being compensated for by good veno-occlusive function. Those who have both low maximal PSV and an incomplete erection have *arterial insufficiency*, but their veno-occlusive function cannot be isolated by the study. Patients requiring a large dose of intracorporeal agent to achieve a normal maximal PSV and complete erection have some combination of abnormal erectile tissue, borderline arterial insufficiency, and/or veno-occlusive dysfunction.

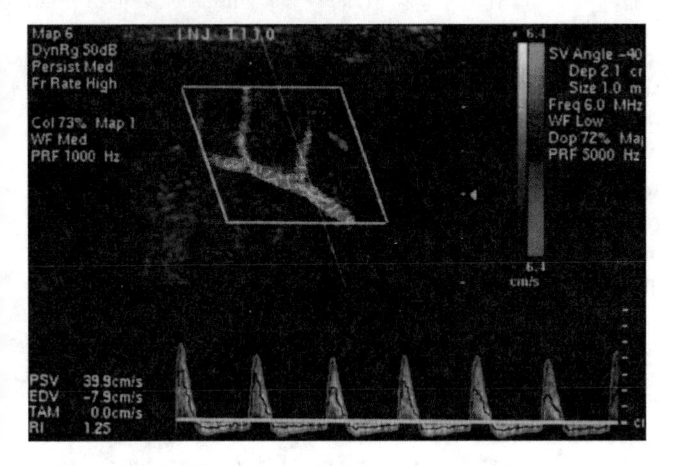

FIG. 10.5. In Phase IV of pharmacologic erection, EDV becomes negative. PSV remains high

Pitfalls of Hemodynamic Studies

In performing a color Doppler ultrasound hemodynamic study, it is important to watch for the following pitfalls:

1. Some authors reported using 5- or 10-min intervals for PSV measurements. Such measurement methods may not be reliably detect the highest PSV. The hemodynamic of an erection is truly a dynamic event. Many patients reach their peak response in less than 5 min. A falsely low maximal PSV could be recorded if measurements do not start within 2–3 min after the injection. Furthermore, the PSV may not be sustained in a normal range for longer than 5 min. A dynamic observation rather than a spot check is preferable.[2,5]
2. PSV values differ with varying sites of measurement. We find that the PSV is generally highest at the proximal cavernosal artery and decreases with more distal sites of measurement. We noted that the PSV at the midshaft is, on average, 68% of that at the penoscrotal junction. Additionally, only 25% of patients having a normal PSV at the proximal penile shaft also have a normal value at the midshaft.[5] Thus, measuring distal sites may give a false low value, making it preferable to measure hemodynamic parameters at a consistent proximal site. We find it technically more difficult to measure the hemodynamic parameters at the proximal crura through the scrotum; therefore, the penoscrotal junction is our preferred site of measurement.

3. Consider the impact of varied vascular anatomy on the measurement of hemodynamic parameters. The cavernosal artery anatomy varies among patients. Some anatomical variations have impact on the hemodynamic parameters.[7] Patients with a bifurcated cavernosal artery or a cavernosal artery that gives out major branches at the proximal shaft tend to have a lower PSV after the bifurcation or branch. Thus, it is better to measure the hemodynamic parameters proximal to the branch. The majority of patients with bifurcated arteries or multiple arteries have different PSV values in each. If it is not possible to measure the hemodynamic parameters proximal to a large branch or bifurcation, it is desirable to measure the hemodynamic parameters from both branches of the artery and interpret the findings cautiously.

   By carefully assessing vascular anatomy, puzzling hemodynamics may be explained. For example, in a patient with a substantially higher PSV at the midpenile shaft than in more proximal sites, we noted a crosscorporal artery at the midshaft which supplies blood flow from the opposite corpora. This helped us to understand the unusual finding.
4. Do not diagnose contralateral arterial insufficiency when only one side of the penis is injected. The pharmacologic agents injected into one side of corpora may have a lower concentration in the opposite corpora. We have noted that patients with low PSV on the contralateral side following the first injection may convert to a normal PSV after an injection is administered to that side.[1,5,6]
5. Be careful in interpreting EDV and RI. An EDV of 0 (or RI of 1) is commonly used as an indicator of adequate veno-occlusive dysfunction. High EDV suggests venous leak. However, such diagnostic criteria should be used with caution. Since RI = (PSV – EDV)/PSV, the resistive index result depends on the EDV. When the EDV is 0, the RI is 1. When the EDV is >0, the RI is <1. In general, EDV reflects the intracorporal pressure. Schwartz et al. studied the correlation of EDV and the intracorporal pressure.[3] By placing needles in the corpora to directly measure intracorporeal pressure, they found that the EDV of the cavernosal arteries decreases with increasing intracorporeal pressure. When the pressure reached near systemic diastolic blood pressure, the EDV decreased to 0 (RI = 1). However, we believe that the EDV can also be affected by other factors, such as the status of the corporal artery and poor sinusoidal smooth muscle relaxation. We observed some patients have an EDV of zero, but have a soft penis. In these patients, the 0 EDV (and RI of 1) cannot be explained by the intracorporeal pressure. An EDV of zero with a flaccid or semierect penis is probably caused by an arterial factor rather than intracorporeal pressure, making it a mistake to conclude that a patient has adequate veno-occlusive function based on EDV and RI alone. Furthermore, at a flaccid state of penis, we commonly observe an intermittent cavernosal artery flow with a zero EDV. It reflects the contracted state of the cavernosal artery and does not indicate that the patient has an adequate veno-occlusive function. Thus it is advisable to record the status of the erection to avoid misinterpretation of EDV and RI An EDV of negative value is usually more reliable in reflecting on a high intracavernosal pressure and an adequate veno-occlusive function.[5]

To diagnose veno-occlusive dysfunction using color Doppler ultrasound, we assess the hemodynamic pattern and erectile status rather than relying solely on EDV or RI. It is reasonable to suspect the presence of veno-occlusive dysfunction if a patient has normal arterial flow but an incomplete erectile response and a high EDV after intracorporeal injection of pharmacologic agents. With a careful analysis of the hemodynamic pattern, color Doppler ultrasound provides a global assessment of veno-occlusive dysfunction in a noninvasive manner. For patients with sonographic evidence of veno-occlusive dysfunction further study dynamic infusion or gravity cavernosometry may be necessary to have a more complete evaluation before considering venous ligation surgery.[8–10]

In summary, an erection is a complex and dynamic process. Color Doppler ultrasound studies for erectile dysfunction are best performed with the involvement of a urologist who has a thorough understanding of the hemodynamics of erection. Dynamic studies and careful interpretation of blood flow parameters are necessary to provide an accurate assessment of the hemodynamic abnormalities of erectile dysfunction. Penile arterial anatomy varies among individuals. The value of hemodynamic parameters differs with varied sites of measurement. To obtain a reliable result, hemodynamic parameters should be measured at a consistent proximal site. The variation in vascular anatomy and cavernosal artery pathology should be considered when interpreting color Doppler studies.

Color Doppler Ultrasound Evaluation for Priapism

The literature on color Doppler ultrasound study of priapism is limited. Most reports are related to patients with high flow priapism as a result of cavernosal artery injury. Color Doppler ultrasound is the primary diagnostic tool for the differentiation of high flow (nonischemic) and low flow (ischemic) priapism. However, the diagnostic criterion for high flow vs. low flow priapism is poorly defined. To our knowledge, color Doppler ultrasound hemodynamic studies for priapism patients following surgical shunt treatment have not been previously reported. We found that penile hemodynamic characteristics are important not only for the initial evaluation of priapism but also for the treatment decisions after initial intervention.[11,12]

Procedure

For the evaluation of priapism, color Doppler ultrasound evaluation is performed before penile injection or aspiration. Hemodynamic assessment may be repeated after therapeutic aspiration and penile injection of alpha adrenergic agent or shunt surgery to examine the restoration of cavernosal blood flow which indicates the adequate relief of priapism. With the penis placed toward the abdomen and the transducer placed at the ventral surface of penis, we examine the cavernosal arteries from the penoscrotal junction to the midpenile shaft and measure hemodynamic parameters (PSV, EDV, and resistive index). With the transducer pushing down the scrotum, we also examine the cavernosal arteries at the crura.

Color Doppler Ultrasound Findings and Interpretation for Priapism

Priapism is traditionally divided into ischemic (low flow) and nonischemic (high flow) categories. Color Doppler ultrasound is a useful tool to categorize priapisms. Penile blood gas has also been used to help the diagnosis. It is generally recommended that a low flow (or ischemic) priapism is a medical emergency and requires urgent management for detumescence, while a high flow (nonischemic) priapism does not require urgent management. However, this categorization and the treatment strategies based on such classification have many caveats.

Priapism is a dynamic event and the hemodynamic characteristics may vary at different phases of the condition. Additionally, the hemodynamic characteristics change after therapeutic intervention. For example, a patient who receives an intracavernosal injection of papaverine or prostaglandin E1 typically has high blood flow initially, with their high flow status lasting for a varied length of time. If remains untreated, it progresses to a low flow and ischemic status.[11,13] Metawea et al. noted that if the PSV is greater than 66 cm s^{-1} and the EDV is 0 cm s^{-1} after an intracavernous injection of papaverine/phentolamine, patients have high risk for priapism lasting for >6 h.[14] Secil et al. reported that if the cavernosal arterial flow reaches a phase of undetectable flow by color Doppler ultrasound after intracavernous injection of papaverine, the patient has high risk for persistent priapism.[15] Pharmacologically induced priapism usually go through phases of hemodynamic response, and it is not clear how long and at what point the priapism becomes ischemic.[2,5] When patients are presented at 4–6 h after injection, and a color Doppler ultrasound shows a high cavernosal arterial flow, it would not be safe to inform patients that the cavernosal blood flow is high and they require no treatment until low flow ensues.

Priapism of other etiologies probably has various phases of hemodynamic events as well. To obtain an erection, a high cavernosal arterial flow is usually required. In the case of priapism, it is not clear at what point the high cavernosal arterial flow becomes low. When these patients present for management with 24 h or longer of priapism, most patients show little detectible cavernosal blood flow in the color Doppler ultrasound.

Another caveat of categorizing patients into high flow and low flow priapism is our observation that some patients with low flow priapism may develop high cavernosal blood flow after a successful shunt surgery. Clinically, these patients may appear to have persistent priapism. However, other patients with similar clinical findings may have persistent low flow status if the shunt surgeries have not achieved their goal. We find that the CDU hemodynamic characteristics are important for subsequent treatment decisions following the initial shunting procedure.[11–14] One patient's CDU, who previously failed Winter shunt and Quakle shunt treatments before being referred to us, showed undetectable cavernosal blood flow. We performed a penile cavernosa-dorsal (CD) vein shunt, and his CDU study showed high cavernosal blood flow following surgery (Fig. 10.6). It is not uncommon following initial shunt surgery for patients to have some degree of persistent erections. This could be due to ineffective shunt surgery or postischemic hyperperfusion. If patients have ineffective shunt surgeries without further intervention, they are likely to be impotent subsequently. Thus, color Doppler ultrasound confirmation of priapism resolution is desirable.[11–13]

With these considerations, we believe that to understand the basic hemodynamic abnormality during various phases of priapism is of critical importance in the management of priapism. We believe that the traditional classification of "high flow"/low flow or ischemic/nonischemic requires modification. We classify priapisms according to the hemodynamic abnormality and underlying pathophysiology as follows:

1. *Arteriogenic priapism.* These patients typically have perineal trauma that causes cavernosal artery injury. Color Doppler ultrasound typically shows the presence of arteriosinusoidal malformation (Fig. 10.7). The cavernosal blood flow varies, but a pure arteriogenic priapism without veno-occlusive component seldom has the EDV <0 cm s^{-1}.
2. *Veno-occlusive priapism.* The veno-occlusive mechanism of erection is initially a result of passive compression by

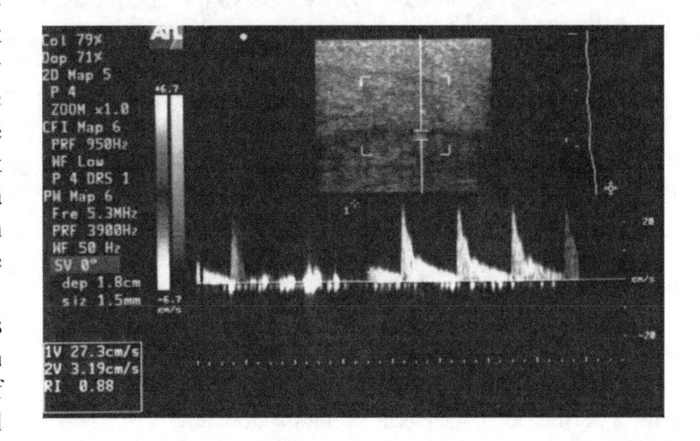

Fig. 10.6. In a patient who previously failed Winter shunt and Quakle shunt, initial CDU shows undetectable cavernosal blood flow. We performed penile cavernosa-dorsal (CD) vein shunt, and his CDU study showed high cavernosal blood flow after surgery

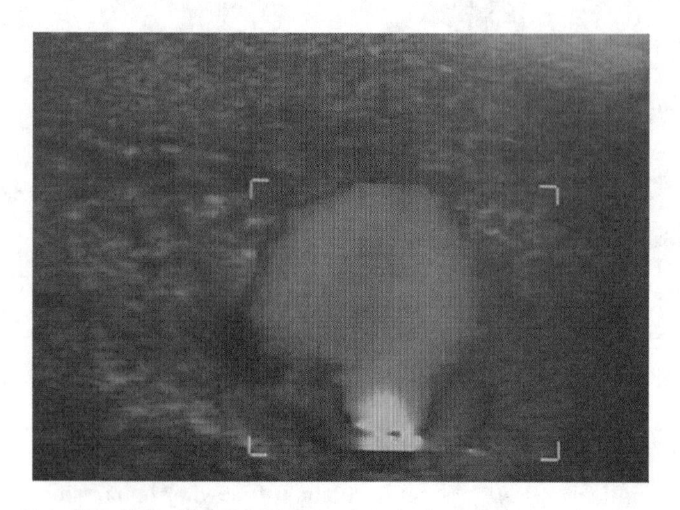

Fig. 10.7. Color Doppler ultrasound typically shows the presence of arterio-sinusoidal malformation

the dilated sinusoids which is induced by smooth muscle relaxation and increased cavernosal arterial blood flow. We hypothesize that after a certain time period of passive compression, thrombosis of emissary veins may develop causing primarily veno-occlusive priapism.

3. *Combined arteriogenic and veno-occlusive priapism.* Priapism induced by an intracorporal injection of erection inducing pharmacological agents typically has both an arteriogenic component and a veno-occlusive component during the initial phases. When the effect of pharmacologic agents on the cavernosal artery subsides, persistent priapism may become solely the veno-occlusive component.

In the course of priapism in an individual patient, the hemodynamics may change at the different phases of their priapism, and they should be managed differently according to their hemodynamic pattern.

The recognition of hemodynamics in priapism is also important in deciding whether priapism patients should receive a second shunt surgery. We believe that an effective shunt should relieve the veno-occlusive status of priapism. In color Doppler ultrasound, restoration of cavernosal blood flow with a positive or zero EDV is usually observed. A negative value of EDV and/or undetectable cavernosal blood flow usually indicates the persistence of veno-occlusive priapism. Patients who were referred to us after having failed previous shunt surgeries typically have veno-occlusive priapism in color Doppler ultrasound study. After we carry out penile CD shunt surgeries for these patients, we commonly observe a restoration of cavernosal arterial blood flow. With our technique of penile CD shunt, the patency of shunt can usually be detected by color Doppler ultrasound.[11–13] Some patients may have a period of high cavernosal blood flow after their penile CD shunt surgery. This is likely related to postischemic hyperperfusion and may be one of our body's repairing mechanisms for the damaged cavernosal tissue. This observation has two significant clinical implications. First, if the color Doppler ultrasound study, performed after a surgical shunt procedure, shows the persistence of undetectable blood flow, one should suspect that that shunt has not achieved its intended purpose to adequately drain the cavernosal blood. Second, if the patient appears to have a persistent priapism following a shunt procedure, but the color Doppler ultrasound reveals high cavernosal blood flow and a patent shunt, it may be part of a recovery phase for priapism after a successful shunt surgery. Thus observation rather than further intervention is recommended. With a management strategy that utilizing penile CD shunt and incorporating color Doppler ultrasound studies before and after shunt surgery, we have noted high rate of potency preservation for priapism patients.[13]

In summary, the hemodynamic of priapism appears to have various phases. Color Doppler ultrasound is useful not only to differentiate arteriogenic priapism from veno-occlusive priapism, but also in monitoring the success of shunt surgery. If color Doppler ultrasound shows a recovery phase of hemodynamics with high cavernosal blood flow and a patent shunt, further surgery is not necessary. In contrast, if following a surgical shunt procedure the cavernosal blood flow remains undetectable or has not improved since before the shunt surgery, it is likely that the shunt surgery has not achieved its purpose and further intervention should be performed without undue delay.

References

1. Lue, T.F., Hricak, H., Marich, K.W., Tanagho, E. Vasculogenic impotence evaluated by high-resolution ultrasonography and pulsed Doppler spectrum analysis. Radiology 155:777–781, 1985
2. Chiou, R.K., Pomeroy, B.D. Erectile dysfunction. Using color Doppler ultrasound hemodynamic studies for evaluation. Cont Urol 10:87–101, 1998
3. Schwartz, A.N., Lowe, M., Berger, R.E., Wang, K.Y., Mack, L.A., Richardson, M.L. Assessment of normal and abnormal erectile function: Color Doppler flow sonography versus conventional techniques. Radiology 180:105–109, 1991
4. Meuleman, E.J., Bemelmans, B.L., Van-Asten, W.N., Doesburg, W.H., Skotnicki, S.H., Debruyne, F.M. Assessment of penile blood flow by duplex ultrasonography in 44 men with normal erectile potency in different phases of erection. J Urol 147(1):51–56, 1992
5. Chiou, R.K., Pomeroy, B.D., Chen, W.S., Anderson, J.C., Wobig, R.K., Taylor, R.J. Hemodynamic patterns of pharmacologically induced erection: evaluation by color Doppler sonography. J Urol 159:109–112, 1998
6. Chiou, R.K., Anderson, J.C., Chen, W.S., Wobig, R.K., Jacobsen, D.D., Matamoros Jr, A., Taylor, R.J. Hemodynamic evaluation of erectile dysfunction and Peyronie's disease using Color Doppler Ultrasound. J Ultrasound Medi 16:S20, 1997
7. Chiou, R.K., Alberts, G.L., Pomeroy, B.D., Anderson, J.C., Carlson, L.K., Anderson, J.R., Wobig, R.K. Study of cavernosal artery anatomy using color and power Doppler sonography: Impact on hemodynamic parameter measurement. J Urol 162:358–360, 1999
8. Lue,T.F., Donatucci, C.F. Dysfunction of the venoocclusive mechanism.In: Alan H. Bennett, Ed. Impotence – Diagnosis and management of erectile dysfunction. 1994, pSaundersp. 197–204

9. Puech-Leao, P., Chao, S., Glina, S., and Reichelt, A.C. Gravity cavernosometry – a simple diagnostic test for cavernosal incompetence. Brit J Urol 65:391, 1990
10. De Meyer, J.M., Thibo, P., Oosterlinck. The evaluation of arterial inflow by gravity cavernosometry. J Urol 158:440–443, 1997
11. Chiou, R.K., Broughton, F.L., Chiou, C.R., Liu, S. Color Doppler Ultrasound Hemodynamic Characteristics of Priapism Patients Before and after therapy and its impact on subsequent Penile Shunt Surgery. Sex Med 4(Suppl 1):85, 2007
12. Chiou, R.K., Henslee, D.L., Anderson, J.C., Wobig, R.K. Color Doppler sonography assessment and saphenous vein graft penile veno-corporeal shunt for priapism. Br J Urol 83:138–139, 1999.
13. Chiou, R.K., Mues, A.C., Chiou, C.R., Broughton, F.L., Yohannes, P. Clinical Experience and Sexual function outcome of Priapism patients treated with Penile Cavernosa-Dorsal Vein (CD) Shunt using saphenous vein graft. J Sex Med 4(Suppl 1): 76–77, 2007
14. Metawea, B., El-Nashar, A.R., Gad-Allah, A., Abdul-Wahab, M., Shamloul, R. Intracavernous papaverine/phentolamine-induced priapism can be accurately predicted with color Doppler ultrasonography. Urol 66:858–860, 2005
15. Secil, M., Arslan, D., Goktay, A.Y., Esen, A.A., Dicle, O., Pirnar, T. The prediction of papaverine induced priapism by color Doppler sonography. J Urol 165:416–418, 2001

Chapter 11
The Physics of Ultrasound and Some Recent Techniques Used

Gert Karlsson

This chapter will focus on understanding the underlying physics of diagnostic ultrasound. This will help ultrasound operators get the best possible performance and understand how simple adjustments can improve the quality of the scanning thus obtaining a better diagnostic tool. To achieve a good performance of the scanning, the examiner needs to know how the adjustments can be used to obtain the best possible diagnostic image.

It is also the aim to go through some frequently seen image artifacts and how to reduce the negative influence of these artifacts, thereby ensuring that the ultrasound can be a real help in the diagnostic session. Finally some more recent technical developments that can influence the future choice of equipment are outlined.

The Piezoelectric Effect

The operation of all ultrasound transducers is based on the piezoelectric effect. The materials used for making crystals for transducers are endowed with a property called the piezoelectric effect.

This effect means that when the material is submitted to a voltage, the piezoelectric material deforms slightly. Inversely, if the material is deformed by external forces, a small voltage change results.

In diagnostic ultrasound, short-duration electrical pulses are applied to the ultrasound crystals during the transmit phase giving rise to short-duration deformations of the crystals. These deformations result in an ultrasound transmit waveform being transmitted into the tissue with a rather constant velocity, estimated on average to be 1,540 m s^{-1} in human tissue. (The velocity is much lower in air and much higher in bone.)

Characteristics of Ultrasound

Ultrasound is characterized by its frequency. The frequencies of ultrasound used for diagnostic purposes in urology are usually in the range from 2 to 20 MHz.

A frequency of 2 MHz means that the ultrasound wave generates 2,000,000 cycles per second.

The lower the frequency of ultrasound, the greater its ability to penetrate deeper into tissue, but because the wavelength becomes longer with decreasing frequency, the resolution will be lower.

The higher the frequency of ultrasound, the poorer its ability to penetrate into deeper parts of the tissue, but because the wavelength becomes shorter with increasing frequency, the resolution will be higher.

Due to this relationship between resolution and penetration, the general rule for ultrasound scanning is that the frequency used should always be as high as possible, taking into account how deep in the tissue the target organ is situated – in other words, how much penetration depth is desired. For very superficial organs, like testis and penis, very high frequencies (>10 MHz) are used. For organs like the kidneys, more penetration is needed; therefore, lower frequencies (3.5–5 MHz) must normally be used.

For prostate scanning, the change in procedure in the last decades (from scanning from the outside, through the bladder, to scanning the prostate using transrectal ultrasound (TRUS)) has meant that much higher frequencies are now used (6–12 MHz instead of 3–5 MHz).

The result of this is a significantly higher image resolution during ultrasound scanning of the prostate.

The Principle of Ultrasound Scanning

The ultrasound waves used in urology are transmitted as a series of short pulses with a duration of a few microseconds. Between these short pulses being sent out, the transducer is receiving the echoes coming back from the different depths of the tissue. The time necessary for receiving an echo depends on the tissue depth.

Ultrasound is reflected when it goes from one kind of tissue to another. How much is reflected depends on the change in impedance between the two kinds of tissue and on the angle

O. Ukimura and I.S. Gill (eds.), *Contemporary Interventional Ultrasonography in Urology,*
DOI: 10.1007/978-1-84800-217-3_11,

of incidence of the ultrasound beam. The reflected part of the ultrasound energy is seen as echoes of different brightness on the ultrasound image.

If most of the incident ultrasound wave is reflected by some structure, the echo on the image will be very bright (hyperechoic) in this part of the ultrasound image.

The time duration for receiving echoes from a specific depth equals (2× depth)/speed of sound; from a depth of 15 cm, the time will be 195 μs.

A-mode scanning (Amplitude mode scanning): In the early days of ultrasound, this was the only way possible to do the scanning. For each echo received, the amplitude of the echo was displayed on a screen, with the amplitude displayed as the *Y*-axis and the time as the *X*-axis.

B-mode scanning (Brightness scanning): In B-mode scanning, the amplitudes are converted into different gray levels, and the gray levels in the different parts of the tissue being scanned are displayed with varying gray scale levels on a map with the depth of the tissue as *Y*-axis and the position along the transducer surface as the *X*-axis.

For a B-mode image, modern equipment usually uses a gray scale resolution of 256 levels. Liquid collections like cysts and the gall bladder will appear black, while areas with many strong reflectors such as bony structures will appear echo-rich or even white.

The Propagation of Sound in Tissue

When an ultrasonic wave is moving down through the tissue, the actual movement is influenced by:

Speed of Sound

Even though the speed of sound in tissue is relatively constant (apart from being very different in air and bone with total reflection as a result), it is slightly lower in fatty tissue than in muscle or normal kidney. Usually the ultrasound system is set up to use a speed of sound of 1,540 m s^{-1}. If the actual speed is different, this has an impact on how accurately a point is displayed and on how accurate measurements are.

Attenuation

The attenuation of the sound wave is very dependent on the frequency used. It will also increase with increasing depth of the tissue. The attenuation is due to the absorption and reflection of sound energy in tissue, in particular when most of the energy is reflected due to a big difference in impedance. When the ultrasonic wave meets air or bony structures, it is almost completely reflected. As a result, a shadow artifact appears behind the area where air or bone is encountered.

This phenomenon means that for good image quality, it is important to ensure good contact (no air) between transducer and tissue. Ultrasound gel is used to avoid too much impedance difference between the transducer surface and the tissue.

For transrectal scanning of the prostate, it is essential that no air is trapped between the transducer and the rectal wall. In cases where a water-filled balloon is used, air bubbles must be eliminated from the balloon as well.

The attenuation means that it is important to use as high a frequency as possible without sacrificing penetration depth, keeping in mind the depth of the intended organ.

The operator has to use the time gain compensation (TGC) function to compensate for this attenuation in the tissue. Without this, the image will be darker and darker as you go from the transducer surface down through the tissue. All scanners have TGC to allow a depth-dependent gain adjustment in order to compensate for the tissue attenuation.

Focusing the ultrasonic beam

See Fig. 11.1.

During the use of an ultrasound transducer, the operator must try to make sure that the area to be examined is placed within the focal range. With electronic transducers an important adjustment available for the operator is the ability to move the focus as close to the area of interest as possible.

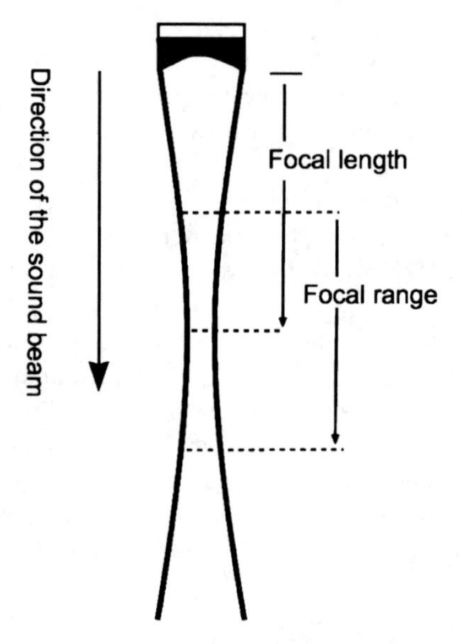

Fig. 11.1. Illustration of the form of the ultrasound beam of an electronic transducer, where the focal range indicates the range of depths giving the best resolution for the transducer. The Focal range is the distance from the transducer array to the depth, where the sharpest focus will be obtained

Limitations of Ultrasound

Resolution

Resolution plays an important part in optimizing the image quality during scanning. Resolution is divided into different categories: axial, lateral, and contrast resolution.

The axial and lateral resolutions are decisive for separation of the different reflecting structures. If the resolution is insufficient, two reflectors may be displayed as one. The minimum displayed lateral size will be equal to the beam width, and the minimum axial dimension will be equal to one-half of the pulse length.

Axial Resolution

This is the resolution in the direction of the ultrasonic beam. It depends very much on the length of the pulse used – a shorter pulse gives a higher axial resolution, but when the pulse becomes shorter, the sensitivity and penetration are reduced. The axial resolution also depends on the ultrasound frequency – higher frequencies correspond to shorter wavelengths. Two points in the tissue cannot be distinguished if they are located within one wavelength of each other.

For the operator, the important adjustments are the choice of transducer and – for a given transducer – the choice of frequency. The pulse form and length is built into the equipment and cannot be changed by the operator.

Some transducers have a fixed frequency, but in most modern equipment, different frequencies can be selected for the same transducers.

In addition to this some recent ultrasound systems have the possibility of using a high frequency in the surface and gradually reducing the frequency in the lower part of the image, thus optimizing the image for high near-field resolution, but keeping an adequate penetration depth.

See Fig. 11.2

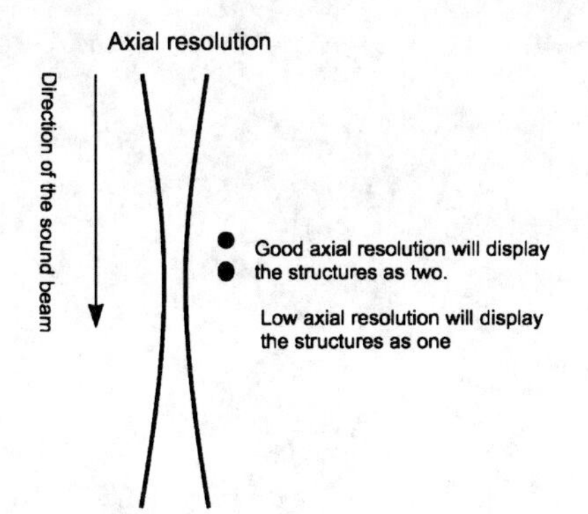

FIG. 11.2. Illustration of the effects of axial resolution. The resolution in the direction of the beam is called the axial resolution and can be adjusted by changing the frequency. Higher frequencies will offer better axial resolution

Lateral Resolution

The lateral resolution of an electronic transducer depends on the width of each ultrasonic beam and on the density of lines in the image. Optimizing the pitch of the transducer and electronic focusing of the beam are the two main ways of optimizing the beam width in the area of interest.

Pitch is a description of the size of each individual crystal in an array. A smaller crystal means a smaller pitch and a finer resolution, but sometimes at the cost of good focus in the deeper part of the tissue. Near-field transducers use high frequency with a finer pitch; abdominal transducers for kidney scanning use a lower frequency with a larger pitch. For the operator, the relevant adjustments affecting the lateral resolution are adjustment of the line density and optimizing the focus position. The sharper the focus and the higher the line density, the better the lateral resolution at that point. The cost of higher lateral resolution is usually the frame rate: in order to optimize the axial resolution, the image frame rate will be reduced (Fig. 11.3).

Contrast Resolution

This term is used as a measure of the system's ability to distinguish between two parts of the tissue with almost – but not completely – identical echogenicity: if the system can distinguish well between tissues that are very similar, the contrast resolution is high. The actual contrast resolution is an integrated characteristic of the combined ultrasound system and transducer.

All ultrasound systems allow the operator to adjust the gray scale and dynamic range. This can be important for creating a diagnostic image, in which it is possible to easily differentiate pathology and normal tissue. It should, however, not be used to compensate for an ineffective adjustment of the monitor.

The monitor must be correctly adjusted before other image adjustments are attempted.

Tissue harmonic imaging can sometimes be used to increase the contrast resolution.

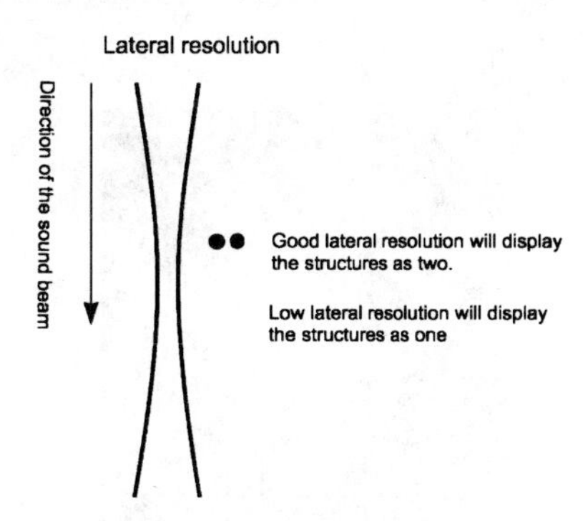

FIG. 11.3. Illustration of the effects of the lateral resolution. The resolution in the image plane perpendicular to the ultrasound beam is called the lateral resolution. In order to obtain a better lateral resolution, a higher line density or a sharper focus can be used

Artifacts in Ultrasound

In ultrasonic imaging, artifacts are areas in the image that are not indicative of the tissue being examined. They can be caused by the instrumentation or related to physical phenomena that the instrument is not able to compensate for.

Examples of artifacts often encountered during a normal scanning situation are:

- Enhancement
- Shadowing
- Reverberation
- Mirror artifacts
- Propagation speed errors

Some artifacts, like enhancement and shadowing, can be very helpful for diagnosing structures like cysts and calculi. Other artifacts, like reverberations or artifacts due to poor contact between transducer and tissue or the presence of strong reflectors, may disturb the image and reduce the diagnostic value of the ultrasound images obtained.

Propagation speed artifacts are due to basic assumptions not being fulfilled. The equipment assumes that sound in tissue travels in straight lines with a uniform velocity of 1,540 m s^{-1}, and that only echoes from the transducer axis are received.

These assumptions unfortunately are not always true.

Enhancement

Increased echogenicity from tissues behind areas with low attenuation. This type of artifact is normally seen behind cystic or other liquid collections. This kind of artifact helps in identifying cystic structures and making sure that the structure is a true cyst (Fig. 11.4).

Shadowing

Shadowing happens due to a decrease of echogenicity from tissues behind a zone with strong reflectivity or attenuation. This artifact occurs behind strongly reflecting structures like calculi or bony structures (for example, the pubic bone). A so-called acoustic shadow behind a strong reflector (for example, the bone or calculus) is the result. In order to have a closer look at the tissue located in the shadow, the transducer must be reoriented so that the shadow does not cover the desired area.

Reverberations

When two or more strong reflectors are present, multiple reflections between these reflectors and the transducer surface may occur. The reverberations are caused by internal re-reflections in the tissue, or between the transducer and a reflector in the tissue. The rectal wall and a water balloon, often used, can form reverberation artifacts if air bubbles or other materials are located between the transducer and the area to be examined (Fig. 11.5).

If the ultrasound beam does not hit an interface at a perpendicular angle, the direction of the beam will be altered. The equipment assumes straight-line propagation when it calculates the image, so a reflector may not be displayed in the correct position. These artifacts can often be avoided by trying to scan at a perpendicular angle.

One troublesome result of refraction is called the anisotropic effect, frequently seen during transrectal scanning of the prostate. Ultrasonic beams hitting the prostate near the neurovascular bundles will hit the prostatic border in a tangential manner. Therefore a significant part of the beam will be reflected in other directions than the direction of the incident ultrasound beam. As a result, a lower intensity will be received by the transducer, and, due to attenuation, the echoes from these areas will be displayed as darker areas. This could be mistaken for suspicious hypoechogenic areas, but is just a result of the attenuation due to hitting these areas in a tangential manner (Fig. 11.6).

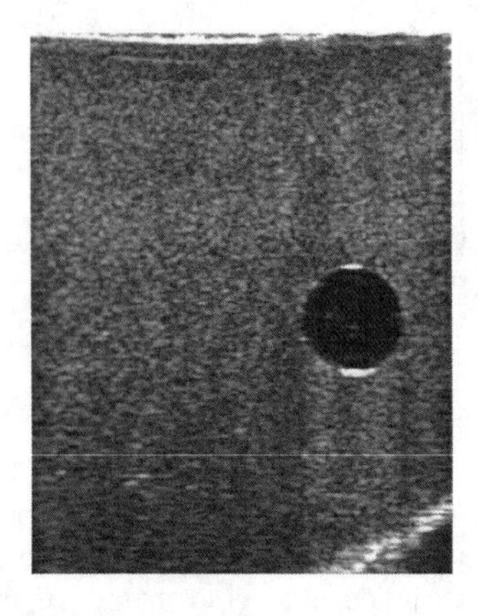

Fig. 11.4. A cystic structure showing enhancement behind the cyst, because the cyst attenuates the beam less than the surrounding tissue does

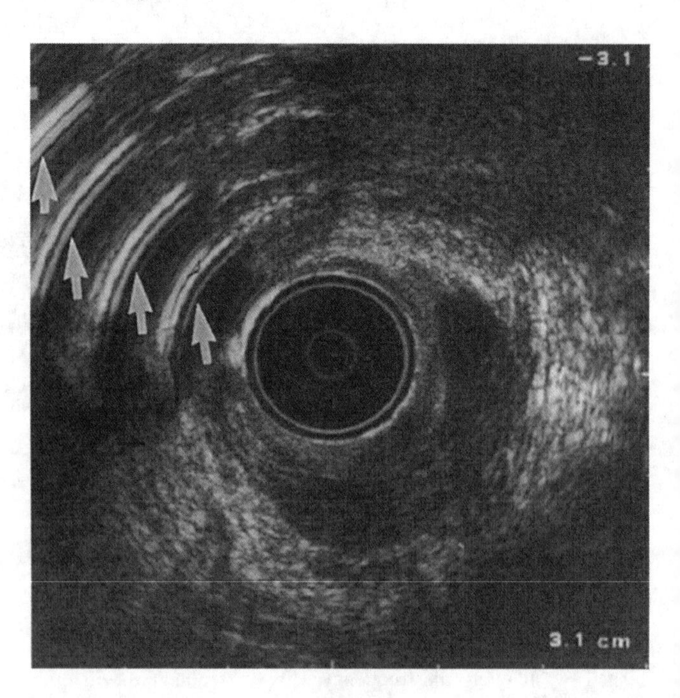

Fig. 11.5. Strong reflection-artifacts (*arrows*) due to air trapped between a water-filled balloon and the rectal wall

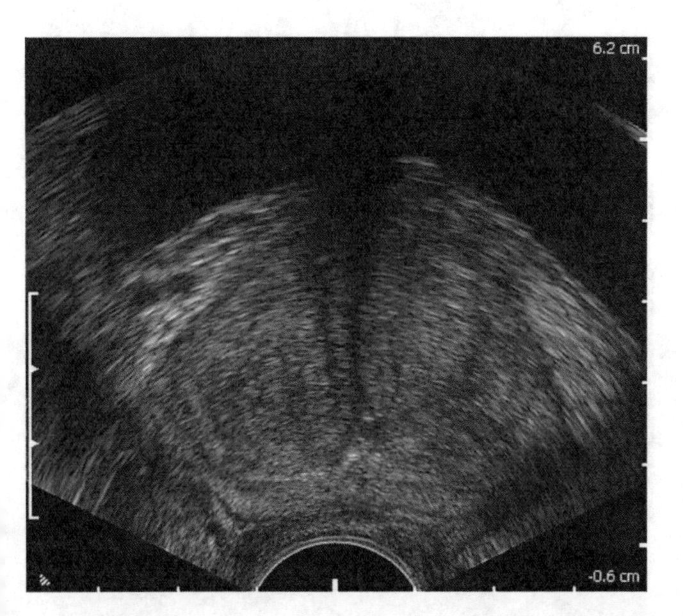

FIG. 11.6. Anisotropic effect demonstrated at the left and right-hand corner of the prostate

Mirror Artifacts

If the ultrasound beam hits a strong reflector, a mirror image of a real structure is seen on the other side of the reflector. This artifact can usually be avoided by changing the position of the transducer.

When scanning the liver and kidneys, this artifact is often seen when the diaphragm is hit at an angle close to 90°.

Propagation Speed Error

The sound speed in tissue is assumed to be 1,540 m s^{-1}. if the actual speed is higher or lower than this, a structure at a certain distance will be displayed as being closer or further from the transducer than it really is.

Newer Techniques and Methods in Urologic Ultrasound

Prostate Harmonic Imaging

When an ultrasound wave passes through tissue, it becomes distorted, and additional frequencies that were not present in the fundamental signal are generated. Multiples of the fundamental frequency are called harmonics, and the second harmonic frequency is of particular interest. The use of this feature – a scanning modality called tissue harmonic imaging – enhances the visibility and detection of hypoechoic structures. It also seems to suppress some of the detrimental effects of the presence of hyperechoic structures.

Propagation of ultrasound in any medium is determined by the Impedance (Z = the density of the medium multiplied by the velocity of ultrasound in that medium) and by the Reflection Coefficient (r = Z/SZ). The ultrasound wave becomes distorted as the tissue expands and compresses in response to the wave. This nonlinear distortion results in the generation of additional frequencies not present in the original waveform.

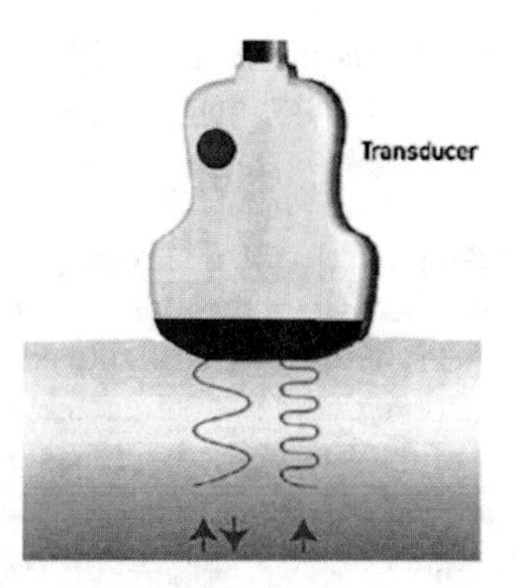

FIG. 11.7. Fundamental and second harmonic frequency

The reflected signal thus not only includes the fundamental frequency but also multiples of this frequency. The frequency that is double the fundamental frequency is called the second harmonic.

The second harmonic frequency for imaging has been used for some time for scanning the liver and kidneys but has now also become an imaging possibility when scanning the prostate.

Harmonic imaging of the prostate combined with random plus targeted biopsies may prove to be advantageous in increasing the sensitivity of transrectal prostate ultrasound (Fig. 11.7).

Grating Lobes

In ultrasound it is assumed that all energy is transmitted from the transducer in the expected direction of the ultrasound beam. Unfortunately this is not true. The main part of the energy is transmitted in this manner – this is called the main lobe. Part of the energy is, however, transmitted in other directions – called the side lobes. Energy falling outside the main lobe in the sound beam from an array transducer is a result of the active transducer aperture being split into elements. This phenomenon is called Grating Lobes (or Side Lobes). The energy in these lobes is substantially less than the energy in the central ultrasound beam (the main lobe) but is inversely proportional to the radius of curvature of an array probe.

A prostate ultrasound probe will always tend to have a small radius of curvature in order to keep the outer diameter of the probe a reasonable size, and therefore side lobes can sometimes create artifacts and degrade the image quality.

Grating lobes are particularly disturbing in prostate ultrasound. The lobes will extend almost laterally out from the probe because of the small radius of curvature. When passing through the periprostatic fat tissue, the grating lobes will eventually hit the inferior side of the pelvic bone, where the difference in impedance to the ultrasound is very high. This shift in impedance will cause an almost 100% reflection of the energy in the grating lobes, hence the energy will bounce back across the prostate ultrasound image, resulting in a degradation of the image quality.

Strong second harmonic signals are generated in a region of high sound pressure, and accordingly only weak signals are found in the region where the grating lobes are being generated. But with almost total reflection, the lobes are disturbing enough.

Using the second harmonic imaging technique not only reduces the effect of the lateral grating lobes but also reduces the angle of the second harmonic lobes. The result is that the lobes are more parallel to the sound beam. Hence the risk of the lobes being reflected from the pelvic structures is also minimized (Fig. 11.8).

The true advantage of prostate harmonic imaging may be the enhancement of any hypoechoic structures combined with

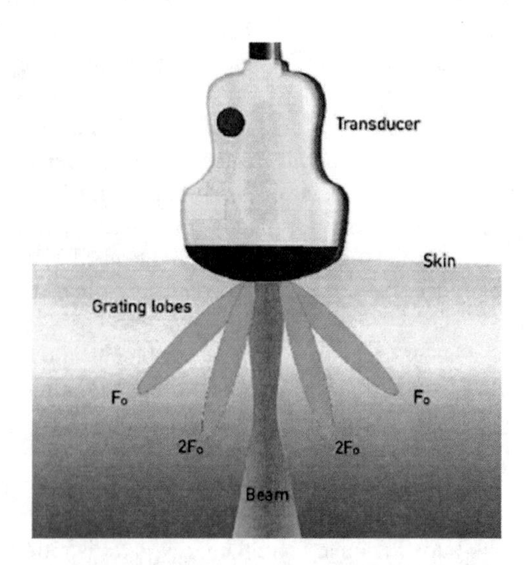

Fig. 11.8. Grating Lobes. F_0 = Fundamental Frequency, $2F_0$ = Second Harmonic Frequency

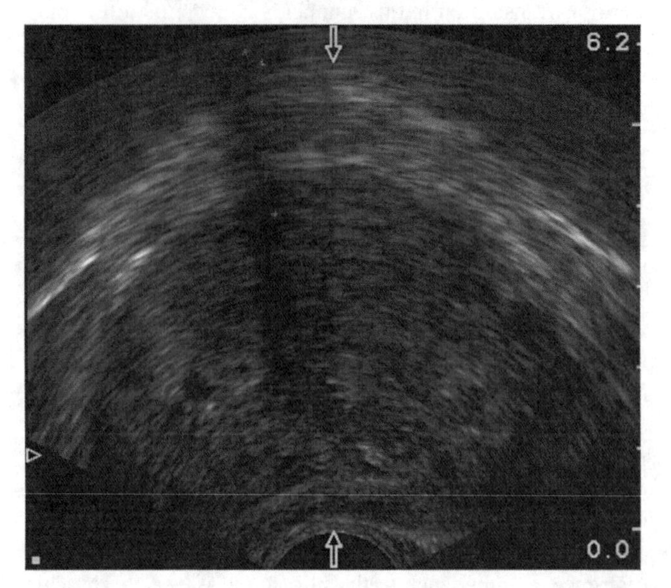

Fig. 11.9. Conventional ultrasound image illustrates a 77-cm^3 prostate without any focal lesion or nodules

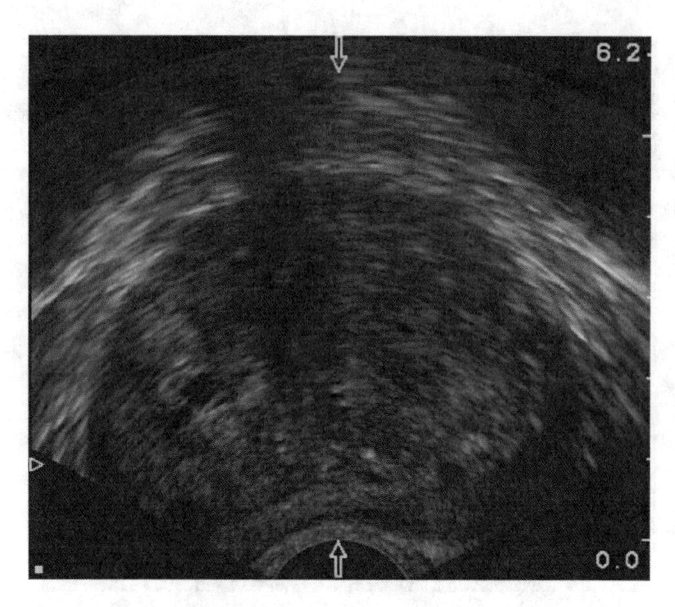

Fig. 11.10. Same patient scanned using harmonic imaging. Note the increased resolution in differentiating between the peripheral zone and the transitional zone

the suppression of hyperechoic phenomena, such as shadowing due to the ultrasound beam being reflected from *corpora amilacia* (Figs. 11.9 and 11.10).

Compared to conventional TRUS, tissue harmonic zoography allows better visualization of malignant lesions resulting in improved differentiation and better detection of small prostate masses. It appears to be a promising tool for improving the diagnostic yield of prostate TRUS.

The transitional zone and the rather compressed peripheral zone are often better seen on the harmonic imaging picture because of reduced grating lobes.

3D Ultrasound

3D ultrasound has been employed in different clinical applications for several years. The acquisition of a 3D data set and the techniques employed are, however, not the same in different applications. The most commonly known version of render mode is *surface render mode*, used extensively to produce early images of the face of a fetus.

Surface render mode only gives good results when a surface is available to render. These techniques fail when a strong surface (a shift in the ultrasound impedance of tissue) cannot be found, as is the case in the subtly layered structures within the anal canal, rectal wall, prostate, etc.

High-resolution 3D ultrasound acquires four to five transverse images per mm of acquisition length. Because of this high resolution, which typically is close to – or equal to – the axial and transverse resolution of the 2D image, 3D postprocessing facilities can reveal significantly more features than can be seen in relatively low-resolution 3D data sets obtained in other applications. Combined with the *volume render mode*, 3D scanning has the potential to give higher spatial resolution for assessing prostatic disease, compared to what is possible using 2D ultrasound.

A 2D ultrasound image has under normal circumstances almost no depth, because of the requirements of keeping the depth of the image as small as possible.

Volume rendering mode techniques use what is called a ray tracing model as the basis of operation. A ray or beam is projected from each point on the viewing screen (the display) back into and through the volume data. As the ray passes through the volume data it reaches the different elements (voxels) in the data set thereby creating the volume render view, making it possible to look deeper into the data set.

This *volume render* effect may in particular be dramatic if a number of vowels inside an acquired 3D data set are produced from scanning hypo echoic structures. A good example is the use of this technique to assess hypo echoic prostate lesions. Voxel values behind, for example, a strongly reflective interface will also result in the illusion of looking into a semitransparent dark cavity in the anatomy.

It is also possible to apply other render mode projections:

Maximum Intensity Projection (MIP) tries to find the brightest or most significant color or intensity along a ray path.

Transparent modes allow the separation of color and intensity data and selective control of the transparency of the two components. Using this method, it is possible to reduce the intensity of the gray scale voxels so that they appear as a light fog over the color information. Color information hidden behind an obstruction can then be made visible.

Furthermore, and possibly more important, acquired 3D data sets open up for completely new postprocessing techniques where, for example, the data block can be made opaque, resulting in additional depth information.

3D acquisitions give access to a new, wider range of viewing planes that are unavailable with 2D scanning. 3D ultrasonography reconstructs a "volume" from 2D scans. This volume can be analyzed using viewing in scan planes not accessible by 2D ultrasound – for example, the new coronal view of the prostate. 3D ultrasonography permits quantitative examinations and excellent measurement capabilities.

A major advantage of working with the 3D system is that images used for diagnosis are totally reproducible. Using the original electronic data, images can be reviewed as many times as needed.

The Specific Benefits of 3D Ultrasonography of the Prostate

3D ultrasonography enables a simultaneous view of the sagittal, transverse, and – particularly important – coronal planes. By providing such variety of different views of the prostate, urologists get an invaluable tool for diagnostics with 3D imaging. They can more easily distinguish the zones of the prostate and see small lesions.

3D prostate imaging makes spatial relationships much clearer, so urologists can better assess the extent of disease. It also provides information that can be valuable for selecting patients for alternative therapies, for example external beam radiation or prostatectomy/radioactive seed implantation. In particular, it may be easier to determine whether the "prostatic capsule" has been penetrated, a key factor in tumor staging. The 3D data set is acquired in a precise, controlled manner, and can be evaluated at any depth, plane, or angle. It can easily be saved for interpretation off-line.

The 3D acquisition is performed using a precision motorized device, and a much higher number of images are interpreted for the total image reconstruction (typically several hundred). This technique has resulted in a much improved spatial resolution.

The 3D volume is constructed from the sequence of acquired images using interactive 3D software built into a 2D ultrasound system. The software allows the 3D image to be sliced in any orientation as well as rotated in any direction. The display software allows up to three surfaces of the prostate to be viewed simultaneously in a 3D volume rendering. Visualization of lesions in three planes appears to allow improved assessment of extracapsular extension. The 3D image is formed with the coronal in addition to the standard sagittal and axial planes, which means that instead of a single transverse or sagittal scan section of the prostate, as seen with 2D transrectal ultrasonography, the 3D images provide an added surface to be visualized. This surface could be the lateral, posterior, anterior, superior, or inferior surface of the prostate, or a through section of the gland where the posterior surface of the prostate shows tumor infiltration beyond the periprostatic fat.

Examples of 3D Ultrasonography of the Prostate

See Figs. 11.11 and 11.12

3D views of a prostatic carcinoma. By manipulating the data, views can be obtained, where capsular penetration is demonstrated. By means of 3D manipulation of the data obtained views

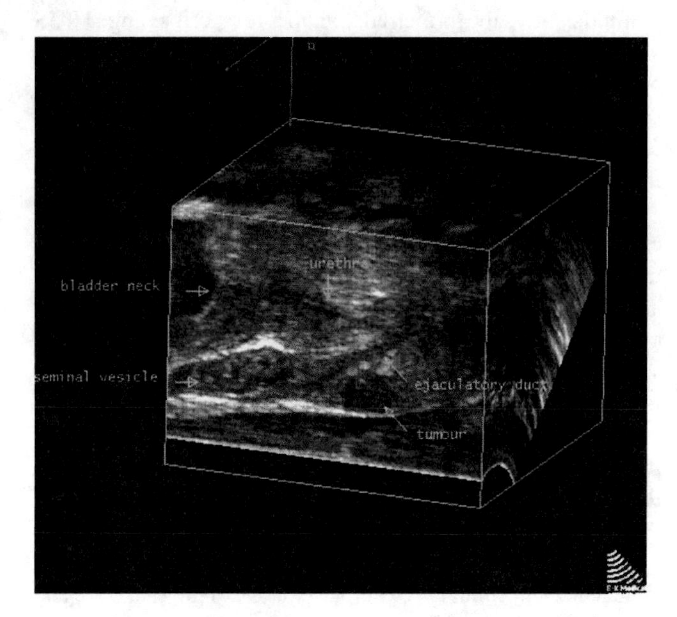

Fig. 11.11. Adjusting the plane and viewing angle of the 3D datas proved the lesion to be penetrating the prostate capsule a fact not seen during the 2D prostate scan

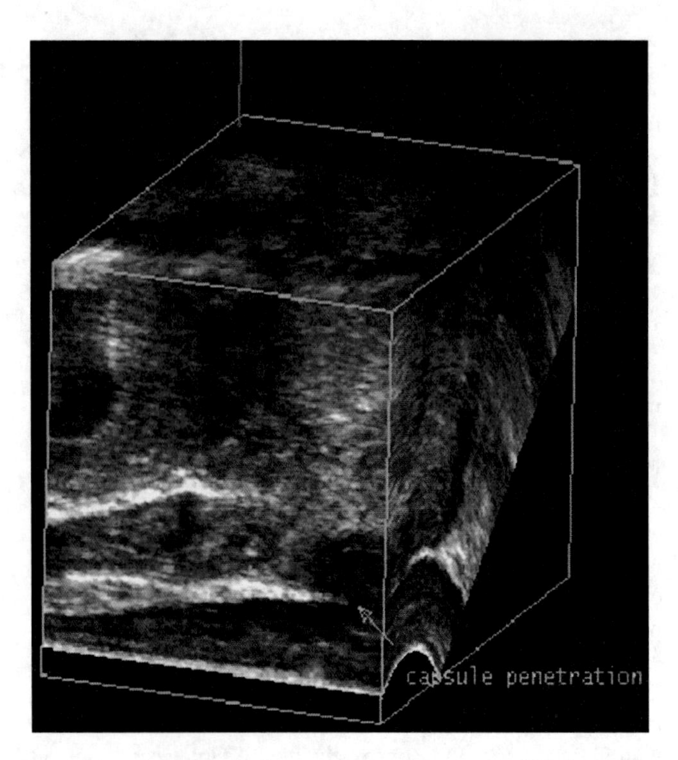

FIG. 11.12. From the 3D image of the prostate a small lesion of the peripheral zone seems not to be penetrating the capsule. This was also the conclusion from the prior 2D prostate scan

not possible to obtain by 2D scannings, e.g., coronal views can be used to obtain additional diagnostic information.

Recent Developments in Transducer-Design for TRUS

Until recently, the preferred method for performing TRUS was either to use an endfire transducer for prostate scanning, or to use the biplanar approach for the scanning. Different scan planes can be visualized using both methods, but until a few years ago none of the scanning methods could visualize more than one scan plane at a time.

A one-plane view of the prostate can make it difficult to carry out a precise biopsy regimen because you can't be certain that you are sampling from the intended targets. This applies particularly when you are attempting to use a strategy of placing some biopsies in very lateral positions. Some recent scientific publications have stated that such a strategy seems to lead to better efficiency for detecting the cancer.

Particularly in patients with the peripheral zone compressed due to BPH, it can be very difficult to be certain that the needle is hitting the intended target in the lateral part of the peripheral zone.

A few years ago a new kind of TRUS transducer made it possible to scan in simultaneous biplane, i.e., scan in transverse and sagittal planes at the same time. Based on the isocenter idea – that the design must make the needle echo visible in both planes in one point (the isocenter) – this concept makes it possible to make sure of the exact placement of the needles (Figs. 11.13–11.15).

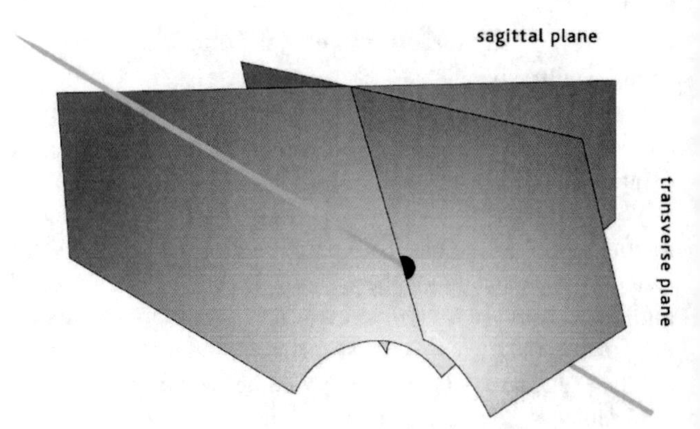

FIG. 11.13. The two simultaneous image planes of the simultaneous biplane transducer. Both image planes are projected nearly perpendicular to the longitudinal axis of the transducer. The transducer is manufactured with a forward tilt of both arrays for better patient tolerance, as the depth of introduction into the *ampulla recti* is correspondingly less

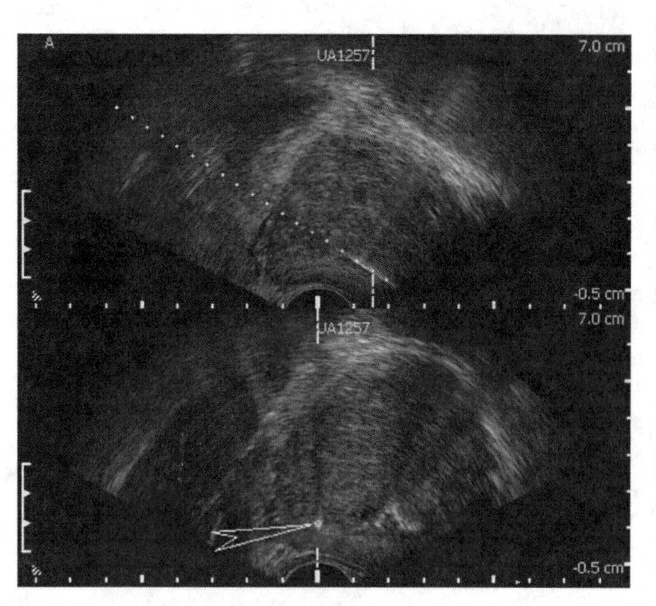

FIG. 11.14. Targeting the right lateral peripheral zone of the prostate ultrasonically guided precision biopsy. The *arrow* on the transverse (*lower*) image points to the marker that indicates the projection of the needle path in the perpendicularly opposite image plane, the sagittal (*upper*) image. Note that this target is exactly in the lateral peripheral zone. Many urologists consider biopsies of this area difficult if they are only based on the sagittal image

The simultaneous biplane view makes it possible to target the areas you intend for biopsies more correctly and with great precision. The combined transverse and sagittal views make it possible for you to see exactly where and how deeply your biopsy needles are placed.

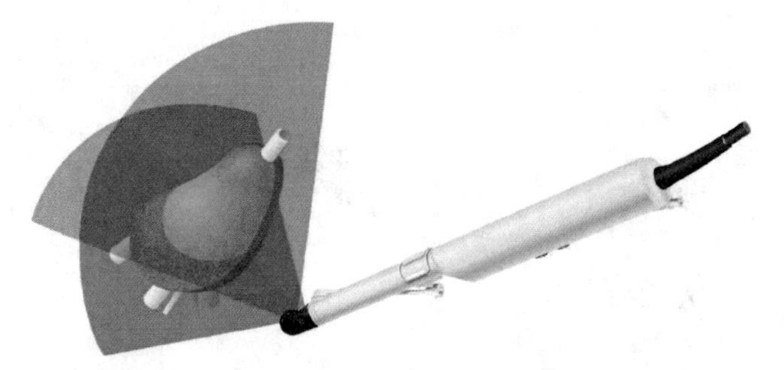

FIG. 11.15. An illustration of the two simultaneous scan planes for scanning the prostate

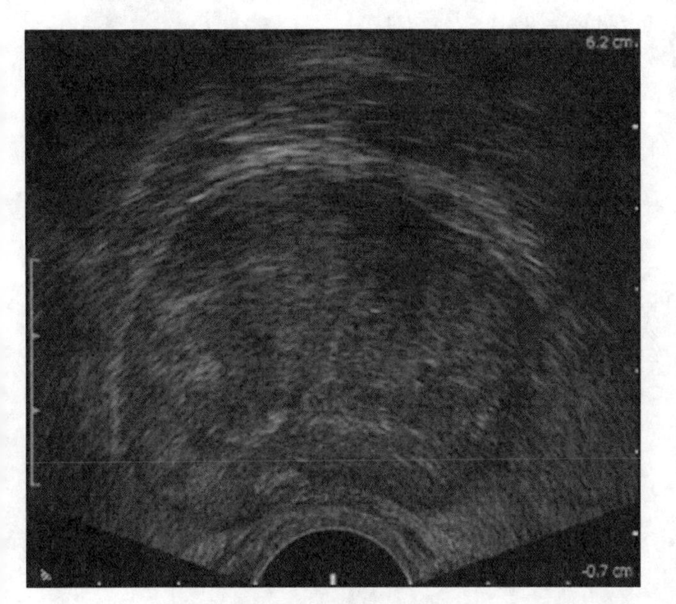

FIG. 11.16. Transverse image of large prostate

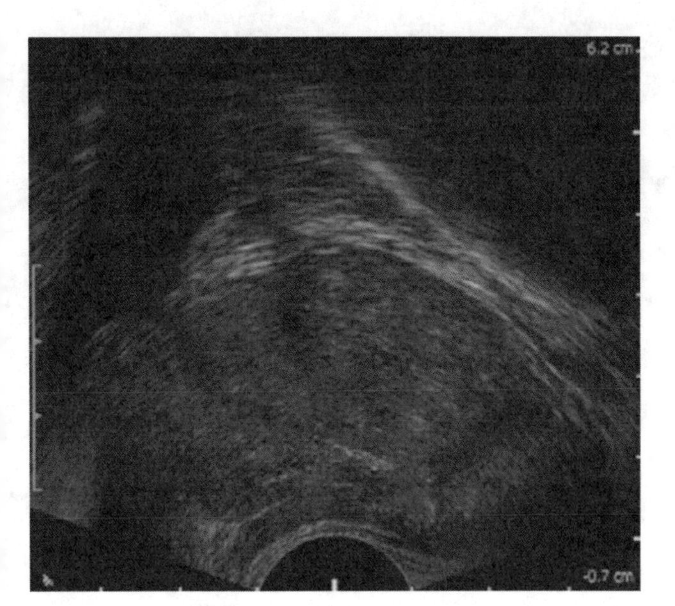

FIG. 11.17. Sagittal image of a large prostate

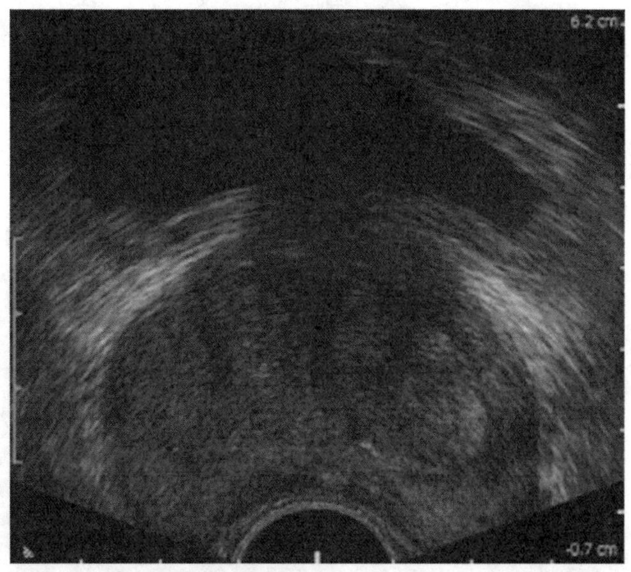

FIG. 11.18. Endfire image of a large prostate

Simultaneous biplane is particularly valuable for targeting more lateral biopsies of the peripheral zone with greater precision because the peripheral zone, certainly in elderly patients with BPH, becomes very thin and difficult to target.

A real-time transverse image together with a real-time sagittal one provides a clear indication that the needle is in the intended area, for quicker and more accurate biopsies.

In some patients, however, simultaneous biplane has some limitations for biopsies in the apical part of the prostate. The biopsy regimen should include biopsies that are from the left and right apical part of the prostate, yet still close to the parasagittal plane.

Endfire imaging, although offering less confidence for the precise placement of the lateral biopsies, is ideal for taking apical biopsies, because the biopsy guide for endfire imaging is placed immediately behind the imaging array.

Thus the ideal transducer for biopsies close to the prostate apex seems to be an endfire type. The ideal transducer for placing lateral peripheral zone biopsies is the simultaneous biplane transducer. By combining the two concepts: real-time simultaneous imaging and the biopsy route through the midcentral transducer finger – and the endfire guidance of the biopsy route, the biopsy technique remains optimal for all individual biopsies of the prostate.

One transducer, using one dual biopsy guide and one insertion, combines the best from endfire scanning with simultaneous biplane scanning.

This scan technique for TRUS combines simultaneous biplane scanning and biopsy with endfire imaging and biopsy in the same transducer. One insertion of the transducer combines the best from endfire scanning with the best from simultaneous biplane scanning.

This new technical development makes it possible to take biopsies in all sections of the prostate with excellent orientation and confidence (Figs. 11.16–11.19).

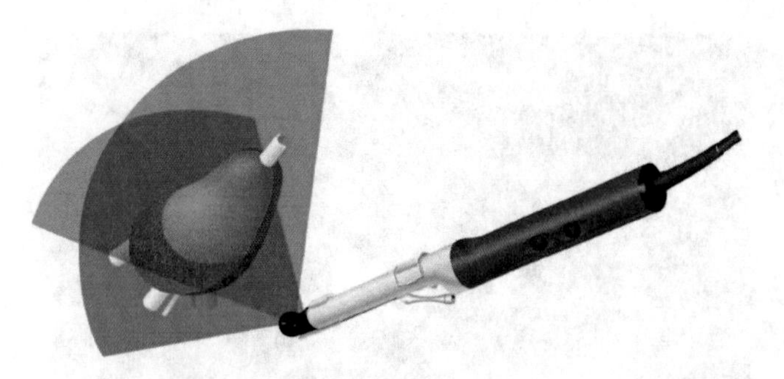

Fig. 11.19. Illustration of the two scan planes when the transducer is used in simultaneous biplane mode

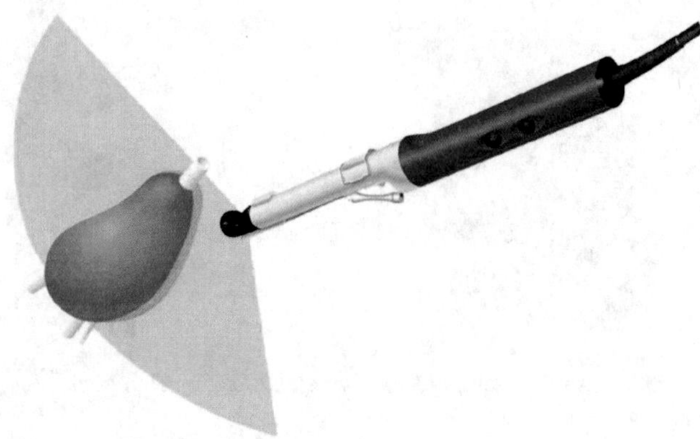

Fig. 11.20. Illustration of the scan plane when the transducer is used in endfire mode

Chapter 12
Contrast-Enhanced Ultrasound for the Prostate

N. Wondergem and J.J.M.C.H. de la Rosette

Introduction

Imaging of the prostate can be performed using different imaging techniques and has several applications in the evaluation of benign and malignant prostate diseases. Many imaging techniques are used to detect and follow up abnormalities of the prostate such as prostatitis, abscesses, benign prostate hyperplasia, and prostate cancer, or to investigate symptoms that can be caused by the prostate such as hemospermia or male lower urinary tract symptoms (LUTS). Other utilities of prostate imaging are guidance of prostate biopsies or to support prostate cancer treatment using image-guided therapy.

One of the most important applications for imaging of the prostate is the detection and staging of prostate cancer. The incidence of prostate cancer is globally increasing, and different disease stages of prostate cancer require different treatment modalities.[1] In 2007, an estimated 220,000 new prostate cancer cases will occur, and it will be the second leading cause of cancer death for men in the United States.[2] To prevent under- or overtreatment as a consequence of incorrect staging, an accurate detection-staging cascade is necessary. Consequently an accurate detection-staging cascade will improve patient selection for the different existing treatment modalities resulting in better treatment outcomes. Sensitivity and specificity of the existing imaging techniques used to date to detect prostate cancer is low. Transrectal ultrasonography (TRUS) of the prostate is the most widely used technique for imaging of the prostate to detect cancer. Even in combination with digital rectal examination and prostate biopsies, however, the sensitivity of TRUS in detecting prostate cancer is low. Sextant transrectal ultrasound-guided biopsies are reported to have a sensitivity of 50–85% in the detection of prostate cancer.[3] O'Dowd et al. found that 26% of men with initial biopsies negative for prostate cancer showed positive biopsies for prostate cancer within 1 year after the first series.[4] That is why *the search for more sensitive and specific imaging techniques for prostate cancer continues*.

The latest development in the detection and staging of prostate cancer is perfusion imaging of the prostate. Tumor growth is associated with angiogenesis, increased vascularity, and abnormal blood flow patterns because of an increased need of oxygen and nutrients due to expansive growth of malignant tissue.[5] Perfusion imaging is able to visualize these hemodynamic properties. This chapter is dedicated to the application of contrast-enhanced ultrasound of the prostate to improve detection, monitoring, treatment, and follow up of prostate cancer. We will address the following questions: What is the contribution of contrast-enhanced ultrasound for the detection and staging of prostate cancer? Can CEUS support the existing imaging modalities and what will future developments bring?

Prostate Cancer Imaging

Ultrasonography

Transrectal grayscale ultrasonography (TRUS) of the prostate is the most widely used technique for imaging of the prostate with its seminal vesicles and vas deferens. TRUS was initially used as a technique to evaluate rectal abnormalities, but in 1963 Takahashi et al. were the first to use this technique for evaluation of the prostate.[6] Nevertheless it lasted until 1971 before Watanabe et al. introduced and improved TRUS as a clinical application for the evaluation of the prostate.[7,8] Today TRUS for imaging of the prostate is a standard and widely used procedure to detect abnormalities of the prostate, guide prostate needle biopsies, and measure prostate volume. The best formula to estimate prostate volume is a combination of the prolate spheroid formula using the transverse diameter as the major axis and the anterioposterior diameter as the minor axis. The formula is expressed as p/6 (transverse diameter)^2 (anterioposterior diameter).[9] There is a considerable variation in repeated measurements of prostatic volume, and the variation is greatest for two observers compared to one observer.[10]

TRUS is universally used as the initial investigation in case of suspicion for prostate cancer and to guide needle biopsies of the prostate. Prostate cancer does not present as a solitary round mass, but is known to be a multifocal disease and that is what makes diagnosing prostate cancer difficult. TRUS turned

O. Ukimura and I.S. Gill (eds.), *Contemporary Interventional Ultrasonography in Urology*,
DOI: 10.1007/978-1-84800-217-3_12,

out to be more accurate to detect cancers greater than 0.2 cc in volume and located in the peripheral zone, but sensitivity and specificity remain low.[11] At least one-quarter of the prostate carcinomas is isoechoic, and consequently not all tumors are identified on TRUS.

Since the introduction of ultrasound-guided sextant biopsies as a standard technique in 1989 by Hodge et al., detection of prostate cancer improved significantly.[12] But even a combination of TRUS with needle-guided prostate biopsies has a low sensitivity of 50–85% in detecting prostate cancer.[3] Up to 56% of carcinomas are found in areas that appeared normal on TRUS and hypoechoic lesions have a 17–57% chance of being malignant.[13] However, it remains important to take biopsies of a prostatic lesion identified by TRUS because prostatic lesions are almost twice as likely to show cancer compared to normal areas of the prostate. These cancers are of higher grade and volume and more clinically significant.[14,15]

We can conclude that sensitivity and specificity of TRUS alone or in combination with biopsies to detect prostate cancer are low. TRUS alone lacks distinguishing benign from malignant tissue, and prostate biopsies often miss the cancer because cancer foci may be small and spread throughout the prostate.

TRUS of the prostate has multiple clinical supporting applications. Ukimura et al. used real-time intraoperative TRUS guidance during laparoscopic radical prostatectomy to enhance intraoperative surgical precision and improve functional and oncological outcomes.[16–18] In 1993 Onik et al. were the first to use TRUS to guide percutaneous radical cryosurgical ablation of the prostate and monitor the whole treatment.[19] Gelet et al. used TRUS for a high-intensity focused ultrasound (HIFU) experiment on benign prostatic hypertrophy.[20] Currently TRUS is also used to support HIFU treatment for prostate cancer.[21] Wallner et al. described TRUS as a technique for verification of proper needle placement in the prostate at the time of I-125 seed implantation.[22]

Color and Power Doppler Ultrasonography

Sensitivity and specificity of TRUS can be improved by using color or power Doppler ultrasound. The technique of both methods differs, but both use ultrasound waves reflected from moving objects (red blood cells) to detect abnormal vascularity of the prostate. Rifkin et al. found three different flow patterns using color Doppler that may be associated with prostate cancer: diffuse flow, focal flow, and surrounding flow. Up to 85% of men with prostate cancers greater than 5 mm in size have visible increased flow in the area of tumor involvement.[23]

Power Doppler allows comparison of the vascular anatomy of the normal prostate with that of a prostate with diseases such as prostate cancer and benign prostatic hyperplasia.[24] Malignant tissue generally grows faster and more irregular with an altered and increased blood flow, and hypervascularity correlates with increased Gleason score.[25]

Doppler imaging has significant limitations because benign lesions and inflammatory foci also can cause hypervascularity. Although some authors claim that Doppler has a high negative predictive value and may help to reduce the number of unnecessary biopsies, Halpern et al. concluded that grayscale and Doppler ultrasonography fail to identify many malignant lesions found on sextant biopsy. Therefore a strategy that relies on a limited number of Doppler-targeted biopsies will miss some malignant lesions.[26,27]

Color and power Doppler ultrasonography increase the sensitivity of TRUS, but cannot avoid the necessity of random biopsies. As a result we can say that Doppler ultrasound imaging can be useful in addition to conventional grayscale TRUS, but both sensitivity and specificity are low.

Three-Dimensional Ultrasonography

Three-dimensional transrectal ultrasound (3D-US) enables the physician to interpret the aspect of the prostate in every desired direction and view the images in sagittal, transverse, and coronal planes simultaneously. Volume measurement with 3D-US has lower variability and higher reliability than conventional 2D ultrasound, but it is hard to make it clinically applicable because it is labor intensive and time consuming.[28] 3D-US is a good technique to image the transitional zone in case of benign prostate hyperplasia.[29] In the detection of prostate cancer 3D-US has an increased sensitivity compared to conventional 2D imaging.[30] This does not result in significant clinical improvement of prostate cancer detection and staging, because specificity decreased.

Elastography

Elastography or strain imaging is based on external tissue compression and was first described by Ophir et al.[31] It is a method for quantitative imaging of strain and elastic modules distributions in soft tissues and is used for the detection of prostate cancer.

Elastography is based on the fact that malignant tissue is less compressible than benign prostate tissue. Therefore it is important that real-time elastography should always be interpreted in combination with conventional ultrasound because harder tissue caused by prostatolithiasis, benign nodes, or prostatitis can lead to pathologic elastograms.

König et al. used real-time elastography in combination with conventional ultrasound. In 127 of 151 cases (84.1%) prostate cancer was detected, and they concluded that it is possible to detect prostate cancer with a high degree of sensitivity using real-time elastography as an additional diagnostic tool.[32] Cochlin et al. demonstrated that adding elastography to conventional ultrasound has real clinical value. Taking targeted biopsies from abnormal prostate areas detected by elastography, in combination with conventional ultrasound-guided biopsies, improved prostate cancer detection.[33] Elastography detects a lot of prostatic cancers, but sensitivity of elastography alone is not enough to replace grayscale imaging.

Cross-Sectional Imaging

(Endorectal) magnetic resonance imaging (MRI) does not play a role in the detection of prostate cancer. Wefer et al. found that endorectal MRI can detect just as much prostate cancers as sextant biopsies, but the additional value is not clear yet because prostate biopsies are still required for confirmation and grading.[34] Sensitivity is low for small prostate cancer foci because MRI is unable to visualize microscopic disease.[35] Recent studies showed promising outcomes claiming that dynamic contrast-enhanced MRI can identify early-stage prostate carcinoma with high sensitivity and specificity.[36] Currently, the major clinical indication for MRI is the detection of extracapsular extension and seminal vesicle invasion. MRI is a promising and useful technique for local staging of prostate cancer but reproducibility, interobserver variability, and high costs play an important role.

Computer tomography (CT) has no clinical value in the local staging of prostate cancer. CT does not show tumor in the prostate, cannot define margins with any great accuracy, and overestimates the prostate volume. CT can be used for staging of pelvic and distant metastases, but should not be used as a routine investigation before radical prostatectomy because sensitivity is low.[37]

Scintigraphy and positron emission tomography (PET) only play a role in detecting local recurrence after treatment, or in advanced disease to determine the amount of metastases.[38]

Contrast-Enhanced Ultrasonography

Contrast Agents

Contrast-enhanced ultrasonogaphy (CEUS) was first used in echocardiography after a coincidental finding of ultrasound signal increase caused by small bubbles formed at a catheter tip.[39] CEUS uses gas-filled microbubbles that are administered intravenously to the circulation as a bolus, or constantly by means of an infusion pump to reach a steady state. Depending on the kind of contrast agent, stabilizing shells consist of denaturated albumin, surfactants, or phospholipids. The gasses consist of air or perfluoro gas.[40] Microbubbles with heavy gas cores are likely to last longer in circulation because heavy gasses are less water soluble. Because of their stabilizing shell the microbubbles can withstand hydrostatic pressure within the vascular system and acoustic pressure from the ultrasound wave. As a result they remain stable passing the pulmonary capillaries without being excreted. The encapsulated gas bubbles, varying in size from 1 to 4 mm, remain in the blood pool for a few minutes until they dissolve. Their size makes them smaller than erythrocytes, which allows them to move through the microcirculation without difficulty.

Contrary to contrast agents used for CT and MRI that diffuse into the tissue, microbubble contrast agents remain intravascular as blood-pool markers of the microcirculation. (Abnormal) Blood perfusion of the target organ (micro) circulation can be visualized. Microvessels originating from malignant lesions can be visualized by the intense reflected signal from the microbubbles. Microbubble destruction, caused by an increased mechanical index of the ultrasound beam, is used for a total depletion of contrast microbubbles in the targeted imaging area. Imaging the inflow of new contrast microbubbles after the destruction may reveal aberrant flow patterns correlated to prostate cancer.

Safety

Several papers have been published concerning the safety of ultrasound contrast agents.[41–43] Adverse events with ultrasound contrast agents are usually minor, rare, and transient. Complications like nephrotoxicity, which can occur with iodine-containing contrast media in use for CT or the gadolinium chelates used in MRI, have never been reported. After use in thousands of patients the most frequently reported side-effects of microbubble contrast agents are headache, altered taste, local pain at the injection side, a warm facial sensation, and a general flush.[43] Controlled studies revealed that the symptoms may not be related to the ultrasound contrast agents because they have also been observed in the placebo-controlled groups. No cases of an allergic reaction have been reported to date, but a single case of general flush with erythema and papules has been observed. Generalized allergy-like or hypersensitivity reactions occur only rarely.

Because the gaseous content of the microbubble agents is eliminated by the lungs, it is of importance to evaluate whether impaired pulmonary function could be a contraindication for the use of microbubbles. In a study with Sonovue (Bracco) in patients with Chronic Obstructive Pulmonary Disease, CEUS appeared to be as safe and well tolerated as in a healthy control group.[44]

Theoretically there is an improved risk of biochemical effects, such as cavitation. In the expansion part of the ultrasound cycle, dissolved gas in fluids can form cavities in the form of gas bubbles. This “acoustic cavitation” is only described in in vitro situations and never in human blood. Other in vitro studies also showed that CEUS can cause hemolysis and platelet aggregation, but this has never been seen in humans. Animal studies showed myocardial ischemia, which was not associated with histopathological evidence of myocardial damage, and several sorts of arrhythmias.[42] These effects were seen after direct echocardiography with a high mechanical index. Recently, some cardiac events occurred in patients previously known with severe heart problems after use of Sonovue. Although relationship with the injection of the contrast agent cannot be proven, the use of this microbubble agent has since been restricted to noncardiac imaging and patients without serious cardiac morbidity.

In 2004 general safety guidelines for the use of ultrasound contrast agents were published.[45] One should remember that ultrasound contrast agents are new products and that it may take several years of accurate surveillance to document possible adverse reactions. Significant differences in safety between the different contrast agents have not been published.

Technique

Different techniques are used for contrast-enhanced ultrasonography. The first contrast-enhanced ultrasound images were made with regular B-mode ultrasound.[39] Sensitivity of this B-mode ultrasound was improved with Doppler technique. The imaging technique used to date is based on the nonlinear behavior of the microbubble contrast agents: Harmonic imaging. The effect of this technique depends on the fact that encapsulated gasses are compressible unlike normal tissue resulting in altered ultrasound frequencies. The nonlinear behavior of the microbubbles is used to emphasize the difference between tissue and contrast.

With harmonic imaging the signal returned from the body includes not only the initial transmitted ultrasound frequency coming from tissue (like conventional ultrasonography) but also a harmonic frequency which is twice the initial frequency (coming from contrast microbubbles). Because of acoustic impedance the pulse transmitted by the ultrasound probe bounces off the interface between the bubble and surrounding tissue with the initial frequency (as in conventional ultrasonography). As a result of the shock from the ultrasound pulse the bubble starts vibrating, generating a harmonic signal twice the frequency of the initial ultrasound pulse. Only the signals returning from the body with twice the initial frequency are coming from places where the microbubbles are located. Microvessels, originating from malignant lesions, may be visualized by the intense reflected signal from the microbubbles within the vessels. Harmonic imaging provides image information in three configurations: tissue-only, contrast agent-only, or tissue in combination with contrast agent. *This makes simultaneous viewing of tissue-only and contrast-only images possible.*

Applications

CEUS has been evaluated for many indications. The main field in which CEUS has been used is echocardiography for the evaluation of left ventricular function and assessment of myocardial perfusion.[46] CEUS is the dynamic imaging modality of choice for the diagnosis and characterization of hepatocellular carcinoma and other liver lesions, and it can be used for monitoring of ablative therapies of liver masses.[47,48] Several studies describe the use of CEUS to evaluate tumor angiogenesis in breast lesions and to establish the response of breast cancer therapy.[49,50] Other applications are imaging of acute cerebrovascular disease, sentinel lymph node detection, assessment of splenic abnormalities, and abdominal trauma.[51–54] Applications of CEUS in diagnosis, treatment, and follow up of renal diseases are discussed in the next chapter of this book.

Contrast-Enhanced Ultrasonography of the Prostate

Detection of Prostate Cancer

CEUS of the prostate detects lesions that cannot be seen on grayscale ultrasound or found with systemic biopsies, because *CEUS allows the assessment of angiogenesis, increased vascularity, and abnormal blood flow associated with prostate cancer.*[55]

Sedelaar et al. correlated images, obtained by CEUS in 70 patients with biopsy-proven prostate cancer, to the histopathological outcomes of their radical prostatectomies.[56] Their purpose was to determine the characteristics of malignant lesions on CEUS. The results indicated that the detection of prostate tumors with a maximum diameter >5 mm varied between 68 and 79%, depending on the interobserver differences. Of the tumors <5 mm an average of 31% was detected. CEUS was found to improve the sensitivity of detecting malignant tissue in a group of prostate cancer patients. Other studies showed that CEUS has the potential to visualize lesions with increased microvessel density, which seems to be associated with higher grade prostate cancer.[57] Goossen et al. demonstrated that time enhancement curves, derived from the CEUS signal, can localize prostate cancer most accurately in either the right or the left lobe using the minimal time to peak.[58] They could not discriminate between malignancies in either the dorsal or ventral side of the prostate because of anatomical differences between dorsal and ventral areas of the prostate.

Better visualization of prostate cancer with CEUS will increase diagnostic accuracy because biopsies can be taken targeted instead of randomly. CEUS-guided targeted biopsies may detect a larger number of prostate cancers with fewer needle biopsy cores, compared to grayscale ultrasound-guided biopsies. Using CEUS, Frauscher et al. detected the same amount of cancers, with higher Gleason scores, with almost fewer than half the number of biopsies compared to conventional grayscale ultrasound-guided systematic core biopsies. The detection rate for targeted biopsies (10.4%) was significantly better than for systemic biopsies (5.3%). It was concluded that CEUS-targeted biopsies is a reasonable approach for detecting a greater number of clinically significant cancers, decreasing the number of prostate biopsies.[59,60] Halpern et al. found a significant improvement in sensitivity from 38 to 65% in detecting prostate cancer using CEUS. Sextant biopsies were scored prospectively as benign or malignant with grayscale imaging and again for CEUS. Specificity was similar for both conventional grayscale ultrasound and CEUS.[61] Roy et al. proposed to use CEUS for repeat biopsies in patients after a first negative routine biopsy protocol because CEUS improves the positive biopsy rate of prostate cancer with directed core biopsies.[62]

Doppler ultrasound can be used to enhance the contrast signal. Adding microbubble contrast agents to three-dimensional power Doppler imaging offers an increased detection of prostate cancer. Sensitivity increased from 38 to 85% using microbubble contrast agents during needle-guided prostate biopsies. Specificity did not change.[63]

Our clinic is investigating the role of CEUS of the prostate in the detection of prostate cancer and follow up after treatment. Figure 12.1 shows a contrast-enhanced ultrasound image of a prostate in a man with biopsy-proven prostate cancer in combination with histology of the resected prostate. Abnormalities of the blood flow detected with CEUS correspond to the cancer foci in the prostate seen on histology. Figure 12.2 shows grayscale, color Doppler, and contrast-enhanced ultrasound images of a prostate with a large tumor on the right side.

Support of Prostate Cancer Treatment

Like conventional grayscale imaging, *CEUS can support treatment of prostate cancer*. CEUS has a higher sensitivity in detecting prostate cancer, resulting in a higher certainty to predict where and how extensive the tumor is. This information can be used to determine the right treatment modality or to support treatment. One could decide to spare one neurovascular bundle on the side without aberrant vascularity on CEUS, assuming there is no malignant tissue on that site. In case of suspicion of capsular invasion based on CEUS, one could decide to resect or freeze the prostate more radically. Figure 12.3 shows a CEUS image of a prostate in a man with biopsy-proven prostate cancer in combination with histology of the resected prostate. Based on CEUS there was a suspicion of extraprostatic growth, confirmed by histology of the resected prostate.

With radiotherapy it is possible to increase the radiation dose on the areas of the prostate with aberrant vascularity, correlated to malignancy. Zaider et al. used magnetic resonance spectroscopic imaging (MRSI) to optimize dose distributions for permanent I^{125} seed implantation.[64] They increased the radiation dose on those places where intraprostatic lesions were seen. Calculation of the tumor control probability showed a minimum increase of 25% compared to the standard treatment

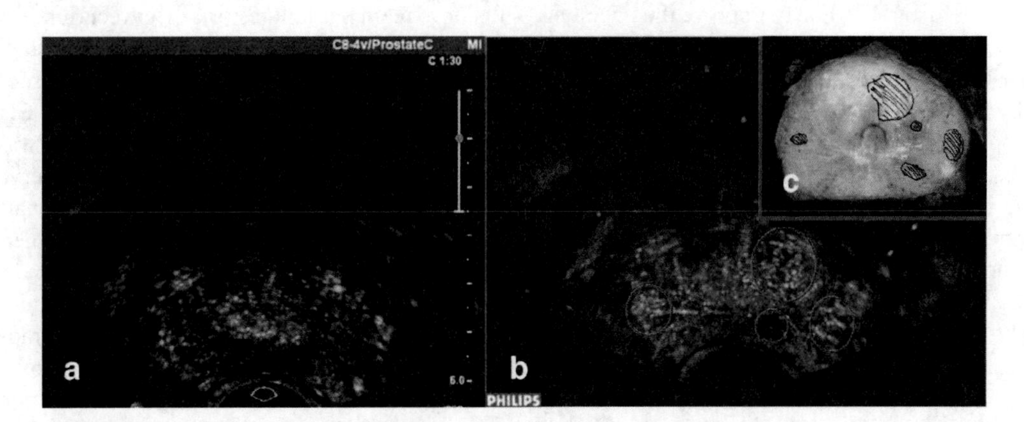

FIG. 12.1. A contrast-enhanced ultrasound (CEUS) image of a prostate in a man with biopsy-proven prostate cancer. Conventional grayscale ultrasound showed no abnormalities. Real-time CEUS showed four areas with significant abnormal vascularization suspicious for malignant tissue, corresponding to histology after prostatectomy (*colored areas* (**c**)). In contrary to the dynamic investigation, the static real-time image does not show any abnormalities (**a**). Microvessel imaging technique (**b**) suggests the four abnormal areas that were demonstrated more clearly during real-time investigation (*encircled areas*)

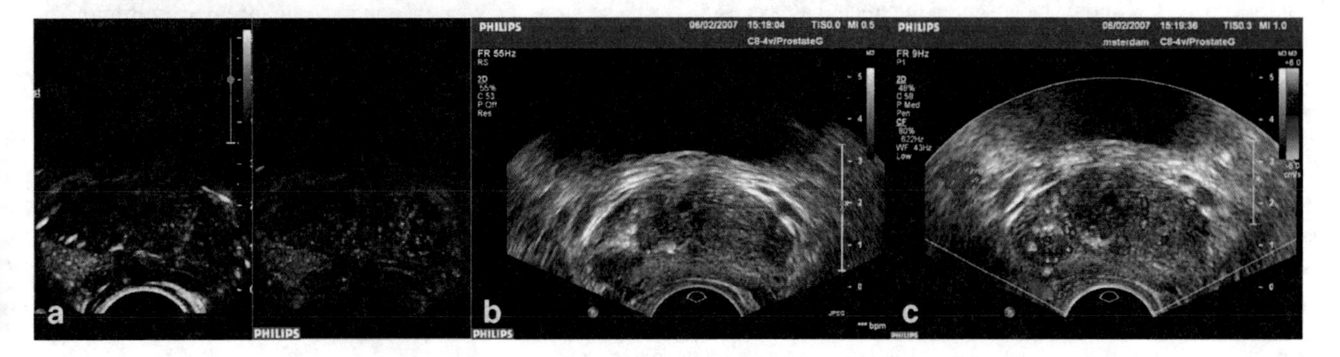

FIG. 12.2. A CEUS image of a prostate in a man with biopsy-proven prostate cancer (**a**). The right side of the prostate (*left side* of the image) shows a high amount of contrast enhancement, corresponding to malignant tissue. Conventional grayscale ultrasound shows a hypodens lesion corresponding to the lesion seen on CEUS. Color Doppler ultrasonography already showed hypervascularization of the hypodens lesion (**c**)

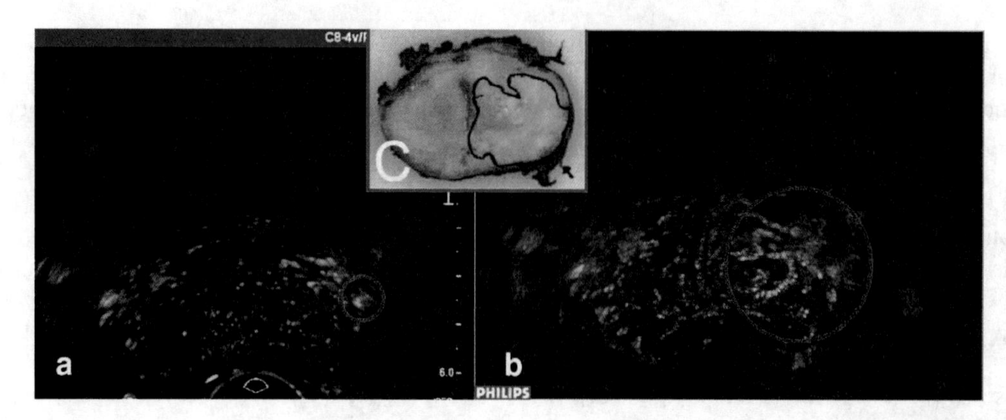

Fig. 12.3. A CEUS image of a prostate in a man with biopsy-proven prostate cancer. Conventional grayscale ultrasound showed no abnormalities. During real-time CEUS imaging an extension of abnormal vascularization beyond the prostate was seen, suspicious for extraprostatic invasion (encircled area Fig. 2a). Microvessel imaging technique showed an abnormal vascularization on the same side of the prostate, extending outside the prostate (Fig. 2b). The suspicion of a tumor extending outside the prostate was confirmed by the histology of the resected prostate (Fig. 2c)

plan. They concluded that a prostate cancer brachytherapy planning system, based on MRSI, may improve the oncological outcome for patients with organ-confined prostate cancer. As for MRSI, CEUS could support prostate cancer brachytherapy planning by detecting intraprostatic lesions. These data can be used to optimize dose distributions and improve oncological outcomes.

During active surveillance of prostate cancer CEUS can be used to image and follow up the possible tumor foci. In case of an increase in contrast enhancement during follow up, associated with more clinical significant prostate cancer, treatment can be adjusted to the new situation.

Follow up of Prostate Cancer Treatment

CEUS can be used for several purposes in the follow up of prostate cancer, using the absence of blood signals as an indicator of treatment outcomes. Both high-intensity focused ultrasound (HIFU) and cryosurgery are treatments causing ablation of tissue by very high or very low temperatures, respectively.[21] After successful prostate cancer treatment with HIFU or cryosurgery, blood flow should be absent in the treated area caused by direct thermal and indirect physiological effects of treatment. At this moment follow up after HIFU or cryotherapy is based on digital rectal examination, prostate specific antigen (PSA), and in some cases prostate biopsies to determine biochemical and pathological disease-free survival. CEUS can be used as an extra surveillance, to detect treatment failures or recurrence of prostate cancer. Sedelaar et al. consider CEUS as a promising method to determine the size of the defect after HIFU therapy for prostate carcinoma. The absence of blood flow after treatment reflected the affected tissue.[65] As for HIFU, CEUS can be used to determine the size of the affected tissue after treatment after treatment with cryotherapy. CEUS after optimal treatment will show a total absence of contrast enhancement in the prostate, meaning an absence of blood perfusion. Treatment failures or cancer recurrence will be shown by areas of contrast enhancement, corresponding to remaining vital (tumor) tissue. This way CEUS can be used as a verification of the used therapy. Figure 12.4 shows a CEUS image of a prostate, next to a conventional grayscale ultrasound image, 2 weeks after prostate cancer treatment with cryotherapy.

CEUS can be used to monitor the hormonal treatment of prostate cancer. Eckersley et al. found by means of CEUS that the vascular enhancement of the carcinoma declined with therapy, similar to PSA. The demonstrated reduction in vascularity produced by antiandrogen hormone therapy can be used to monitor therapy.[66] The same should be possible with follow up after radiotherapy treatment. Radiotherapy kills cancer cells, theoretically resulting in a reduction of vascularization of prostate cancer foci, found by means of CEUS.

The role of angiogenesis inhibitors in the treatment of cancer is increasing. Angiogenesis inhibitors put a stop to cancer angiogenesis. Monitoring of treatment can be performed by CEUS and is important to see if, and how long the patient benefits from therapy. In case of successful therapy CEUS will show a decrease of contrast enhancement in tumor foci during the use of angiogenesis inhibitors. Lamaruglia et al. used CEUS to evaluate angiogenesis inhibitors in renal cancer and concluded that it might be an effective tool for evaluating antiangiogenic drugs.[67]

Future Development

CEUS will benefit from technical improvements like three-dimensional (3D) imaging and quantification of enhancement. 3D CEUS imaging enables the assessment of the prostate in sagittal, transverse, and coronal plane simultaneously and could improve the detection of prostate cancer.

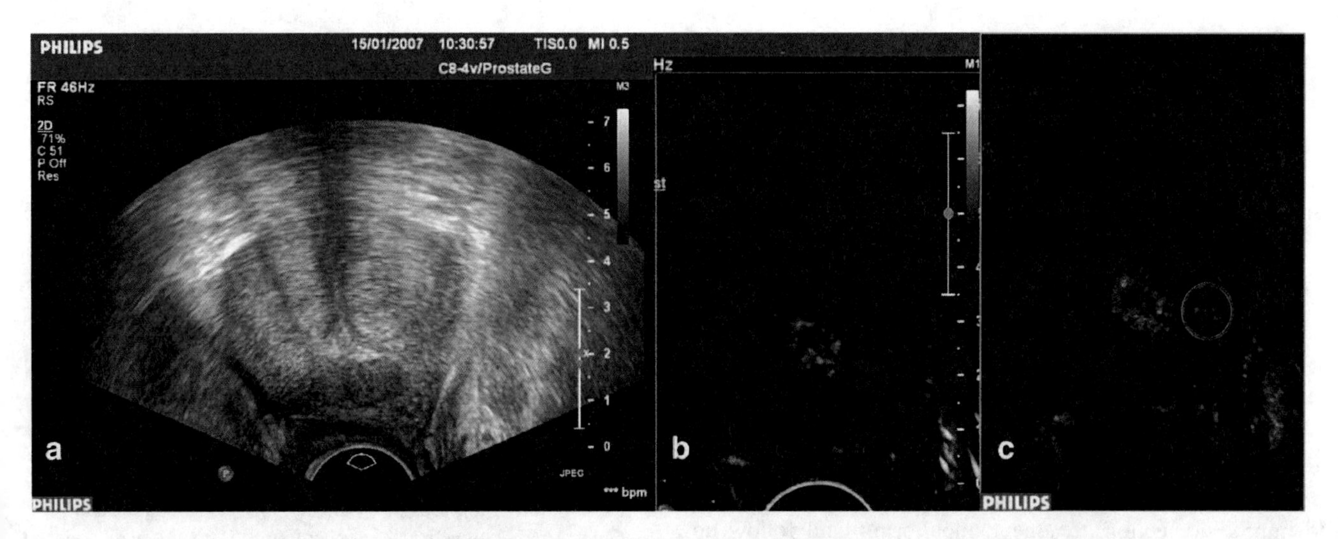

FIG. 12.4. A transrectal grayscale ultrasound (TRUS) image of a prostate, next to the CEUS image, 2 weeks after prostate cancer cryotherapy. TRUS shows no abnormalities or treatment effects (Fig. 3a). CEUS shows a complete absence of contrast enhancement, meaning an absence of blood perfusion in the prostate with its carcinoma (Fig. 3b,3c). Only the urethra, which was protected from freezing damage, shows contrast enhancement, corresponding to vital tissue. The small areas with minimal contrast enhancement (*encircled white spots*) show that total avascularity of the prostate is not reached yet after 2 weeks

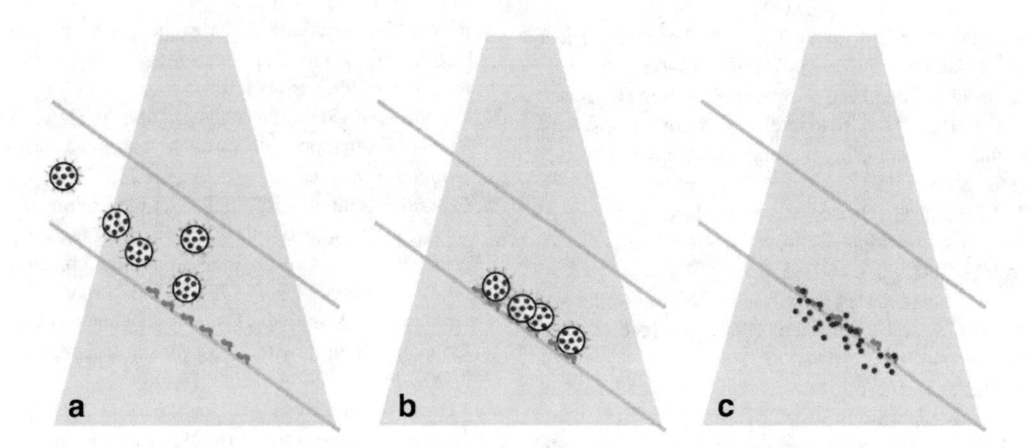

FIG. 12.5. This figure shows the mechanism of therapeutic imaging. Drug- or gene-loaded microbubbles with ligands (**a**) bind to a selected cell type (**b**). Microbubble destruction, caused by increasing the mechanical index of the ultrasound beam, releases and delivers the drug or gene at the desired place (**c**)

A computerized method for quantification of microbubbles makes an objective grading of contrast enhancement possible, to detect areas of the prostate with abnormal contrast enhancement. The development of, and search for, new ultrasound contrast agents for better reflection of ultrasound signals continues. Also new imaging techniques could improve ultrasound contrast agent detection.

The latest development in using ultrasound microbubble contrast agents is targeted and therapeutic contrast-enhanced imaging.[68,69] Therapeutic imaging uses drug- or gene-loaded microbubbles with ligands that bind to a selected cell type. Using the right ligands for the right receptor, microbubbles can be used for the delivery of any drug or genetic material, to any desired location in the body. Microbubble destruction, caused by increasing the mechanical index of the ultrasound beam, releases and delivers the drug at the desired place. Figure 12.5 shows the mechanism of therapeutic imaging.

Targeted imaging uses microbubbles with ligands that bind to a selected cell type to detect pathophysiologic conditions. Because microbubbles remain intravascular, targeted contrast-enhanced ultrasound focuses on intravascular diseases such as inflammation, thrombus formation and angiogenesis.[70] Maybe in the future targeted and therapeutic contrast-enhanced ultrasound can improve the detection and treatment of prostatic diseases.

Conclusion

CEUS imaging of the prostate is easy to perform, not time consuming and increases the visibility of abnormal microvascular blood flow correlated with malignancy. CEUS of the prostate shows promising results in cancer detection by improving sensitivity of TRUS and targeted biopsies. It can be useful in tumor staging, treatment support, monitoring of prostate cancer therapy, and discovering tumor recurrence after initial treatment.

CEUS of the prostate is a rather new imaging technique and ultrasound imaging techniques are still improving. More applications of contrast-enhanced ultrasound for the prostate are to be discovered, and more studies are necessary to determine the exact role of CEUS for prostate cancer. The aim is to improve detection, treatment, monitoring, and follow up of prostate cancer with better cancer-specific outcomes and lower patient morbidity.

References

1. Aus G, Abbou CC, Bolla M et al. EAU guidelines on prostate cancer. Eur Urol 2005; 48(4):546–551.
2. Jemal A, Siegel R, Ward E, Murray T, Xu J, Thun MJ. Cancer statistics, 2007. CA Cancer J Clin 2007; 57(1):43–66.
3. Norberg M, Egevad L, Holmberg L, Sparen P, Norlen BJ, Busch C. The sextant protocol for ultrasound-guided core biopsies of the prostate underestimates the presence of cancer. Urology 1997; 50(4):562–566.
4. O'Dowd GJ, Miller MC, Orozco R, Veltri RW. Analysis of repeated biopsy results within 1 year after a noncancer diagnosis. Urology 2000; 55(4):553–558.
5. Folkman J. How is blood vessel growth regulated in normal and neoplastic tissue? G.H.A. Clowes memorial Award lecture. Cancer Res 1986; 46(2):467–473.
6. Takahashi H, Ouchi T. The ultrasonic diagnosis in the field of urology. Proc Jpn Soc Ultrasonics Med 1963; 3:7–8.
7. Watanabe H, Kaiho H, Tanaka M, Terasawa Y. Diagnostic application of ultrasonotomography to the prostate. Invest Urol 1971; 8(5):548–559.
8. Watanabe H, Igari D, Tanahasi Y, Harada K, Saito M. Development and application of new equipment for transrectal ultrasonography. J Clin Ultrasound 1974; 2(2):91–98.
9. Terris MK, Stamey TA. Determination of prostate volume by transrectal ultrasound. J Urol 1991; 145(5):984–987.
10. Bates TS, Reynard JM, Peters TJ, Gingell JC. Determination of prostatic volume with transrectal ultrasound: A study of intra-observer and interobserver variation. J Urol 1996; 155(4):1299–1300.
11. Terris MK, Freiha FS, Mcneal JE, Stamey TA. Efficacy of transrectal ultrasound for identification of clinically undetected prostate-cancer. J Urol 1991; 146(1):78–84.
12. Hodge KK, Mcneal JE, Terris MK, Stamey TA. Random systematic versus directed ultrasound guided trans-rectal core biopsies of the prostate. J Urol 1989; 142(1):71–75.
13. Sedelaar JPM, Vijverberg PLM, de Reijke TM et-al.. Transrectal ultrasound in the diagnosis of prostate cancer: State of the art and perspectives. Eur Urol 2001; 40(3):275–284.
14. Beerlage H, de Reijke TM, De la Rosette JJMC. Considerations regarding prostate biopsies. Eur Urol 1998; 34(4):303–312.
15. Toi A, Neill MG, Lockwood GA, Sweet JM, Tammsalu LA, Fleshner NE. The continuing importance of transrectal ultrasound identification of prostatic lesions. J Urol 2007; 177(2):516–520.
16. Ukimura O, Gill IS, Desai MM et al. Real-time transrectal ultrasonography during laparoscopic radical prostatectomy. J Urol 2004; 172(1):112–118.
17. Ukimura O, Gill IS. Real-time transrectal ultrasound guidance during nerve sparing laparoscopic radical prostatectomy: Pictorial essay. J Urol 2006; 175(4):1311–1319.
18. Ukimura O, Magi-Galluzzi C, Gill IS. Real-time transrectal ultrasound guidance during laparoscopic radical prostatectomy: Impact on surgical margins. J Urol 2006; 175(4):1304–1310.
19. Onik GM, Cohen JK, Reyes GD, Rubinsky B, Chang ZH, Baust J. Transrectal ultrasound-guided percutaneous radical cryosurgical ablation of the prostate. Cancer 1993; 72(4):1291–1299.
20. Gelet A, Chapelon JY, Margonari J et al. High-intensity focused ultrasound experimentation on human benign prostatic hypertrophy. Eur Urol 1993; 23:44–47.
21. Aus G. Current status of HIFU and cryotherapy in prostate cancer – A review. Eur Urol 2006; 50(5):927–934.
22. Wallner K, Chiutsao ST, Roy J, Rosenstein M, Smith H, Fuks Z. A new device to stabilize templates for transperineal I-125 implants. Int J Radiat Oncol Biol Phys 1991; 20(5):1075–1077.
23. Rifkin MD, Sudakoff GS, Alexander AA. Prostate – Techniques, results, and potential applications of color Doppler US scanning. Radiology 1993; 186(2):509–513.
24. Leventis AK, Shariat SF, Utsunomiya T, Slawin KM. Characteristics of normal prostate vascular anatomy as displayed by power Doppler. Prostate 2001; 46(4):281–288.
25. Cornud F, Hamida K, Flam T et al. Endorectal color Doppler sonography and endorectal MR imaging features of nonpalpable prostate cancer: Correlation with radical prostatectomy findings. Am J Roentgenol 2000; 175(4):1161–1168.
26. Halpern EJ, Strup SE. Using gray-scale and color and power Doppler sonography to detect prostatic cancer. Am J Roentgenol 2000;174(3):623–627.
27. Remzi M, Dobrovits M, Reissigl A et al. Can power Doppler enhanced transrectal ultrasound guided biopsy improve prostate cancer detection on first and repeat prostate biopsy? Eur Urol 2004; 46(4):451–456.
28. Tong SD, Cardinal HN, McLoughlin RF, Downey DB, Fenster A. Intra- and inter-observer variability and reliability of prostate volume measurement via two-dimensional and three-dimensional ultrasound imaging. Ultrasound Med Biol 1998; 24(5):673–681.
29. Strasser H, Janetschek G, Reissigl A, Bartsch G. Prostate zones in three-dimensional transrectal ultrasound. Urology 1996; 47(4):485–490.
30. Sedelaar JPM, van Roermund JGH, van Leenders GLJH, Hulsbergen-van de Kaa CA, Wijkstra H, De la Rosette JJMC. Three-dimensional grayscale ultrasound: Evaluation of prostate cancer compared with benign prostatic hyperplasia. Urology 2001; 57(5):914–920.
31. Ophir J, Cespedes I, Ponnekanti H, Yazdi Y, Li X. Elastography – A quantitative method for imaging the elasticity of biological tissues. Ultrasonic Imaging 1991; 13(2):111–134.
32. Konig K, Scheipers U, Pesavento A, Lorenz A, Ermert H, Senge T. Initial experiences with real-time elastography guided biopsies of the prostate. J Urol 2005; 174(1):115–117.

33. Cochlin DL, Ganatra RH, Griffiths DFR. Elastography in the detection of prostatic cancer. Clin Radiol 2002; 57(11):1014–1020.
34. Wefer AE, Hricak H, Vigneron DB et al. Sextant localization of prostate cancer: Comparison of sextant biopsy, magnetic resonance imaging and magnetic resonance spectroscopic imaging with step section histology. J Urol 2000; 164(2):400–404.
35. Kirkham APS, Emberton M, Allen C. How good is MRI at detecting and characterising cancer within the prostate? Eur Urol 2006; 50(6):1163–1175.
36. Hara N, Okuizumi M, Koike H, Kawaguchi M, Bilim V. Dynamic contrast-enhanced magnetic resonance imaging (DCE-MRI) is a useful modality for the precise detection and staging of early prostate cancer. Prostate 2005; 62(2):140–147.
37. Flanigan RC, Mckay TC, Olson M, Shankey TV, Pyle J, Waters WB. Limited efficacy of preoperative computed tomographic scanning for the evaluation of lymph node metastasis in patients before radical prostatectomy. Urology 1996; 48(3):428–432.
38. Carey BM. Imaging for prostate cancer. Clin Oncol 2005; 17(7):553–559.
39. Gramiak R, Shah PM. Echocardiography of the aortic root. Invest Radiol 1968; 3(5):356–366.
40. Cosgrove D. Ultrasound contrast agents: An overview. Eur J Radiol 2006; 60(3):324–330.
41. Correas JM, Bridal L, Lesavre A, Mejean A, Claudon M, Helenon O. Ultrasound contrast agents: properties, principles of action, tolerance, and artifacts. Eur Radiol 2001; 11(8):1316–1328.
42. Jakobsen JA, Oyen R, Thomsen HS, Morcos SK. Safety of ultrasound contrast agents. Eur Radiol 2005; 15(5):941–945.
43. Wink MH, Wijkstra H, De la Rosette JJMC, Grimbergen CA. Ultrasound imaging and contrast agents: A safe alternative to MRI? Minim Invasive Ther Allied Technol 2006; 15(2):93–100.
44. Bokor D, Chambers JB, Rees PJ, Mant TG, Luzzani F, Spinazzi A. Clinical safety of SonoVue, a new contrast agent for ultrasound imaging, in healthy volunteers and in patients with chronic obstructive pulmonary disease. Invest Radiol 2001; 36(2): 104–109.
45. Albrecht T, Blomley M, Bolondi L, et al. Guidelines for the use of contrast agents in ultrasound. Ultraschall Med 2004; 25(4):249–256.
46. Lang RM, Mor-Avi V. Clinical utility of contrast-enhanced echocardiography. Clin Cardiol 2006; 29(9 Suppl 1):I15–I25.
47. Catalano O, Nunziata A, Lobianco R, Siani A. Real-time harmonic contrast material-specific US of focal liver lesions. Radiographics 2005; 25(2):333–349.
48. Meloni MF, Livraghi T, Filice C, Lazzaroni S, Calliada F, Perretti L. Radiofrequency ablation of liver tumors: the role of microbubble ultrasound contrast agents. Ultrasound Q 2006; 22(1):41–47.
49. Forsberg F, Goldberg BB, Merritt CRB et al. Diagnosing breast lesions with contrast-enhanced 3-dimensional power Doppler imaging. J Ultrasound Med 2004; 23(2):173–182.
50. Rizzatto G, Martegani A, Chersevani R et al. Importance of staging of breast cancer and role of contrast ultrasound. Eur Radiol 2001; 11:E47–E51.
51. Postert T, Braun B, Meves S et al. Contrast-enhanced transcranial color-coded sonography in acute hemispheric brain infarction. Stroke 1999; 30(9):1819–1826.
52. Wisner ER, Ferrara KW, Short RE, Ottoboni TB, Gabe JD, Patel D. Sentinel node detection using contrast-enhanced power Doppler ultrasound lymphography. Invest Radiol 2003; 38(6):358–365.
53. Tafuto S, Catalano O, Barba G et al. Real-time contrast-enhanced specific ultrasound in staging and follow-up of splenic lymphomas. Front Biosci 2006; 11:2224–2229.
54. Thorelius L. Contrast-enhanced ultrasound in trauma. Eur Radiol 2004; 14:43–52.
55. Pelzer A, Bektic J, Berger AP et al. Prostate cancer detection in men with prostate specific antigen 4 to 10 ng/ml using a combined approach of contrast enhanced color Doppler targeted and systematic biopsy. J Urol 2005; 173(6):1926–1929.
56. Sedelaar JPM, van Leenders GJLH, Goossen TEB et al. Value of contrast ultrasonography in the detection of significant prostate cancer: Correlation with radical prostatectomy specimens. Prostate 2002; 53(3):246–253.
57. Sedelaar JPM, van Leenders GJLH, Hulsbergen-van de Kaa CA et al. Microvessel density: Correlation between contrast ultrasonography and histology of prostate cancer. Eur Urol 2001; 40(3):285–293.
58. Goossen TEB, De la Rosette JJMC, De Kaa CAHV, van Leenders GJLH, Wijkstra H. The value of dynamic contrast enhanced power Doppler ultrasound Imaging in the localization of prostate cancer. Eur Urol 2003; 43(2):124–131.
59. Frauscher F, Klauser A, Halpern EJ, Horninger W, Bartsch G. Detection of prostate cancer with a microbubble ultrasound contrast agent. Lancet 2001; 357(9271):1849–1850.
60. Frauscher F, Klauser A, Volgger H et al. Comparison of contrast enhanced color Doppler targeted biopsy with conventional systematic biopsy: Impact on prostate cancer detection. J Urol 2002; 167(4):1648–1652.
61. Halpern EJ, Rosenberg M, Gomella LG. Prostate cancer: Contrast-enhanced US for detection. Radiology 2001; 219(1):219–225.
62. Roy C, Buy X, Lang H, Saussine C, Jacqmin D. Contrast enhanced color Doppler endorectal sonography of the prostate: Efficiency for detecting peripheral zone tumors and role for biopsy procedure. J Urol 2003; 170(1):69–72.
63. Bogers HA, Sedelaar JPM, Beerlage HP et al. Contrast-enhanced three-dimensional power Doppler angiography of the human prostate: Correlation with biopsy outcome. Urology 1999; 54(1):97–104.
64. Zaider M, Zelefsky MJ, Lee EK et al. Treatment planning for prostate implants using magnetic-resonance spectroscopy imaging. Int J Radiat Oncol Biol Phys 2000; 47(4):1085–1096.
65. Sedelaar JPM, Aarnink RG, van Leenders GJLH et al. The application of three-dimensional contrast-enhanced ultrasound to measure volume of affected tissue after HIFU treatment for localized prostate cancer. Eur Urol 2000; 37(5):559–568.
66. Eckersley RJ, Sedelaar JPM, Blomley MJK et al. Quantitative microbubble enhanced transrectal ultrasound as a tool for monitoring hormonal treatment of prostate carcinoma. Prostate 2002; 51(4):256–267.
67. Lamuraglia M, Escudier B, Chami L et al. To predict progression-free survival and overall survival in metastatic renal cancer treated with sorafenib: Pilot study using dynamic contrast-enhanced Doppler ultrasound. Eur J Cancer 2006; 42(15):2472–2479.
68. Lindner JR. Evolving applications for contrast ultrasound. Am J Cardiol 2002; 90(10A):72J–80J.
69. Weller GER, Wong MKK, Modzelewski RA et al. Ultrasonic imaging of tumor angiogenesis using contrast microbubbles targeted via the tumor-binding peptide arginine-arginine-leucine. Cancer Res 2005; 65(2):533–539.
70. Lindner JR. Molecular imaging with contrast ultrasound and targeted microbubbles. J Nucl Cardiol 2004; 11(2):215–221.

Chapter 13
Contrast-Enhanced Ultrasound of the Kidneys

Patricia Beemster, Pilar Laguna Pes, and Hessel Wijkstra

Introduction

Several imaging techniques can be used for visualization of the kidneys dependent on the indication. Ultrasound (US), computerized tomography (CT), and magnetic resonance imaging (MRI) are most commonly used. US is a safe, relatively inexpensive, noninvasive, and widely available imaging method. It is therefore often used as a screening tool, especially for nephrolithiasis, hydronephrosis, renal masses, and perirenal processes. Often, in case of an abnormal finding, a CT or MRI follows for more detailed information about the extent, the anatomical landmarks, and eventually surgical treatment planning.

US is commonly used for identification of stones and hydronephrosis. However, US does not provide optimal information about both stone size and location which are important parameters in the therapeutic decision.[1] Additional imaging with CT or intravenous urography has to be done to answer these questions. US is highly accurate in the diagnosis of hydronephrosis, with sensitivity ranging from 90 to 100% and specificity ranging from 90 to 98%.[2] It is also a good instrument to monitor the development, progression, or resolution of hydronephrosis – not only in patients with ureteral stones who are being observed, but also in the postoperative period after surgery of the urinary tract.

Cystic lesions of only a few millimeters in diameter can be detected by US, while solid renal masses are better seen when approaching 2 cm.[2] Although the differentiation between simple cysts and solid renal lesions can be made with an accuracy of approximately 98%, US fails to differentiate malignant masses from benign masses like oncocytoma or angiomyolipomas with low fat content.[2] In case of a complicated cyst or a solid mass a contrast-enhanced CT is indicated for further characterization.

US is a sensitive modality for demonstrating perirenal fluid collections, such as lymphoceles, urinomas, hematomas, and abscesses, although no differentiation can be made between the different types of fluid collections.[2]

Another important application for ultrasonography is its intraoperative use. Especially in minimally invasive nephron-sparing surgeries like laparoscopic partial nephrectomy, cryoablation, and radiofrequency ablation (RFA), laparoscopic ultrasonography is essential.[3] It allows for real-time three-dimensional visualization of the tumor and thus for better excision or better placement of cryoprobes or RFA electrodes. Also, the presence of satellite lesions may be identified.

Another more experimental treatment option for renal tumors is high-intensity focused ultrasound (HIFU). For this extracorporeal and thus noninvasive technique to ablate renal tumors gray-scale ultrasound can be used for identification and real-time targeting of the tumor.[4]

Although US certainly has its advantages over CT and MRI, it also has certain limitations. One of these limitations arises from the lack of detailed visualization of perfusion. Although Doppler US can visualize blood flow in large arteries like the renal artery and vein, perfusion of the microvasculature of the kidney parenchyma cannot be assessed by Doppler ultrasound. However, by using contrast-enhanced ultrasound (CEUS) also the blood flow in the microvasculature can be imaged.

CEUS has been evaluated for many indications. The main field in which CEUS has been used is echocardiography where it is used for evaluation of left ventricular function and assessment of myocardial perfusion.[5] CEUS is the dynamic imaging modality of choice for the diagnosis and characterization of hepatocellular carcinoma and other liver lesions, and it can be used for monitoring of ablative therapies of liver masses.[6,7] As described in the previous section, CEUS is nowadays investigated for the detection of prostate cancer and for taking targeted biopsies.

This chapter will describe the use of CEUS in diagnosis and follow up of renal diseases. Also, new developments and future perspectives are discussed.

Ultrasound Contrast

Ultrasound contrast agents consist of gas-filled microbubbles with a diameter smaller than red blood cells (~8 mm in diameter) which are injected intravenously. They act as *selective blood pool agents* and significantly increase the number of

O. Ukimura and I.S. Gill (eds.), *Contemporary Interventional Ultrasonography in Urology*,
DOI: 10.1007/978-1-84800-217-3_13,

reflectors in the vascular space, making, e.g., Doppler imaging more sensitive. Nowadays, more sensitive CEUS techniques have been developed that are capable of detecting single microbubbles. In this way, *real-time imaging of the (micro-)vasculature is possible* and makes CEUS an attractive alternative to other imaging modalities.

Contrast agents and their mechanism of action have been described in detail in the previous section. In short, the newest CEUS imaging techniques make use of so called nonlinear behavior of the injected microbubbles. In this way, the reflections of the microbubbles can be separated from the tissue reflections, and simultaneous and real-time viewing of a tissue-only and a contrast-only image is possible. With a short-lasting pulse of a high mechanical index the microbubbles can be destroyed which allows repeated and detailed real-time imaging of inflow of microbubbles.[8] With this so called destruction-replenishment imaging information about the dynamics of perfusion within a tissue can be obtained. The microbubbles used for CEUS imaging of the kidneys travel through the renal microvasculature and are not subjected to renal filtration or excretion like the iodinated contrast agents used in CT or the gadolinium chelates used in MRI. Therefore, specific information about the perfusion of the kidney can be obtained. In addition, the tolerance for ultrasound contrast agents in clinical practice is excellent and *no renal toxicity* has been reported.[8,9] The administration of contrast can be repeated even in patients with renal failure. This makes CEUS the perfect tool for renal imaging.

Diagnosis

The added value of CEUS to conventional US is detailed visualization of the renal microvasculature. *This means that CEUS can especially improve the detection of renal diseases that disrupt or alter the architecture of (small) blood vessels.*

Renal Artery Stenosis

Renal artery stenosis is the most common cause of potentially curable secondary hypertension. The use of CEUS improves the visualization of the main renal artery substantially and reduces the number of unequivocal examinations.[10] Multicenter trials have shown the accuracy in detection of renal artery stenosis with Doppler US to increase from approximately 65 to 78–84% with the use of US contrast, including patients with obesity and renal dysfunction.[10] Also, the examination can be done twice as fast and with less technical failures.[11] The follow up of the treatment of renal artery stenosis with percutaneous transluminal angioplasty can also be done with CEUS, and preliminary studies show promising results.[10]

Renal Perfusion Defects

Detection of focal renal perfusion defects can be important in the differential diagnosis of pyelonephritis, renal infarction, segmental renal artery stenosis, and intravascular thrombosis or in detecting rejection of a transplanted kidney. For this purpose CT, MRI, angiography, scintigraphy, or Doppler US can be used. Color and pulsed Doppler are sensitive means to detect significant segmental infarcts in the superficial renal cortex of the kidney. However, the diagnosis of small or distal perfusion defects remains difficult because of the lack of sensitivity, particularly when the kidney is deep, hypoperfused, or moving with breathing.[12] Several animal studies indicate that CEUS improves the detection of focal perfusion defects[12–14]; they are seen as flow defects with sharp edges and correspond closely to perfusion defects seen on angiography. In one of these studies the combination of gray-scale and contrast-enhanced Doppler US allowed the differentiation of renal ischemia from renal infarction.[13] It is critical to differentiate these two since treatment and prognosis for these conditions differ.

Renal Trauma

The published literature on the value of CEUS in renal trauma such as contusions and lacerations is very scarce. Theoretically, the presence of active hemorrhage could be confirmed by extravasation of contrast agent on ultrasonography. One study in a porcine model explored the detection of renal hemorrhage when using a contrast agent injected either intravenously (iv) or intra-arterially (ia).[15] After contrast administration, a crescent-shaped area of increased echogenicity became apparent within the perinephric space at the site of injury. Dependent on the observer, the detection improved significantly from 54 to 64% before contrast to 70–74% after ia contrast; however, there was no significant improvement after iv injection of contrast.

Ureteropelvic Junction Obstruction

Research on congenital hydronephrosis caused by obstruction of the ureteropelvic junction (UPJ) suggests that the cause may lie in a disturbance in pelvic peristalsis due to an abnormal orientation of muscle fibers at the UPJ.[16] The incidence of vessels crossing the UPJ is much greater in the population with UPJ obstruction than in the general population, and they might add to the obstruction.[16] To avoid vascular injuries during endourologic UPJ repair, preoperative detection of crossing vessels is critical.[16] Frauscher et al.[16] compared the detection of crossing vessels using color Doppler US with and without a contrast agent to the number of vessels found during laparoscopic repair. In 29 patients with a total of 26 vessels found during laparoscopy, all but one vessel were detected with CEUS, while unenhanced color Doppler US only detected 15. In addition the mean examination time was significantly decreased from 23 to 14 min using contrast. In another study, Frauscher et al. found that the postoperative assessment of the position and displacement of the crossing vessels is also possible with CEUS.[17]

Cystic Renal Masses

With the use of gray-scale US simple cysts are easily identified and do not need further evaluation or treatment. However, a complicated cyst needs to be differentiated from a malignant renal tumor. This is not always an easy task, and contrast-enhanced CT or MRI is usually required for further evaluation. US findings suggestive of a cystic or pseudocystic renal neoplasm include a thick irregular peripheral wall, mural nodule(s), multiple thick septations, and a heterogeneous thick content.[12,18,19] The diagnosis of cystic renal cell carcinoma (RCC) relies on the demonstration of vascular flow within the solid component or septa of the lesion on CT or MR imaging. Since CEUS is particularly useful for visualization of renal vasculature, this imaging technique might be especially helpful in differentiating benign from malignant complicated cysts (Fig. 13.1).

In a preliminary study of 13 complicated cysts contrast-enhanced power Doppler US showed best visualization of tumor vascularity compared with CT and conventional power Doppler US.[18] However, limitations can result from strong enhancement of the surrounding vessels or normal parenchyma that should not be confused with thick wall enhancement.[12]

Solid Renal Masses

Detection

The early detection and the characterization of solid renal masses are of great importance for their accurate diagnosis, treatment planning, and prognosis. Up to 83% of asymptomatic renal tumors are detected incidentally with the use of conventional US.[20] However, US is less sensitive than CT in detecting renal lesions <2 cm, particularly if they are endophytic and isoechogenic compared with the surrounding parenchyma.[19] Especially in these cases, contrast agents may substantially improve detection by ultrasonography. An alteration of the normal cortical thickness and renal pyramid spacing, abnormal vascular architecture, and necrotic areas are all suggestive of renal cell cancer.[19,21] Other features that can be indicative of tumor are a heterogeneous enhancement pattern, and a different speed of uptake and vascular washout of the contrast agent compared to the normal parenchyma[22,23] (Fig. 13.2). Renal cell carcinomas may be less vascular, hypervascular, or similar in vascularity to adjacent normal parenchyma on CEUS, findings that correlate to the measured Houndsfield units (an objective measurement of enhancement) on CT.[19,22]

One study compared the diagnostic accuracy of gray-scale US and CEUS for RCC. Based on 20 RCCs features were identified that were regarded as positive findings for RCC, namely: heterogeneous enhancement, intratumoral anechoic areas, and presence of a pseudocapsule. If a mass showed two of these features, it was regarded as an RCC. For CEUS they found a sensitivity, specificity, and accuracy for RCC of 97, 93, and 95%, respectively. On gray-scale US they found these to be 70, 86, and 78%, respectively, all significantly different compared to CEUS.[24]

In another study, the usefulness of CEUS was evaluated in the diagnosis of solid renal tumors in 29 patients compared to contrast-enhanced CT.[21] These diagnoses were also compared to histopathologic diagnoses from the resected lesions. Based on hypervascularity, positive predictive values for CEUS and contrast-enhanced CT in the diagnosis of renal tumor were 100 and 82%, respectively.

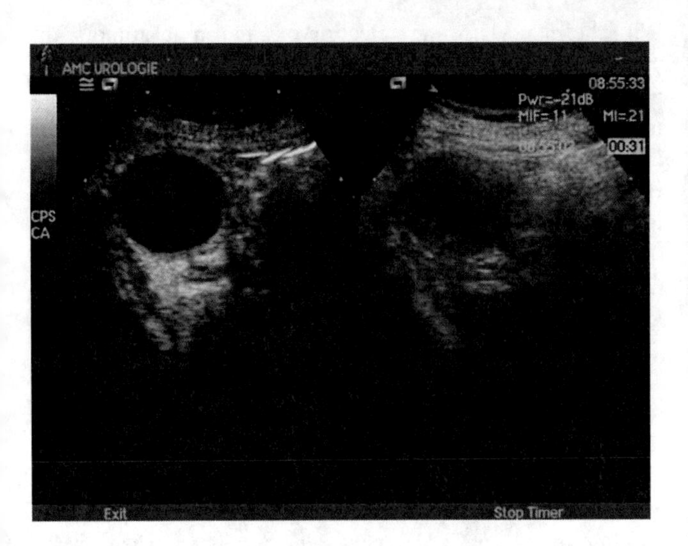

FIG. 13.1. *Cystic lesion.* Two images of a cystic renal mass: on the right the B-mode ultrasound image and on the left the contrast-enhanced image at the exact same moment. The image on the right shows a hyperechoic rim in the periphery of the cyst – indicative of a complicated cyst. However, the contrast-enhanced image shows a nonenhancing and sharply demarcated simple cyst without perfusion

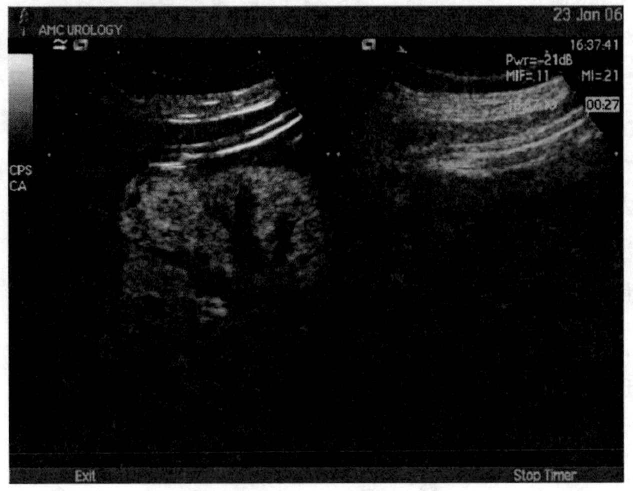

FIG. 13.2. *Solid renal mass.* A contrast-enhanced (*left*) and B-mode ultrasound image (*right*) of a solid renal mass. The regular ultrasound image shows a hyperechoic renal mass in the midsegment of the kidney. The contrast-enhanced image shows that the normal vasculature of the kidney is interrupted by the mass and that it takes up more contrast. In real time the mass also enhanced quicker than the surrounding parenchyma

Differentiation and Characterization

A large study has shown that 12.8% of solitary renal masses treated with radical nephrectomy or nephron-sparing surgery turns out to be benign on pathological examination.[25] For lesions <4 cm this is even increased to 23%.[25] The reason for this is that benign masses like oncocytoma, angiomyolipoma, and pseudotumors may appear similar to renal cell carcinoma, even on CT or MRI. Thus, better differentiation is crucial since this can prevent unnecessary surgery.

Various features of oncocytomas have been described using different imaging modalities such as a homogeneous, well-demarcated lesion, a vascular "spoke-wheel" pattern, and a stellate central scar.[26,27] However, specific criteria for a confident preoperative diagnosis have not been established, and approximately 73% of excised renal masses that turn out the be benign consist of oncocytomas.[25] Whether CEUS can help significantly in diagnosing oncocytomas is unclear since only small numbers have been evaluated.[21] In this study, one of two oncocytomas did show vessels in a spoke-wheel configuration on CEUS which were not seen on CT imaging, leading to a correct preoperative diagnosis of oncocytoma.

On ultrasonography an angiomyolipoma with a low fat content is difficult to differentiate from a malignant tumor since both may appear as hyperechoic lesions. Gray-scale US has a low specificity for characterizing such lesions. Studies have shown that CEUS does not improve this diagnostic (in)accuracy; therefore, differential diagnosis still relies on CT or MRI.[28]

With conventional US pseudotumors such as a prominent column of Bertin and persistent fetal lobulation can be mistaken for a renal neoplasm. CEUS can be helpful in the characterization of these normal variants since in those cases the enhancement is not different from the normal cortex during the overall transit of the microbubbles.[12,19,28]

Reflux

Vesicoureteral reflux is the most common urinary tract abnormality in children. It is usually investigated by means of voiding or radionuclide cystography, both involving the use of radiation. Contrast-enhanced voiding ultrasonography has been used in children to reduce the radiation dose. After introducing microbubbles into the bladder using a catheter, the upper urinary tract is assessed for echoes refluxing from the bladder, including determination of reflux grade. The sensitivity and the specificity of contrast-enhanced voiding US in the detection of vesicoureteral reflux range from 69 to 100% and from 87 to 97%, respectively.[29]

Follow up

Transplant Kidneys

The visualization of tissue perfusion is an important component of the diagnostic evaluation of kidney grafts. Acute rejection of a kidney graft primarily involves the capillary and interstitial area, and also other vascular problems such as allograft artery occlusion or thrombosis can occur in the postoperative period – the added value of CEUS in these situations is already discussed. Later, progressive remodeling of small arteries and arterioles compromises renal function and accounts for the majority of allograft failures.[30]

Color and spectral Doppler sonography are the most commonly used noninvasive diagnostics, whereby perfusion is estimated by measuring the resistance and perfusion index. However, such techniques allow the assessment of renal perfusion only in segmental and interlobar renal arteries and do not give information regarding the preglomerular arterioles.

Recently a study was conducted whereby perfusion of transplant kidneys in the early postoperative period (i.e., the first 10 days) was evaluated by CEUS and compared to conventional US.[31] Specifically, using special software inflow and washout curves of different regions of interest of the allograft were assessed. These preliminary results show that CEUS might be superior in the diagnosis of early kidney allograft dysfunction. Perfusion defects due to acute rejection were better seen using CEUS, and the extent of perirenal hematomas could be better evaluated.

Chronic allograft nephropathy (CAN) is recognized as the main cause of renal allograft failure following the first year after transplantation.[32] In a pilot study quantitative determination of renal blood flow with CEUS was shown to provide significantly higher diagnostic accuracy for the detection of loss of renal function due to CAN compared with conventional color Doppler resistance indices (85% vs. 73% resp.).[30]

Ablation Techniques

With the increase in the detection of small renal tumors, the use of nephron-sparing surgery is becoming more and more popular. Besides partial nephrectomy the two most common approaches are cryoablation and RFA. Another option is HIFU, although currently still in an experimental setting.[4] Because the tumor remains in situ in these treatments, imaging is crucial to evaluate treatment success and possible recurrence. Besides destruction of the tumor itself, these treatments rely on the destruction of tumor-nourishing vessels. Thus, follow up is done by assessing the (absence of) perfusion in the ablated area (Fig. 13.3).

Case studies have reported on the CEUS findings the first weeks after cryoablation.[33,34] One day after ablation single feeding vessels at the rim of the ablated lesion could be assessed with CEUS, with CT or MRI showing peripheral enhancement accordingly. In one patient with a persisting feeding vessel on CEUS, persistent tumor was seen on CT scan 10 weeks later. In two other patients where the feeding vessels disappeared, no recurrent lesion was identified on MRI of CT up to 6 months.

Cryotherapy can be monitored using standard ultrasonography intraoperatively because the iceball that is created is

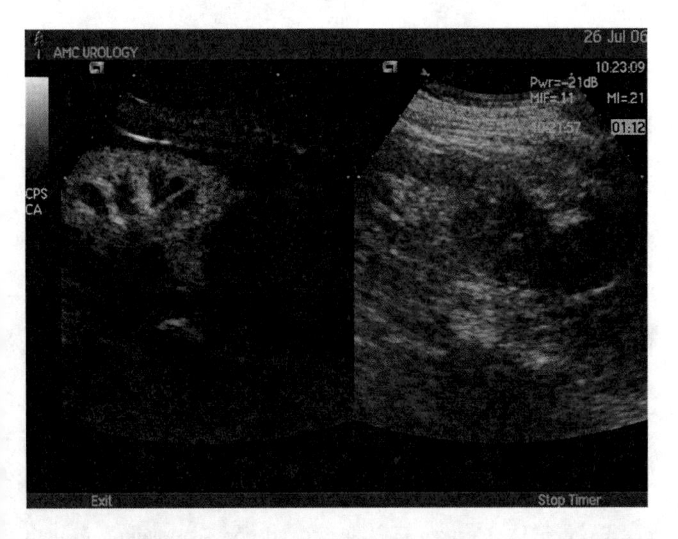

FIG. 13.3. *A cryoablated renal mass.* The left image shows the CEUS image of a kidney tumor 2 weeks after cryoablation. The ablated area is nonenhancing and well demarcated, indicating that the vasculature in that part of the kidney – and thus the tumor – is completely ablated

hypoechoic. However, in RFA such determination of initial treatment success is not possible. Two studies have reported on the use of CEUS directly after RFA in a porcine model.[35,36] Porcine kidneys were assessed for a contrast void corresponding to the area of ablated tissue on gross pathology. The appearance and the size of the lesions seen by CEUS closely mirror the ablation defect apparent on gross examination; on average the CEUS measurements of the lesion diameters were within 3 mm of those seen on gross examination. In addition, the unenhanced area also corresponded with microscopic regions of cell death.[36]

The utility of CEUS for real-time imaging of RFA remains to be assessed.

Future

Treatment Monitoring

Antiangiogenic drugs are under investigation for treatment of RCC.[37] These drugs rely on decreasing the (micro)vascularization of the tumor. Recently, it was shown that the histopathological microvessel density in proven renal cell carcinomas correlates to color pixel ratio – a measure for the vascularization – as measured by contrast-enhanced power Doppler ultrasonography.[38]

In our own institution a clinical trial is in progress to assess the usefulness of CEUS in monitoring the treatment of renal cell cancer with an antiangiogenic drug. Prior to partial or radical nephrectomy patients receive treatment with the drug for 8 weeks. CEUS is done before, halfway, and at the end of the treatment. These images are compared to contrast-enhanced CT images and the final histological specimen. So far, CEUS images showed a strong decrease in enhancement in renal masses reacting to the treatment with the antiangiogenic drug (Fig. 13.4), while tumors not reacting still showed strong enhancement. This corresponded to both CT images and histopathology. So indeed, CEUS could be an excellent tool for determining the efficacy of antiangiogenic drugs and possibly also for predicting survival.

Targeted Imaging

Although the diagnostic value of ultrasound has been improved by the use of microbubbles, research is ongoing to improve this even more. With the use of so called targeted imaging correct and detailed diagnosis, including special information about lesion extent will become available. This technique relies on the selective targeting and retention of a contrast agent and the subsequent US enhancement at specific sites of disease.

Targeting of contrast agents can be accomplished in two ways.[39] The first approach is by selecting certain microbubble shell constituents that facilitate their attachment to cells in regions of disease. An example of this is the attachment of specific phospholipids in the shell of the microbubble to activated leukocytes in regions of inflammation. The second strategy is to attach disease-specific ligands such as monoclonal antibodies, peptides, and peptidomimetics to the microbubble shell surface. Since microbubbles are pure blood pool agents, this limits the choice for potential target cells and antigens. Until now, microbubbles have been developed for evaluating inflammation, angiogenesis, and thrombus formation.[39] Studies to date have primarily focused on testing feasibility of the technique.

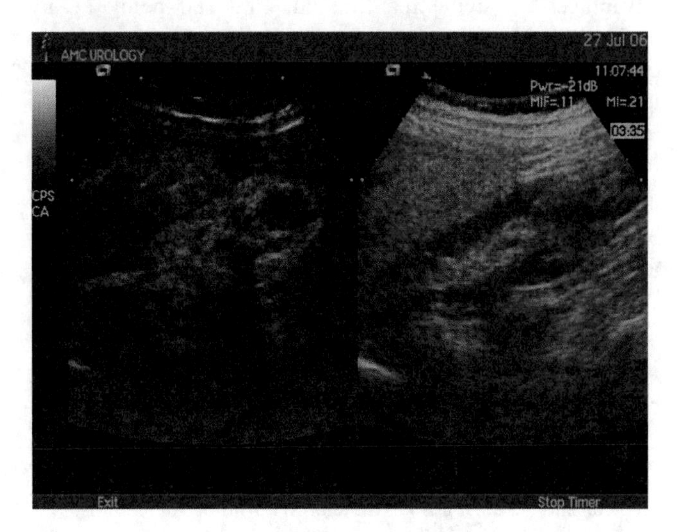

FIG. 13.4. *Antiangiogenic drugs in RCC.* A B-mode (*right*) and CEUS image of a renal tumor 4 weeks after treatment with an antiangiogenic drug. The contrast-enhanced image shows that the mass has a nonenhancing center which was not there prior to treatment; indicating that the antiangiogenic drug has disrupted the tumor vasculature

Targeted Drug and Gene Delivery

Another very interesting application of microbubbles is their potential use as carriers of therapeutic agents such as certain pharmaceuticals or even genes because they can be stored inside or on the surface of the microbubble.[40] The fact they remain stable in a low mechanical index ultrasound field but can be intentionally disrupted by a high mechanical index makes targeted delivery to a specific area of interest possible. In addition, the ultrasound energy itself has certain effects that can help targeted delivery. First, the acoustic force of US can push materials into a tissue. Second, US increases cell permeability and thereby enhances cellular uptake of the therapeutical compound. Last, US can change the chemical properties of the drug, for example, activation of light-sensitive materials. The great advantages of targeted drug delivery are minimizing toxic side effects, lowering the required dose amounts, and decreasing the costs.

The clinical application of gene and drug delivery by means of microbubbles is currently still in its infancy. First, several requirements have to be met. For example, microbubbles have to be developed capable of efficiently carrying payload while still maintaining the ability to be destroyed by acoustic energy. Also, the methods to conjugate antibodies or binding ligands to the surface of microbubbles need to be refined and specificity of microbubbles for sites of disease should be improved.

Conclusion

Studies with contrast ultrasound imaging for the kidney show promising results and more and more applications are being developed. Compared to other imaging techniques it has the advantages of giving real-time imaging and being highly available, relatively inexpensive, without the need for X-ray exposure, non-nephrotoxic, and relatively easy to do by the urologist himself. In addition, the technique of perfusion imaging is still improving, and new techniques as targeted imaging and drug delivery are under development.

Although most series only show preliminary results and definitive conclusions about the value of CEUS cannot be drawn yet, we expect that the impact of CEUS for imaging of the kidney will further increase during the next decade.

References

1. Heidenreich A, Desgrandschamps F, Terrier F. Modern approach of diagnosis and management of acute flank pain: review of all imaging modalities. Eur Urol 2002; 41(4):351–362.
2. McAchran SE, Dogra V, Resnick MI. Office urologic ultrasound. Urol Clin North Am 2005; 32(3):337–52, vii.
3. Anderson JK, Shingleton WB, Cadeddu JA. Imaging associated with percutaneous and intraoperative management of renal tumors. Urol Clin North Am 2006; 33(3):339–352.
4. Wu F. Extracorporeal high intensity focused ultrasound in the treatment of patients with solid malignancy. Minim Invasive Ther Allied Technol 2006; 15(1):26–35.
5. Lang RM, Mor-Avi V. Clinical utility of contrast-enhanced echocardiography. Clin Cardiol 2006; 29(9 Suppl 1):I15–I25.
6. Catalano O, Nunziata A, Lobianco R, Siani A. Real-time harmonic contrast material-specific US of focal liver lesions. Radiographics 2005; 25(2):333–349.
7. Meloni MF, Livraghi T, Filice C, Lazzaroni S, Calliada F, Perretti L. Radiofrequency ablation of liver tumors: the role of microbubble ultrasound contrast agents. Ultrasound Q 2006; 22(1):41–47.
8. Wink MH, Wijkstra H, De La Rosette JJ, Grimbergen CA. Ultrasound imaging and contrast agents: a safe alternative to MRI? Minim Invasive Ther Allied Technol 2006; 15(2):93–100.
9. Jakobsen JA, Oyen R, Thomsen HS, Morcos SK. Safety of ultrasound contrast agents. Eur Radiol 2005; 15(5):941–945.
10. Drelich-Zbroja A, Jargiello T, Drelich G, Lewandowska-Stanek H, Szczerbo-Trojanowska M. Renal artery stenosis: value of contrast-enhanced ultrasonography. Abdom Imaging 2004; 29(4):518–524.
11. Jakobsen JA, Correas JM. Ultrasound contrast agents and their use in urogenital radiology: status and prospects. Eur Radiol 2001; 11(10):2082–2091.
12. Correas JM, Claudon M, Tranquart F, Helenon AO. The kidney: imaging with microbubble contrast agents. Ultrasound Q 2006; 22(1):53–66.
13. Park BK, Kim SH, Moon MH, Jung SI. Imaging features of gray-scale and contrast-enhanced color Doppler US for the differentiation of transient renal arterial ischemia and arterial infarction. Korean J Radiol 2005; 6(3):179–184.
14. Taylor GA, Barnewolt CE, Claudon M, Dunning PS. Depiction of renal perfusion defects with contrast-enhanced harmonic sonography in a porcine model. AJR Am J Roentgenol 1999; 173(3):757–760.
15. Schmiedl UP, Carter S, Martin RW et al. Sonographic detection of acute parenchymal injury in an experimental porcine model of renal hemorrhage: gray-scale imaging using a sonographic contrast agent. AJR Am J Roentgenol 1999; 173(5):1289–1294.
16. Frauscher F, Janetschek G, Helweg G, Strasser H, Bartsch G, zur ND. Crossing vessels at the ureteropelvic junction: detection with contrast-enhanced color Doppler imaging. Radiology 1999; 210(3):727–731.
17. Frauscher F, Janetschek G, Klauser A et al. Laparoscopic pyeloplasty for UPJ obstruction with crossing vessels: contrast-enhanced color Doppler findings and long-term outcome. Urology 2002; 59(4):500–505.
18. Kim AY, Kim SH, Kim YJ, Lee IH. Contrast-enhanced power Doppler sonography for the differentiation of cystic renal lesions: preliminary study. J Ultrasound Med 1999; 18(9):581–588.
19. Robbin ML, Lockhart ME, Barr RG. Renal imaging with ultrasound contrast: current status. Radiol Clin North Am 2003; 41(5):963–978.
20. Helenon O, Correas JM, Balleyguier C, Ghouadni M, Cornud F. Ultrasound of renal tumors. Eur Radiol 2001; 11(10):1890–1901.
21. Tamai H, Takiguchi Y, Oka M et al. Contrast-enhanced ultrasonography in the diagnosis of solid renal tumors. J Ultrasound Med 2005; 24(12):1635–1640.
22. Reichelt O, Wunderlich H, Weirich T, Schlichter A, Schubert J. Computerized contrast angiosonography: a new diagnostic tool for the urologist? BJU Int 2001; 88(1):9–14.
23. Kim JH, Eun HW, Lee HK, et al. Renal perfusion abnormality. Coded harmonic angio US with contrast agent. Acta Radiol 2003; 44(2):166–171.

24. Park BK, Kim SH, Choi HJ. Characterization of renal cell carcinoma using agent detection imaging: comparison with gray-scale US. Korean J Radiol 2005; 6(3):173–178.
25. Frank I, Blute ML, Cheville JC, Lohse CM, Weaver AL, Zincke H. Solid renal tumors: an analysis of pathological features related to tumor size. J Urol 2003; 170(6 Pt 1):2217–2220.
26. Ambos MA, Bosniak MA, Valensi QJ, Madayag MA, Lefleur RS. Angiographic patterns in renal oncocytomas. Radiology 1978; 129(3):615–622.
27. Goiney RC, Goldenberg L, Cooperberg PL et al. Renal oncocytoma: sonographic analysis of 14 cases. AJR Am J Roentgenol 1984; 143(5):1001–1004.
28. Ascenti G, Zimbaro G, Mazziotti S, Gaeta M, Settineri N, Scribano E. Usefulness of power Doppler and contrast-enhanced sonography in the differentiation of hyperechoic renal masses. Abdom Imaging 2001; 26(6):654–660.
29. Valentini AL, De Gaetano AM, Destito C, Marino V, Minordi LM, Marano P. The accuracy of voiding urosonography in detecting vesico-ureteral reflux: a summary of existing data. Eur J Pediatr 2002; 161(7):380–384.
30. Schwenger V, Korosoglou G, Hinkel UP et al. Real-time contrast-enhanced sonography of renal transplant recipients predicts chronic allograft nephropathy. Am J Transplant 2006; 6(3):609–615.
31. Fischer T, Filimonow S, Dieckhofer J et al. Improved diagnosis of early kidney allograft dysfunction by ultrasound with echo enhancer – a new method for the diagnosis of renal perfusion. Nephrol Dial Transplant 2006; 21(10):2921–2929.
32. Yates PJ, Nicholson ML. The aetiology and pathogenesis of chronic allograft nephropathy. Transpl Immunol 2006; 16(3–4): 148–157.
33. Wink MH, Lagerveld BW, Laguna MP, De La Rosette JJ, Wijkstra H. Cryotherapy for renal-cell cancer: diagnosis, treatment, and contrast-enhanced ultrasonography for follow-up. J Endourol 2006; 20(7):456–459.
34. Zou KH, Tuncali K, Warfield SK et al. Three-dimensional assessment of MR imaging-guided percutaneous cryotherapy using multi-performer repeated segmentations: The value of supervised learning. Acad Radiol 2005; 12(4):444–450.
35. Johnson DB, Duchene DA, Taylor GD, Pearle MS, Cadeddu JA. Contrast-enhanced ultrasound evaluation of radiofrequency ablation of the kidney: reliable imaging of the thermolesion. J Endourol 2005; 19(2):248–252.
36. Slabaugh TK, Machaidze Z, Hennigar R, Ogan K. Monitoring radiofrequency renal lesions in real time using contrast-enhanced ultrasonography: a porcine model. J Endourol 2005; 19(5):579–583.
37. Lamuraglia M, Escudier B, Chami L et al. To predict progression-free survival and overall survival in metastatic renal cancer treated with sorafenib: pilot study using dynamic contrast-enhanced Doppler ultrasound. Eur J Cancer 2006; 42(15):2472–2479.
38. Kabakci N, Igci E, Secil M et al. Echo contrast-enhanced power Doppler ultrasonography for assessment of angiogenesis in renal cell carcinoma. J Ultrasound Med 2005; 24(6):747–753.
39. Behm CZ, Lindner JR. Cellular and molecular imaging with targeted contrast ultrasound. Ultrasound Q 2006; 22(1):67–72.
40. Liu Y, Miyoshi H, Nakamura M. Encapsulated ultrasound microbubbles: therapeutic application in drug/gene delivery. J Control Release 2006; 114(1):89–99.

Chapter 14
The Integration of Computed Topography Imaging in Ultrasound Diagnosis: Real-Time Virtual Sonography

Tsuyoshi Mitake and Osamu Arai

Abstract Ultrasound imaging in medicine is a noninvasive and convenient examination method. The probe for the ultrasound scanner is manipulated freehand during examination, so the cross-sectional image is a little less objective compared to other modalities. In addition, the cross-sectional image is not parallel to the body, and hence it is difficult to compare ultrasound images and computed tomography (CT) images. When the doctor makes the comparison between these two kinds of images for diagnosis or interventional operation, he feels some stress. We thought this situation should be improved, so we developed a new technology that combines CT images to ultrasound images. This system enables side-by-side display of CT multiplanar reconstruction (MPR) images obtained from CT volume data and the same cross-sectional ultrasound images in real time. We named it as real-time virtual sonography (RVS).

Keywords: Ultrasound imaging, CT images, MPR.

When diagnosing hepatic cancer, for example, CT is often the first choice, and then ultrasound imaging is used to reduce the patient's exposure to radiation. A technician performs ultrasound imaging while confirming the site of the hepatic cancer using several CT images previously taken at a right angle to the axis of the body. However, since cross-sectional ultrasound images differ from cross-sectional CT images, the diagnosis often depends on the experience and knowledge of the technician when comparing the positioning of images obtained by both modalities.

We developed a new technology called Real-time Virtual Sonography which combines ultrasound images and CT imaging to solve this problem. A method was established to display the same cross-sectional images of an organ with essentially different physical characteristics side by side. We believe that combining both modalities in this way increases the amount of information available and helps with the interpretation of the images.

Introduction

Medical ultrasound imaging enables observation of the morphology and blood flow of various organs by transmitting ultrasound to the targeted organ and receiving the reflected signals. It is currently used at many hospitals and clinics because real-time images can be obtained noninvasively at the bedside. The quality of the images was dramatically improved by digital ultrasound diagnostic equipment which underwent rapid development in the middle of the 1990s after being introduced in the latter half of the 1980s. Much more information is now available when making clinical diagnosis. However, the use of the reflected echoes of ultrasound makes it difficult to capture images through bone, gas, or air. Furthermore, the position of cross-sectional images may not be objective because the images of the site for observation are obtained with a probe for transmitting and receiving ultrasound which is manipulated freehand by a technician, as shown in Fig. 14.1.

Background

The basic concept of this technology was reported in 1996 by Oshio et al. who at the time were conducting research at Harvard Medical School.[1] CT volume data are required for this technology, but only a single-slice helical CT scanner was available at the time. To obtain volume data for the entire liver, a 15-cm section was scanned along the body axis during breath holding for 30 s, but even so, the thickness of each CT image slice was approximately 5 mm. With volume data from such thick slices, it was not practical to construct MPR images.

Today, however, the use of multidetector CT (MDCT) enables scanning of the entire liver in slices of less than 1 mm in thickness during a short period of breath holding. Furthermore, developments in PC technology make it possible to process data for MPR reconstruction using a commercially available PC.

O. Ukimura and I.S. Gill (eds.), *Contemporary Interventional Ultrasonography in Urology*,
DOI: 10.1007/978-1-84800-217-3_14,

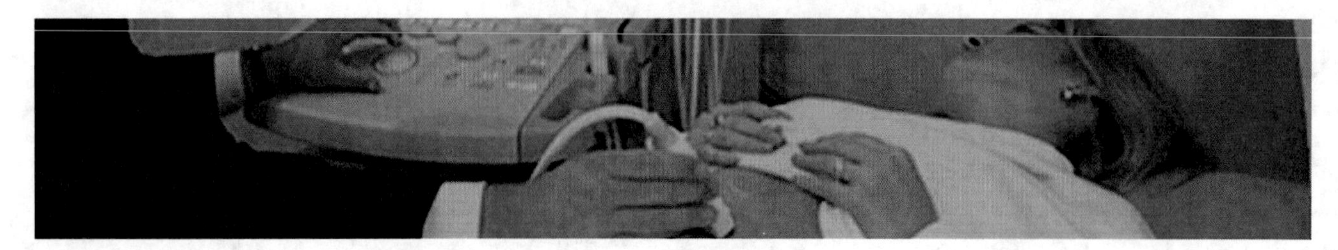

FIG. 14.1. Example of how an ultrasound scanner is used

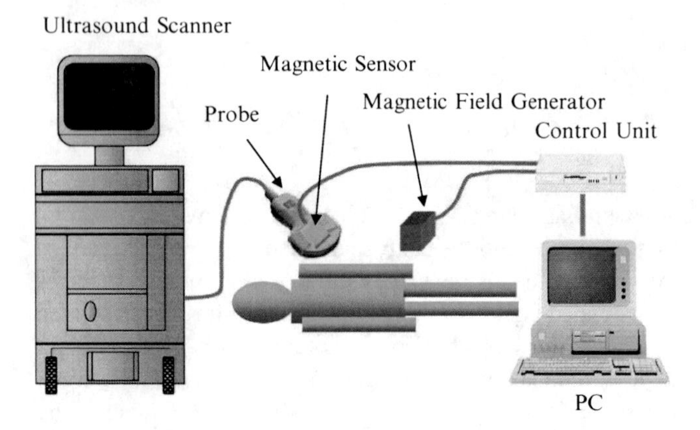

FIG. 14.2. Configuration of the system

TABLE 14.1. Specifications of the magnetic positioning sensor.

Item	Specification
Degrees of freedom	6 (position and orientation)
Translation range	Model 800: ±76.2 cm in any direction
Angular range	All Attitude: ±180° Azimuth and Roll, ±90° Elevation
Static accuracy:	Position: 1.8 mm RMS Orientation: 0.5° RMS
Static resolution:	Position: 0.5 mm Orientation: 0.1° @ 30.5 cm

Source from miniBIRD product brochure by Ascension Technology Corporation

Configuration of the Entire System and Operation of Each Part

Figure 14.2 shows the overall configuration of the system. It consists of ultrasound diagnostic equipment, a probe for transmitting and receiving ultrasound, a PC, and a magnetic positioning sensor unit for detecting the position of probe.

The CT volume data obtained in advance are transferred to the PC via storage media such as CD-ROM or LAN. A magnetic positioning sensor unit (miniBIRD of Ascension, U.S.) is connected to the PC to obtain information on the position of the probe. It consists of the control unit, a magnetic field generator, and a magnetic sensor. The magnetic field generator is placed near the patient, and the magnetic sensor is attached to the probe. Table 14.1 shows the major specifications of the magnetic positioning sensor.

When the ultrasound diagnostic equipment starts scanning and ultrasound cross-sectional images are displayed on the monitor, Real-time Virtual Sonography processing program in the PC detects the position of the probe, and displays cross-sectional images corresponding to its position and angle as MPR images reconstructed from CT volume data.

Obtaining CT Volume Data

The format for the Digital Imaging and Communication in Medicine (DICOM) standard is used to upload multiple images generated by a CT scanner to the PC. This standard is supported by most CT scanners, and the volume data consist of CT images of multiple slices.

For clinical application of this developed technology, it is important to obtain images of extremely thin slices in a short time using MDCT. In case of a CT scanner called a 16-array detector that is currently available for use in clinical settings, it is possible to acquire images of 16 slices in one rotation, and the entire liver can be scanned in around 0.6-mm thick slices during breath holding of less than 20 s. The DICOM format is very useful for MPR image reconstruction because the position and the thickness of each slice are written on the file names and header section of the nearly 300 images acquired.

Obtaining Information on the Position of the Probe

Information on the position of the probe is acquired by the magnetic positioning sensor which is connected to the PC via an RS232C interface. The information obtained by the PC from the magnetic positioning sensor is limited to the spatial position (x, y, z) and the angle (rotation angle to the x-axis, y-axis, z-axis) in the magnetic field generated by the magnetic generator. This means that only information on the position and angle of the magnetic sensor in relation to the magnetic generator is obtained at the ultrasound examination. For this reason, it has to be viewed in relation to the coordinate system of the CT volume data obtained in advance, and the coordinate system executing the ultrasound imaging. This procedure is sometimes called as registration.

Registration of Coordinate Systems

To reconstruct CT MPR whose cross section is the same as ultrasound images, it is necessary to make registration of coordinate systems. Several methods were considered to make the registration of relationship between CT volume space and the practical space of ultrasound imaging. They are:

(1) One-point registration
(2) One cross section registration
(3) Three-point registration

In case of one-point registration, it is easier because of the usage of just only one fiducial point which is located on the surface of body. However, in this case, the patient has to lie down straight in the bed of CT and the bed for the ultrasound. And the magnetic field generator has to be placed to the patient in a right angle. Before starting RVS, it is necessary to settle a point as fiducial in CT volume data space by the software. After that, actually, the probe with the magnetic sensor should be placed on the fiducial point which seems to be located on the same as CT volume data. Then, the software reconstructs and displays MPR image in real time. It seems very helpful to observe this MPR image and real-time ultrasound image simultaneously (Fig. 14.3).

CT Volume data space is defined as
Memory address in data set.

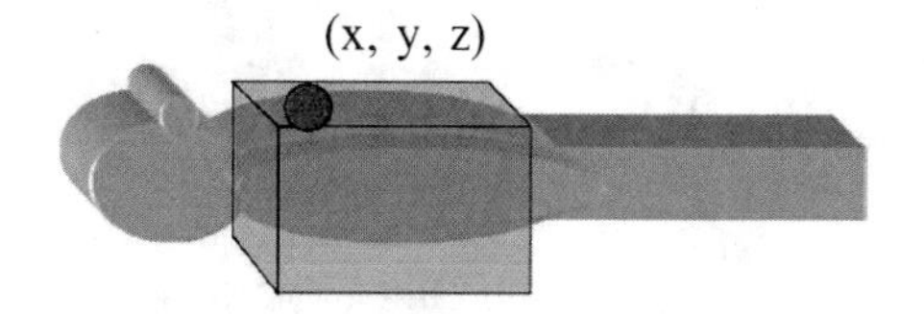

Ultrasound examination space is
captured by magnetic sensor

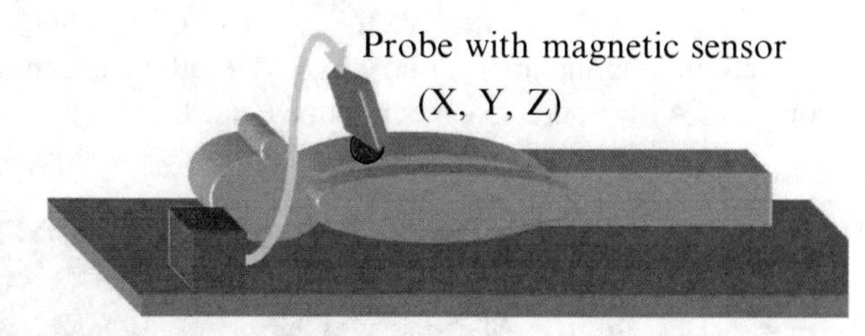

Magnetic Field generator

FIG. 14.3. One-point registration

The aforementioned method is used only for one fiducial. If we will use three points as fiducial, it is possible to avoid the limitation of body position of patient. However, the magnetic positioning sensor has the effect from the metal which is located in the examination room. As a result, the accuracy of position matching between MPR and ultrasound image sometimes may be decreased. In such a case, we propose to use one cross-section registration. At first, an MPR image near the observation point, which is easy to find out with a similar ultrasound image, should be chosen. And, a similar cross section in ultrasound image is found by moving the probe. By pushing the key when the good matching is observed, the software makes the registration and starts to reconstruct MPR. This method is easy to use and it is possible to repeat during examination.

RVS of Phantom is shown in Fig. 14.4. The right image is reconstructed from CT volume data. The right image is ultrasound

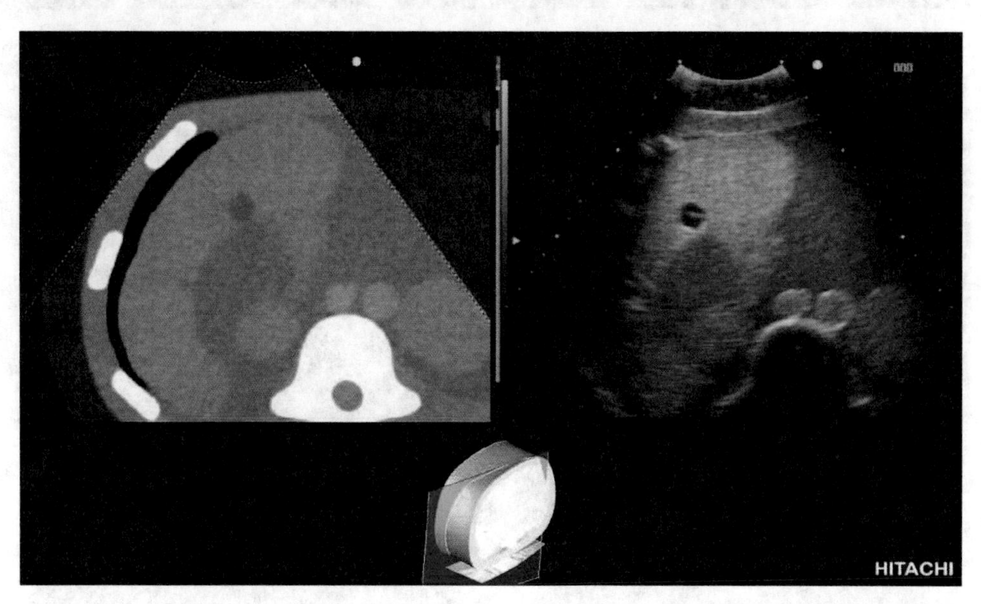

MPR from CT
(Real-time Virtual Sonography)

Ultrasound Image

FIG. 14.4. Image of phantom

image. The bottom image shows the cross section of ultrasound image on CT 3D image.

Clinical Images

This technology is meaningful because it enables more objective diagnosis by freehand ultrasound imaging. It will also be a useful tool for technicians and physicians with little experience. And our concept has been evaluated in Radiological Society of North America scientific assembly and annual meeting.[2,3]

In addition, it will be effective for intraoperative monitoring or determining the therapeutic efficacy of radio frequency ablation (RFA) for hepatic cancer, kidney cancer, and so on, which are increasingly performed under ultrasound guidance. For RFA treatment, a puncture needle is inserted in the site of the cancer under real-time observation using ultrasound images while referring to CT images obtained before surgery. Radio waves are then transmitted from the tip of the needle to cause thermocoagulation of the affected area. At present, this method is often performed while referring to CT images taken vertically to the body axis, but using this system would make the procedure easier to understand and enable more objective diagnosis.

Two cases of kidney in which this developed technology is applied are shown in Figs. 14.5 and 14.6.

Figure 14.5 is the case of the hydrocalycosis with the renal calculus. It was possible to confirm that the puncture needle was inserted just near the renal calculus.

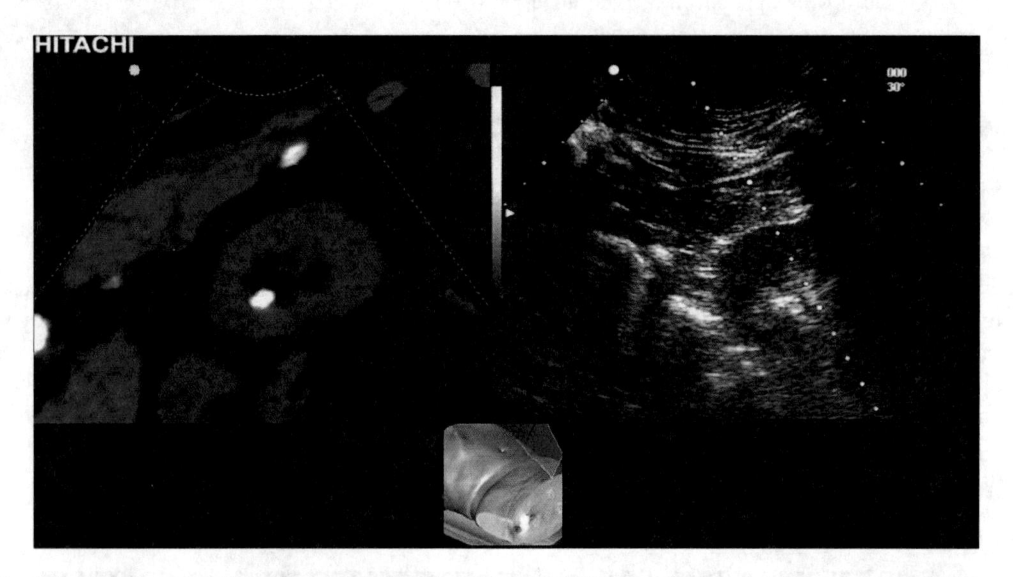

Fig. 14.5. RVS in the hydrocalycosis with the renal calculus (Courtesy of Dr. Ukimura, University Hospital, Kyoto Prefectural University of Medicine, Japan)

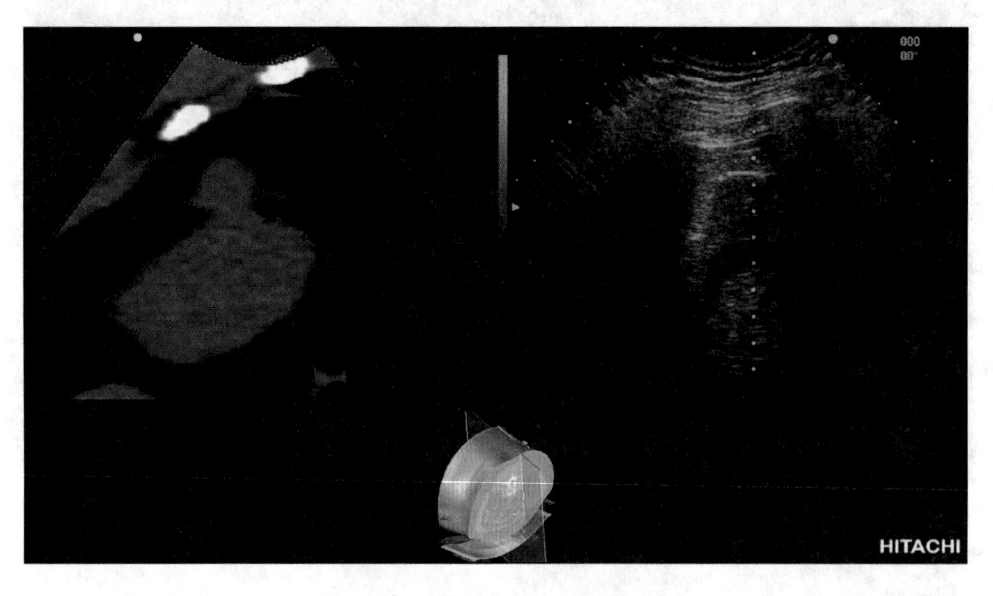

Fig. 14.6. RVS at the puncture from intercostals (Courtesy of Dr. Ukimura, University Hospital, Kyoto Prefectural University of Medicine, Japan)

Figure 14.6 is the case of the puncture from the intercostal in renal cancer. There is some blind area because of costae. However, by using RVS, it is easier and safer to make the operation.

Conclusion

We established a technology called Real-time Virtual Sonography that combines ultrasound information and CT information.

The usefulness of this system has been confirmed by the results of experimental use in a clinical setting. And, the functionality of RVS was integrated into Ultrasound Scanner itself for convenience, so it is not necessary to connect the external PC. Further improvements are planned to correct position aberration of images due to the breathing of the patient during CT scanning and ultrasound diagnosis, and to achieve higher calibration accuracy. In addition, we have the plan to combine not only CT but also MRI, PET, and so on. We strongly hope that our effort will be the way for the next step.

Acknowledgments. We would like to thank Dr. Kiyoshi Okuma, Dr. Hiroshi Shinmoto, and Dr. Koichi Oshio of the Department of Radiology, School of Medicine, Keio University, and Dr. Takao Iwasaki of the Department of Gastrointestinal Medicine, Tohoku University Hospital for their advice and evaluation of this system from a clinical viewpoint during its development.

References

1. Oshio K., Shinmoto H. Simulation of US imaging by using a 3D CT data set. Radiology 1996; 201(Suppl.):517.
2. Arai O., Mitake T., Oshio K., Ookuma K., Shinmoto H., Iwasaki T. Integration Computer tomography in ultrasound diagnosis named virtual sonography (abstr). In: Radiological Society of North America scientific assembly and annual meeting program. Radiological Society of North America 2003; 807.
3. Iwasaki T., Mikami E., Shimosegawa T., Arai O., Mitake T. Real-time virtual sonography: a novel navigation tool in percutaneous radiofrequency ablation of hepatocellular carcinomas (abstr). In: Radiological Society of North America scientific assembly and annual meeting program. Radiological Society of North America 2004; 805.

Chapter 15
Elastography

Katharina Koenig

Introduction

It is well known that cancer of, e.g., prostate or breast is palpable as a stiffer mass in comparison to the normal soft tissue of the organ. There are mechanical characteristics of a tissue that depend on several conditions such as the molecular building blocks (collagen, cells, fat, etc.), the microscopic and macroscopic structural organization, and the metabolic activity. To display the mechanical properties only one parameter is required. This parameter is known as the *shear modulus, elastic modulus, or Young modulus*. Krouskop et al. investigated the elastic moduli of benign prostate tissue, benign hyperplasia, and prostate carcinoma. They found prostates with BPH are significantly softer than normal tissue and cancer is significantly stiffer than the surrounding tissue.[1] Phipps et al. tested mechanically prostate tissue chippings from transurethral resection of the prostate (TURP). They confirmed the significant mechanical differences between benign and malignant prostate tissue. Furthermore they found a significant correlation between prostatic tissue morphology and mechanical characteristics.[2]

The observation of the mechanical differences led to a new approach in the detection of prostate cancer described by Sperandeo et al.[3] Prostatic tissue was compressed using a transrectal probe during conventional sonography. The nondeformable lesions were diagnosed based on fine needle biopsy. A high correlation between nondeformable lesions and prostate cancer was found. 62 of 68 cases (92.6%) of the nondeformable lesions proved to be adenocarcinomas. 75% of the prostatic carcinomas showed these stiffer characteristics.

Sonoelastography

Since the eighties, investigators aimed to provide images that showed elastic differences in organs. One approach was first described by Lerner et al.[4] The *sonoelastography uses realtime Doppler techniques to provide an image that showed the change of vibration patterns*. A low-frequency (less than 1 kHz) vibration is provided by an external source. This is brought into close contact to the organ. There is a local decrease in the peak vibration when a hard lesion is present compared to soft, homogeneous tissue. These amplitudes are mapped on a gray scale where high vibration is bright and lower vibrations are dark.[5,6]

Taylor et al. reported about 3D sonoelastography in 19 patients with prostate cancer. They used a Logiq-7 ultrasound system from GE Medical systems. Color Doppler was used to display the vibration differences. The Doppler images were overlaid on the gray-scale image. Transverse scans were used in 1-mm steps to create a 3D image. They found a *sensitivity of 41–71%* according to the Grading of the tumor. The positive predictive value was 71 and 60%, respectively.[7]

Elastography

1. Method
2. Practice
3. Studies

Method

Another method was first described by Ophir et al. in 1991.[8] *Elastography or strain imaging* is a technique where small displacements between ultrasonic image pairs acquired under axial deformation are compared. The backscattered ultrasound signal does not change their characteristic pattern if the tissue is only slightly compressed (i.e., approximately up to 2%). Time or space differences between local regions of interest within two subsequent images are recorded under different compression. Displacement estimates within corresponding A-lines are obtained by the evaluation of the radiofrequency (RF)-data set. For each pixel of the image a value is calculated from two subsequent images. The value of the shift between corresponding A-lines is dependent on the elastic or Young modulus of the tissue. This value is not absolute but relative since it is dependent on the surrounding tissue and the applied

O. Ukimura and I.S. Gill (eds.), *Contemporary Interventional Ultrasonography in Urology*,
DOI: 10.1007/978-1-84800-217-3_15,

compression force. This is the so-called inverse problem. Stiff tissues like carcinomas are more elastic than softer tissue, so the displacement time difference is smaller (Figs. 15.1 and 15.2). The calculated differences of each pixel of the image can be visualized in colors side by side to the conventional B-mode image or overlaid on the B-mode image on the screen of the ultrasound system (Fig. 15.3).[9–12] The colors can be freely chosen. Examples of color schemes are black for hard tissue, red and yellow for intermediate, and blue for very soft areas (Fig. 15.4). The compression of the tissue can be evaluated by inflation of a balloon.[13] More often the investigator performs a slight compression of the tissue using the probe to apply the force.[14]

Practice

There are some *criteria* which the investigator should pay attention to avoid misinterpretation. First, if the compression is applied by the probe, it is important to make sure that the *organ is compressed at a right angle*. If this is not done correctly, artifacts can easily occur which may lead to misinterpretation. Only a slight compression in the order up to 2% is necessary. The strength and duration of the manually induced *movement should be adjusted by visual control* using the video screen of the ultrasound system for *optical feedback*. The *compression should be performed at least two times* so that the *elastographic image is reproducible*. Calculi and nodules of benign prostate hyperplasia (BPH) may occur stiffer than normal tissue; therefore, the strain image should always be *interpreted together with standard ultrasound*. This is done in order to define these stiffer alterations from tumors. Therefore, the examiner needs experience with conventional ultrasound, which should always be used additionally. Another

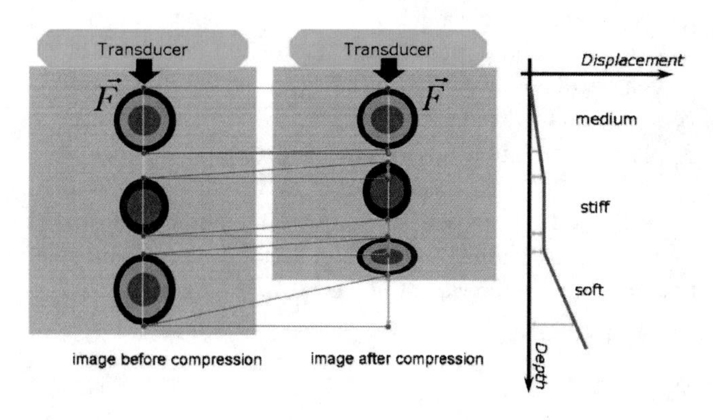

Fig. 15.1. Principles of elastography: Measurement of the displacement between tissue before and after compression. The displacement in stiffer tissue, which is more elastic, is much smaller than in softer tissue

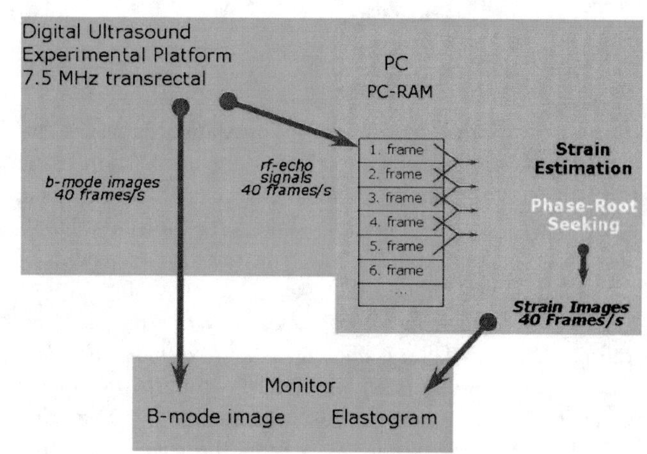

Fig. 15.3. The RF-data are captured by the probe (i.e., a 7.5-MHz probe for investigation of the prostate). At least 20 frames are necessary to obtain a stable image. The displacements between two frames are directly processed by a fast estimation algorithm. The calculated strain images are shown side by side with the conventional B-mode image on the monitor of the ultrasound system

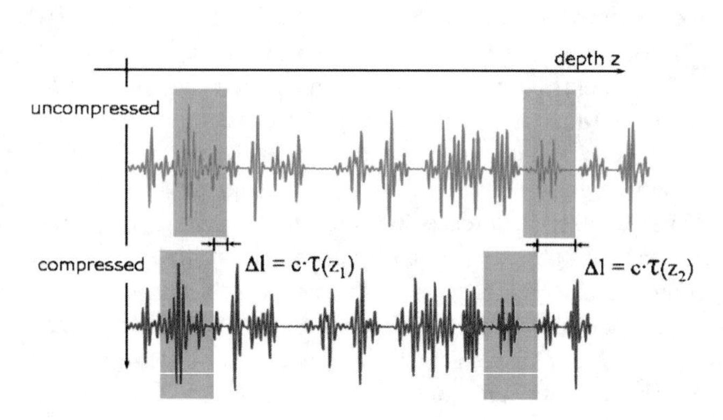

Fig. 15.2. One possibility is the measurement of the time shift between two identical RF-data sets before and after compression. A smaller time shift means a stiffer tissue

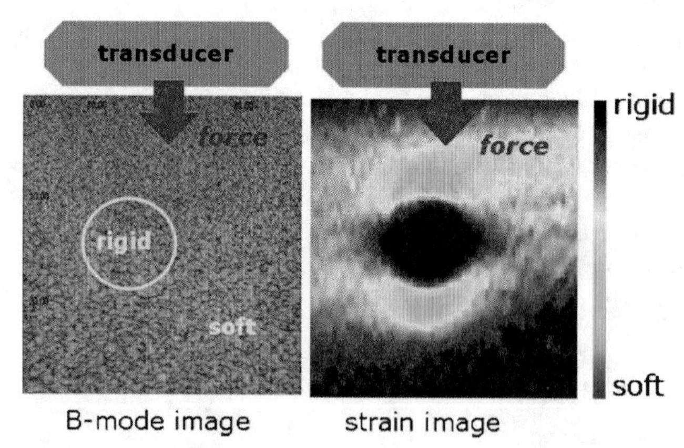

Fig. 15.4. *Left side*: Conventional ultrasound of a phantom. This is constructed by injection of agar–agar in a soft sponge. The inclusion is not visualized because it is isoechoic. On the right side the harder area is clearly shown by elastography. The border to the stiffer area is clearly marked by the halo effect

criterion is that at the *boundary between stiffer and softer tissue,* the softer tissue near the hard area often seems to be much softer than the surrounding soft tissue. The border to an area of different stiffness is often marked by a *small ribbon (halo-effect)* above and under the stiffer area (Fig. 15.4). Furthermore, the border of the organ and between the central and peripheral gland is often visualized. This phenomenon can be explained by the fact that the computation of the elasticity is not absolute but relative. It cannot be marked laterally because of the comparison along the A-lines. This halo effect is not always seen clearly, but it can be considered a facultative sign of malignancy.

A *problem of classification* is found in patients with chronic prostatitis, fibrosis after multiple biopsies or after surgery of the prostate. In these patients often a diffuse increase of the elastic modulus is seen. Thus, it is hardly ever possible to detect a focus. Furthermore, prostates with a T4 carcinoma, which infiltrate the whole gland, often show a "normal," homogeneous elastogram, although the elastic modulus is increased. This is because of the so-called inverse problem. The calculated values for each pixel of the strain image are relative, and therefore the real elastic modulus is not be imaged.

Studies

Kallel et al. reported in vitro elastography of canine prostates which showed the ability to produce consistent images of normal prostate tissue.[15] It has been shown that those macroscopic invisible differences in the cellular organization, i.e., between the central and the peripheral zone results in a stiffness contrast that was elastographically measurable. *Even small parts of the prostate,* i.e., the verumontanum (in canine prostate about 3 -mm wide) which is a stiffer tissue *could be visualized.*

Several clinical studies have been performed to evaluate the use for detection of cancer in soft tissue. Most interesting are tumors of the breast and the prostate as they are often isoechoic and consequently invisible in standard ultrasound imaging.

Based on the principles of elastography described by Ophir et al.,[8,9] Lorenz and Pesavento developed the *real-time elastography.*[10–12] A new fast crosscorrelation technique and improved computer hardware made it possible to perform real-time elastography during the standard ultrasound examination. In a first study, Koenig et al. examined 277 patients elastographically with histological evidence of prostate cancer prior to radical prostatectomy (Combison 530, Kretz, Austria). Three transversal scans per gland (apical, mid, basal) were performed, and the location of the tumor was laid down by the investigator. The elastogram was interpreted together with the conventional B-mode image. After surgery, the glands were cut in transversal slices, and the tumors were outlined with a color-marking pen. The histological findings were matched to the elastograms (Figs. 15.5 and 15.6). In 217/277 (*78.3%*) patients *prostate cancer was detected by real-time elastography* [Koenig K, unpublished work].

The next step was the evaluation of real-time elastography-guided biopsies of the prostate (Voluson 730, GE, Medical systems). 404 patients with elevated PSA underwent standard sextant prostate biopsy. Each biopsy core was separately examined and compared to the elastographic findings. In 151 of 404 patients (37.4%) the diagnosis of prostate cancer was histologically confirmed. In *84.1% of the subjects, pathological alterations were seen in real-time elastography.* The sensitivity was dependent on the Gleason score, where highest sensitivity (86.7%) was seen in the patient group with Gleason score between 5 and 6.[16]

29 patients with histological proven, but untreated prostate cancer were examined by Miyanaga et al.[17] The prostates were manually compressed with the probe. They measured spatial differences before and after tissue compression. *Elastography detected 93% of the prostate cancers successfully.*

Pallwein et al. found an increased finding of prostate cancer in biopsies using contrast-enhanced ultrasound and elastography.[18] Frauscher et al. reported about 15 patients with histological confirmed prostate cancer who underwent elastography prior to surgery (Voluson 730, GE, Medical systems). 32 areas of carcinoma were found histologically. 28 of them (*sensitivity of 88%*) were detected by elastography. No patient with prostate cancer showed a normal, nonpathological elastogram.[19]

Ives reported about 40 patients undergoing prostate biopsy.[20] They were evaluated with conventional ultrasound as well as color Doppler, and elastography (Hi-Vision 8500, Hitachi medical system). In 8 of 14 subjects prostate cancer was diagnosed by elastography.

Souchon et al. reported about 31 patients with prostate cancer who underwent HIFU therapy (Combison 311, Kretz, Austria). The compression of the prostate was performed using a balloon. The compression was 15–20% of the initial dimension of the prostate and displacement step was chosen at 0.25 mm. Three elastograms in parallel imaging planes at the apex, midgland, and base were performed prior to and after the therapy of one lobe and both lobes. They found a *possibility to visualize prostate cancer and HIFU lesions during therapy.*[13] As the patients did not undergo surgery and consequently no histology was available, they performed a second study in which they compared elastographic findings with MRI. In some patients a good correlation between elastography and MRI measurements was found, but elastography was unable to predict MRI in a single individual. Nevertheless, they found *a potential of elastography for monitoring HIFU lesions.*[21]

Future Directions

These first studies are very promising. Mechanical artifacts and the lack of no absolute values available lead to a long learning curve and misinterpretation. To control whether the compression is performed accurately, it is possible to compare echo signal sets during compression. If the *compression*

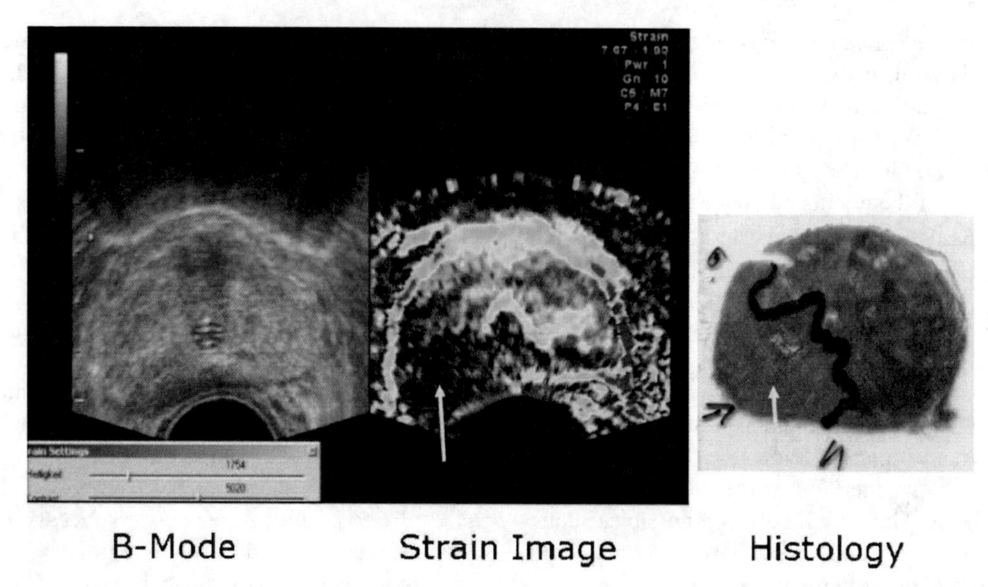

FIG. 15.5. Conventional ultrasound (*left*) and elastography (*right*) of a patient with prostate cancer prior to radical prostatectomy. The tumor can be clearly identified by the elastogram. The histology confirms the localization in the right lobe. The urethra (*blue*) and the verumontanum (*red/black*) are represented in the strain image. The border of the gland is shown with a small ribbon

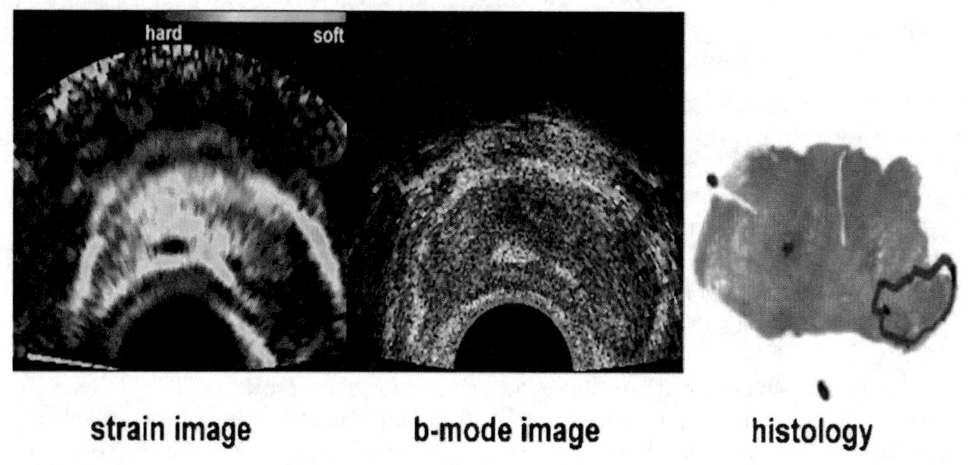

FIG. 15.6. The localization of the tumor in the left lobe can be seen in elastography. A stiffer mass which is in the right lobe can be judged a calculi if the elastogram is compared to the conventional B-mode image

is performed accurately, sets can be found again. Hitachi implemented this calculation and made it visible by *a number scale*. The number "one" represents very accurate compression, and every number higher than "one" represents an increase in artifacts. Stiffer areas in the prostate which are not visible by conventional ultrasound, i.e., chronic prostatitis or scars after surgery (TUR-P) remain a problem in the differential diagnosis. One way to solve the problem is the calculation of the *region of interests*. For example, the fat in the axils can be used as the reference for suspicious areas in the mamma. Since the elastic modulus of fat should always be the same, the relative stiffness of another tissue can be estimated. Unfortunately, there is a lack of reference tissue for the prostate.

To eliminate operator-dependent artifacts Salcudean et al. developed a new system, the so-called *vibro-elastography*. Therefore, the transducer is connected with a vibration mechanism which can impart to it radial vibratory motion. The maximum displacement of the endorectal probe can be set in the range ±0–5 mm, while experiments showed that exitations ±2 mm are sufficient. Elastograms were calculated from the captured RF-data. The first results with a phantom and three patients undergoing brachytherapy for prostate cancer showed significant and repeatable details, including stiff regions within the prostate.[22]

Yinbo and Hossacker measured elasticity by controlled water inflation of a sheath placed over a modified transrectal ultrasound transducer. It was to produce repeatable, accurate measurements of elasticity in order to reconstruct 3D imaging of the prostate.[23]

One effort to solve the so called *inverse problem* is the *reconstruction of elastograms*. Therefore, the calculated displacement or strain is used for an estimation of appropriate material properties. This approach tries to reduce the mechanical artifacts and leads to more quantitative information. Khaled et al. reported about a direct method versus an iterative approach to calculate the shear modulus.[24] The experimental results with a phantom showed additional quantitative information, but the iterative reconstructive method seems to be more sufficient.

Luo et al. developed an iterative approach based upon the stress–strain relations in the polar coordinates for elasticity distribution reconstruction.[25] Simulation results showed that the radial stress decay and the target-hardening artifact in strain images could be greatly reduced after a few iterations.

Elasticity imaging techniques are still in development. The advancement of fast algorithms and fast acquisition hardware promise increase improvement of a very cost effective and noninvasive technique. This technique may be a diagnostic tool with a wide variety of clinical applications in future.

Overview

In the last 15 years many efforts have been made to measure and visualize the elastic modulus of tissues. Methods dealing with ultrasound waves are safe for the patient and cost effective. Clinical studies showed the potential of elastography and elastosonography in the detection of cancer. Prostate cancer can be detected with a high sensitivity rate up to 84.1%. Other tumors for example of the mamma are under investigation. The method has also a place in the surveillance of therapy in the treatment of cancer. The technique is still in development. Furthermore larger clinical studies are recommended and technical problems have to be resolved.

References

1. Krouskop TA, Wheeler TM, Kallel F, Garra BS, Hall T: Elastic moduli of breast and prostate tissue under compression. Ultrason Imaging 20 (1998), 260–274
2. Phipps S, Yang THJ, Habib FK, Reuben RL, McNeill SA: Measurement of tissue mechanical characteristics to distinguish between benign and malignant prostate disease. Urology 66 (2) (2005), 447–450
3. Sperandeo G, Sperandeo M, Morcaldi M, Caturelli E, Dimitry L, Camagna A: Transrectal ultrasonography for the early diagnosis of adenocarcinoma of the prostate: A new maneuver designed to improve the differentiation of malignant and benign lesions. J Urol 169 (2003), 607–610
4. Lerner RM, Parker KJ, Holen J, et al. Sono-elasticity: medical elasticity images derive from ultrasound signals in mechanically vibrated targets. Acoustical Imaging, Vol 19, (1988), pp. 317–327Proc. 16th Int. Symp.
5. Taylor LS, Porter BC, Rubens DJ, et al. Three-dimensional sonoelastography: principles and practices. Phys. Med. Biol. 45 (2000), 1477–1494
6. Parker KJ, Taylor LS, Gracewski S, et al. A unified view of imaging the elastic properties of tissue. J Acoust Soc Am 117(5) (2005), 2705–2712
7. Taylor LS, Rubens DJ, Porter BC, et al. Prostate cancer: Three-dimensional sonoelastography for in vitro detection. Radiology 237 (2005), 981–985
8. Ophir J, Cespedes I, Ponnekanti H, Yazdi Y, Li X, Elastography A: Quantitative method for imaging the elasticity of biological tissues. Ultrason Imaging 13 (1991), 111–134
9. Ophir J, Garra B, Kallel F, et al. Elastographic imaging. Ultrasound Med Biol 26 (Suppl. 1) (2000), S23–S29.
10. Pesavento A, Lorenz A, Ermert H: System for real-time elastography. Electronic Lett 35(Nr. 5) (1999), 941–942
11. Pesavento A, Lorenz A, Siebers S, Ermert H: New real-time strain imaging concepts using diagnostic ultrasound. Phys Med Biol 45 (2000), 1423–1435
12. Lorenz A, Pesavento A, Garcia-Schuermann MJ, Sommerfeld HJ, Senge T: New results with real time strain imaging. Frequenz 55 (2001), 21–24
13. Souchon R, Rouviere O, Gelet A, et al. Visualisation of HIFU lesions using elastography of the human prostate in vivo: preliminary results. Ultrasound Med Biol. 29 (7) (2003), 1007–1015
14. Konofagou EE, Quo vadis elasticity imaging? Ultrasonics 42 (2004), 331–336
15. Kallel F, Price RE, Konofagou EE, Ophir J: Elastographic imaging of the normal canine prostate in vitro. Ultrason Imaging 21 (1999), 201–215
16. Koenig K, Scheipers U, Pesavento A, Lorenz A, Ermert H, Senge T: Initial experiences with real-time elastography guided biopsies of the prostate. J Urol 174 (2005), 115–117
17. Miyanaga N, Akaza H, Yamakawa M, et al. Tissue elasticity imaging for diagnosis of prostate cancer: A preliminary report. Int J Urol 13(12) (2006), 1514–1518
18. Pallwein L, Mitterberger M, Gradl J, et al. Value of contrast-enhanced ultrasound and elastography in imaging of prostate cancer. Curr Opin Urol. 17(1) (2007), 39–47
19. Frauscher F, Klauser A, Pallwein L, Horninger W, Lorenz A: Wertigkeit der Elastographie in der Detektion des Prostatakarzinoms. Ultraschall Med 25 (2004), S1–S30 (abstr)
20. Ives EP, Waldman I, Gomella LG, Halpern EJ: Preliminary experience with prostate elastography and comparison with biopsy results. Prostate Cancer Symp 2005 (abstr)
21. Curiel L, Souchon R, Rouviere O, Gelet A, Chapelon JY: Elastography for the follow-up of high-intensity focused ultrasound prostate cancer treatment: initial comparison with MRI. Ultrasound Med Biol 31(11) 2005, 1461–1468
22. Salcudean SE, French D, Bachmann S, Zahiri-Azar R, Wen X, Morris WJ: Viscoelasticity modelling of the prostate region using vibro-elastography. MICCAI (1) 2006, 389–396
23. Yinbo L, Hossack JA: Combined elasticity and 3D imaging of the prostate. IEEE 3 (2005), 1435–1438
24. Khaled W, Reichling S, Bruhns OT, Ermert H: Ultrasonic strain imaging and reconstructive elastography for biological tissue. Ultrasonics 44 (Suppl. 1) (2006), 199–202
25. Luo J, Ying K, Bai J: Elasticity reconstruction for ultrasound elastography using a radial compression: An inverse approach. Ultrasonics 44(Suppl. 1) (2006), 195–198

Chapter 16
Ultrasonic Tissue Characterization

Ulrich Scheipers

Introduction

This chapter represents the results achieved over a period of several years of research in the field of ultrasonic tissue characterization. *Mainly focusing on the development of a computer-aided diagnostic system for the detection of prostate cancer and on the discussion of the results of the underlying clinical study, this chapter may also be of help to scientists working in the field of ultrasonic tissue characterization and focusing on other organs.*

Eight different groups of tissue describing parameters and features applicable for tissue characterization and typically used by the tissue characterizing community have been evaluated and discussed in this chapter. This discussion may be a valuable overview for scientists approaching the field of tissue characterization and facing the problem of which types of tissue characterization parameters to focus on.

A modern nonlinear classifier, the so-called adaptive network-based fuzzy inference system, is introduced and described to a degree that will facilitate application and usage of the classifier by the reader who intends to establish a higher-order classification system.

Although most parts of the tissue characterization system have been designed for prostate cancer detection, studies on the classification of coronary plaques in intravascular ultrasound, on monitoring of thermal ablation therapy of the liver, on staging of deep venous thrombosis, and on classification of tumors of the parotid gland have recently proven the reliability of the approach described in this chapter.[1]

In the following sections, all details of the multifeature tissue characterization system are discussed. At first, the clinical background is reviewed in detail in section "Clinical Background." Readers with a solid clinical background on prostate cancer diagnostics might want to skip this section and are motivated to go directly to section "Former Work." Former work of the same author and of other groups is presented and discussed here The technical issues of the system will be dealt with in the methods section. The methods section is subdivided into several parts dealing with the acquisition and preprocessing of the radiofrequency (RF) data in Data Acquisition and processing, the parameter or feature extraction steps in section "Parameter Extraction," the classification procedure in section "Classification," and last but not least the data visualization in section "Visualization." In the following section "Results," the underlying clinical study is described and the results of the classification are presented. After a general discussion of the clinical study, the final classification results of the system will be presented in section "Results of Tissue Characterization." In addition to the numerical results, two exemplary cases taken from the 100 patients included in the clinical study are discussed in sections "Case A" and "Case B." Possible applications of the system, including perspectives for the future, are discussed in section "Discussion." The work closes with a few concluding remarks in section "Conclusion."

Clinical Background

There is no doubt about the lack of reliability of the different methods of diagnostics that are used today concerning prostate cancer. Digital rectal examination (DRE), transrectal ultrasound imaging (TRUS), and prostate-specific antigen (PSA) value analysis are relatively insensitive because they rarely detect small well-differentiated tumors (less than 0.1 cm^3).[2] DRE is highly dependent on the physician's skills. Small tumors cannot easily be palpated in surrounding prostate tissue. Due to this, DRE is most seriously limited by its lack of sensitivity. When using TRUS, small tumors may easily be overseen, too.

Using transrectal ultrasound imaging, only approximately two-third of all tumors can be seen, whereas the remaining one-third appears isoechoic and cannot be identified as cancer.[3] Furthermore, conventional B-mode (brightness mode) ultrasound can be applied in different ways. Best diagnostic results are achieved when B-mode ultrasound is applied in a dynamic manner, which means that the insonified organ is compressed manually during the examination by a light force applied by the physician by moving the transducer probe slightly back and forth. As the insonified organs move and

O. Ukimura and I.S. Gill (eds.), *Contemporary Interventional Ultrasonography in Urology,*
DOI: 10.1007/978-1-84800-217-3_16, © Springer-Verlag London Limited 2009

change their shape under varying compressions, different tissue pathologies may be detected. Thus, improved diagnostics in comparison to the static application of B-mode ultrasound alone are possible. The use of conventional transrectal ultrasound as a dynamic modality has always been propagated by experienced radiologists, but as reality shows, only skilled physicians and sonographers apply diagnostic ultrasound in a dynamic way. Nevertheless, transrectal ultrasound imaging can detect some cancers that are not palpable, although the range of sizes of palpable and sonographically visible tumors is similar. However, ultrasound imaging provides a valuable adjunct to DRE.[3]

As the amount of PSA within the patient's blood is correlated with actual tumor size, it is apparent that small tumors are hardly found using PSA value analysis. In addition, the PSA level may often be misleading when taken alone. For example, the PSA level may be elevated because of the presence of benign prostatic hyperplasia (BPH).[4, 5] To a certain degree, the PSA level is dependent on the prostate volume; thus, normalizing measured PSA levels by prostate volume may cope with the BPH dependency. In addition, sexual activity and even riding a bicycle can increase the PSA level in a misleading way. The PSA level also depends on the patient's age and typically is elevated in older patients, which might partly be correlated with the incidence of BPH.

When used in combination with DRE and transrectal ultrasound imaging, however, PSA levels provide useful data, because patients who have abnormal DREs or transrectal ultrasonography findings are much more likely to have cancer if their PSA level is elevated.[2, 6–13] Today, a combination of the three modalities, if available, is recommended and used for prostate cancer diagnostics.[14]

One new diagnostic modality [15] is real-time elastography or strain imaging, which visualizes the local stiffness of tissue using transrectal ultrasound imaging. By using a strain imaging system, the operator or physician is forced to use diagnostic ultrasound in a dynamic way. While manual compression is applied to the insonified organ by slightly pushing and pulling the ultrasound transducer back and forth, image series are recorded at different compression ratios. The applied strain is typically in the range of a few percentages of the insonified organ. Elastography, which was first described by Ophir et al.,[16] was introduced to the field of prostate diagnostics by Lorenz et al.[17–21] Elastography is used today as an adjunct to DRE, transrectal ultrasound imaging, and PSA value analysis in certain clinics. Although the first clinical results of real-time elastography are quite promising,[22–24] elastography is still under clinical evaluation and has not yet been widely introduced.

One feature that digital rectal examination, transrectal ultrasound imaging, and elastography have in common is the dependence of the results on the physician or sonographer conducting the examination. Experienced physicians and sonographers have higher prediction rates than novice physicians due to the fact that one has to learn to apply these modalities.

In addition to diagnostic ultrasound, computed tomography (CT), and magnetic resonance imaging (MRI) have been tested as imaging modalities for prostate cancer diagnostics. Clinical studies on both modalities, CT and MRI, lead to the result that the use of these methods incorporates a diagnostic power, which is too unspecific for clinical use. The contrast between normal prostate tissue and cancerous regions is too low for specific diagnostics, when using conventional CT. MRI is only recommended by some groups for the use in staging high-risk patients with extracapsular prostate cancer.[25–27] As discussed by Jager et al.,[25] only diagnostic reasons prevent the application of MRI for prostate cancer diagnostics. No economic reasons prevent MRI application, as would typically be assumed. Today, both modalities, CT and MRI, are no longer recommended for prostate diagnostics by the American Urological Association.[28]

The use of contrast-enhanced ultrasonography for prostate diagnostics has been investigated in clinical studies, but these only involved small patient contingents.[3, 29] Sedelaar et al.[30, 31] discovered that the microvessel density (MVD) might be an indicative factor for prostate cancer, but the results of only seven patients are not representative enough to provide a final judgment on the question whether contrast-enhanced ultrasound will increase the detection rate of prostate cancer. Nevertheless, it seems that the degree of MVD might be useful in staging prostate carcinoma. In addition, tests for the reproducibility of perfusion parameters have been carried out and found positive after detailed examinations.[32] Potdevin et al.[33] investigated the use of quantitative measures of ultrasound Doppler in 39 patients. The results were dependent on the specific prostate region, but still they were encouraging enough to conduct further studies on the subject. The quantitative estimation of perfusion parameters is considered to be a chance to increase the detection rates for early-stage prostate cancers. *The inclusion of perfusion parameters as an independent group of tissue features in a nonlinear classification system such as the one presented in this chapter is a challenge that still is to be taken.*

Former Work

During the last years, several works dealing with the characterization of prostate tissue using ultrasound have been published. Some approaches are based on video data[34–38] and do not take the depth-dependent diffraction and attenuation into account.[35–38] Some authors tried to characterize prostate tissue by using only a single parameter, e.g., attenuation estimates[39, 40] or backscatter estimates or by combining different parameters using a linear approach or a nearest neighbor technique.[41, 42] Some authors used nonlinear methods such as conventional neural networks[43–48] and Kohonen maps[49–51] to combine tissue parameters and even compared different nonlinear methods with each other.[52, 53] An overview of ultrasonic tissue characterization in general can be found in Refs. [54] and [55]. An overview of prostate diagnostics using ultrasound imaging is given by Sedelaar et al. in Ref. [30].

Basset et al. analyzed video data of 37 images originating from 16 patients by means of texture parameters extracted from co-occurrence matrices. The regions of interest (ROI) applied in the study were too large to allow spatially resolved classification. An accuracy of 78% is reported. No repeated crossvalidation was applied in this study; thus, no error measure is given.[34]

Giesen et al. reported about analyzing video data acquired from 12 patients. Images were analyzed using texture parameters extracted from co-occurrence matrices. A sensitivity of 75% and a specificity of 78% are reported for using needle biopsy results as the gold standard and a partition of the whole dataset into 67% for training and into 33% for evaluation. No error measures are given.[36] In a similar study, based on the same system, Huynen et al. reported a sensitivity of 81% and a specificity of 77%, which was achieved on a dataset of 239 images originating from 51 patients. Again no error measure is given.[35]

Schmitz et al. analyzed RF echo data of 200 datasets originating from 33 patients using Kohonen maps as nonlinear classifiers on parameters extracted from both time domain and frequency domain. A mean sensitivity value of 82% and a mean specificity value of 88% are reported when using leave-one-out crossvalidation. No error measures are reported.[49, 51, 53, 56]

Lorenz et al. evaluated 200 datasets originating from 21 patients using leave-one-out crossvalidation and a nonlinear classifier based on fuzzy inference systems. Four parameters based on spectral and texture estimations are used in the study. Overall classification rates estimated as the mean area under the ROC curve of 61% for isoechoic and 69% for hypoechoic and hyperechoic tumors are reported. Histological prostate slices are used as the gold standard. No error measure is given.[19, 21, 52]

Jenderka et al. reported about work on the extraction of spectrum parameters, especially attenuation estimates, based on RF ultrasound data. No results of a clinical study are reported.[39, 40]

Loch et al. analyzed video data of 61 patients using texture parameters and neural network classifiers based on the multilayer perceptron. From a total of 553 ROIs, 53 ROIs were used for training while the remaining 500 ROIs were used for evaluation. A sensitivity of 79% and a specificity of 99% are reported. However, no details about the methods and no error measures are given in the publications.[37, 38]

Feleppa et al. reported about spectrum analysis of RF echo data. During the first few years, lookup tables were used for classification.[41, 42, 57, 58] Later, conventional neural networks, especially multilayer perceptrons, are used in their work. Feleppa et al. include the so-called level of suspicion (LOS) of the physician conducting the examination as an additional parameter, thus, risking to lose independence from the operator.[43–47] Balaji et al. reported on a clinical study including data from 215 patients and applying the classification system described by Feleppa et al. An area under the ROC curve of 80% with standard deviation of 5% was reported when using needle biopsy results as the gold standard and repeated cross-validation involving 14 partitions with datasets being divided into 70% for training and 30% for evaluation.[48]

Some of the aforementioned works use video data for tissue characterization. By using video data instead of RF data, only a small set of tissue characterization parameters can be calculated, which do not contain the necessary amount of information to classify the data with sufficient accuracy. *Only the use of RF data can provide the information used to calculate parameters that characterize prostate tissue in an adequate way.*[59, 60]

Some of the aforementioned works use linear classifiers. *As different parameters encountered in tissue characterization sometimes have a highly nonlinear interdependence, only a nonlinear model is able to combine these parameters and, thus, lead to reliable classification results.*[1, 37, 38, 49, 51, 61] For this reason, a network-based fuzzy inference system is presented in this chapter.[62–66] Methods based on a linear model have also been evaluated formerly but were found less useful regarding the overall classification results.[1, 67, 68] Most classification approaches only work well if the underlying parameters are statistically distributed. Some parameters used in this approach cannot be assumed to be distributed normally.[69–71] Under these circumstances, a network-based fuzzy inference system, which is quite robust with regard to the distribution of input vectors, still performs well.[72]

Some of the works mentioned do not compensate for depth-dependent diffraction. For the evaluation of spectral parameters, the compensation of depth-dependent diffraction and attenuation effects has been found essential [49, 53, 69–71, 73–76] and is thus performed in the tissue characterization system underlying this chapter.

Some former works only focus on the evaluation of one set of parameters, e.g., co-occurrence parameters [34] or spectral parameters.[42, 43, 46–48, 57] Other works try to combine the results of different sets of parameters.[49, 52, 53, 56]*As the information of tissue characterization parameters of different sets is highly uncorrelated, the combination of parameters originating from different sets can lead to better classification results.* From our point of view, only a combination of different sets of parameters can provide the classification system with enough information to support a precise decision.

During the search for the best tissue parameters, it was found that certain parameters perform better than other parameters for a given depth of the ultrasound echo signal. This observation led to the integration of morphological descriptors, which serve as so-called morphological parameters describing the position of the ROI within the prostate.[1, 67]

Methods

When taking the number of publications into account that are dealing with tissue characterization, it becomes quite clear, that there is not only one exclusive method of tissue characterization out there, but several different methods that sometimes might supplement each other and that sometimes might even contradict each other. *While many methods never left their experimental stage, a few methods have proven successful over the last years.*

In this section, the technical details of the tissue characterization system developed by the author are discussed. While a lot of work on the system for tissue characterization has been done by the author himself, many details and aspects of coworkers and other groups working on tissue characterization have been incorporated in this chapter. References to former publications are given throughout the text. References and discussions are also given for certain parts of the system that might be designed in a different way not strictly following the guidelines provided by the author. *In a fast-changing field like ultrasonic tissue characterization improvements and new ideas can come up every day*; therefore, the following discussion can only be used as a guideline, however, a guideline that presents the current state of the art in ultrasonic tissue characterization.

A typical tissue characterization system is divided into four main parts: data acquisition, parameter extraction, classification, and visualization Fig. 16.1.

All four main parts are discussed in the following subsections. Typically, preprocessing and prefiltering of RF echo data is considered to coincide with the actual data acquisition procedure; hence, both aspects are discussed together in section "Data Acquisition and Preprocessing."

The parameter or feature extraction procedure is rather complex, as parameters can be extracted using different techniques. The section starts with the presentation of an "information model" underlying the system described in this work, and also applicable to tissue characterization in general. Several different parameter groups or methods of parameter extraction are reviewed in separate subsections of section "Parameter Extraction." Following the individual discussions, all parameter groups are discussed again in a concluding overview.

In section "Classification," the classification procedure, which consists of several subprocedures, is discussed systematically. A large part of the section deals with special aspects concerning the training process of tissue characterization systems. An important postprocessing method, the morphological filtering, is also discussed in this section.

Section "Visualization," the last section of the methods section, is devoted to the representation and visualization of the classification results, which, although not directly connected with the tissue characterization procedure itself, plays an important and not negligible role in the system as well.

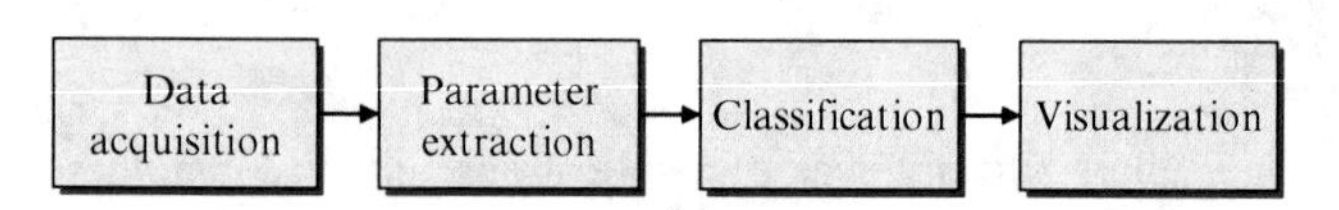

Fig. 16.1. The four main signal processing parts of a typical tissue characterization system as seen from a system developer's point of view

Data Acquisition and Preprocessing

In the system proposed in this chapter, radiofrequency ultrasound echo data of the prostate are captured during the usual transrectal examination of the patient using standard ultrasound imaging equipment. The ultrasound imaging system used in this study was a Kretz Combison™ 330 in combination with the transrectal probe VRW177AK, which consists of a rotating single element transducer with a nominal center frequency of 7.5 MHz and proximal 6 MHz estimated bandwidth. Using this probe, 350 echo lines at an angular spacing of 0.64° were recorded. Thus, the whole image plane comprises 224°. The applied focal depth of the transducer is around 2 cm.

Up to five datasets at different positions of the transducer were recorded per patient. Patient compliance usually was high, as the method does not significantly extend the normal examination time when applying transrectal ultrasound imaging, and the usual examination procedure does not have to be changed in order to apply the system. The system is operator independent, which means that no special knowledge or training is necessary for the successful application of the system. Only typical knowledge of the sonographer or physician of the application of transrectal ultrasound is assumed.

A block diagram of the data acquisition and preprocessing procedure is given in Fig. 16.2. The RF data were captured from the ultrasound imaging system before processing by the ultrasound imaging system's time gain control (TGC) unit. Data are grabbed before being processed by the TGC in order to make sure that data are always amplified with the same time gain control settings and is, therefore, comparable during classification. In fully digital ultrasound systems, sometimes the TGC can be set to a fixed curve, which, when applied during every acquisition, also can assure compatible data.

In the proposed system, the signal is fed into a custom-made hardware TGC with a fixed and known transfer function to compensate for depth-dependent attenuation effects and to provide the following analog-to-digital converter (ADC) with a time signal that uses the whole possible conversion range throughout the sampling time or depth. If ultrasound echo data are grabbed without appropriate depth-dependent amplification, signals originating from deeper positions within the tissue may be too weak to allow a precise analog-to-digital conversion. On the other hand, signals originating from the near field of the transducer might easily overdrive the ADC hardware. The omission of depth-dependent amplification is not recommended, at least not when the product of the center frequency and the desired penetration depth are in the range of the settings for prostate diagnostics.

To ensure that the datasets are comparable, which is quite important for training and classification, a fixed time gain function was forced on the echo data by using custom-made TGC hardware. Later fully digital ultrasound imaging systems allow the reading of the currently applied TGC settings and, thus, if read TGC settings can be interpreted, make grabbing echo data after the imaging system's own TGC unit possible.

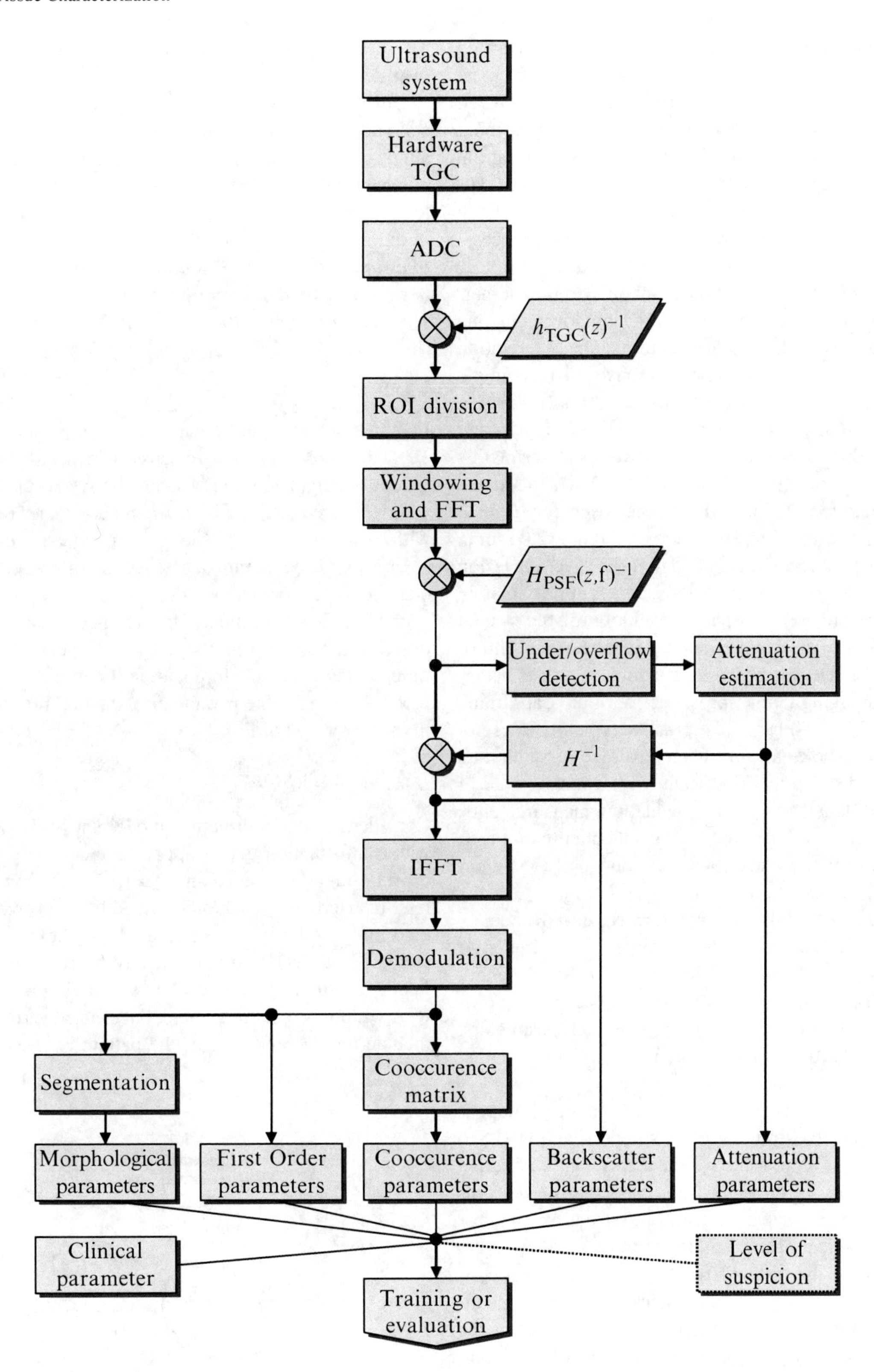

FIG. 16.2. Block diagram of the data acquisition, the preprocessing, and the parameter extraction procedure. The procedure is continued either in the training procedure described in section "Selection of Parameters" or in the evaluation procedure described in section "Evaluation Stage," respectively

After time variant amplification, the data are directly transmitted to a PC workstation and sampled at 33 MHz and 8 bit using a GaGe™ ADC card. For each of the 350 echo lines, 1,536 sample points were recorded. The first 160 sample points of each echo line were discarded due to ring-down artifacts.

During the next step, every echo data line is compensated for the formerly induced TGC amplification, which is an important step, as the tissue attenuation itself is estimated during the feature extraction and used as a tissue describing parameter during classification. During TGC compensation, the word width of the echo data is expanded to 64-bit floating point. The ADC hardware is the part of the system which comprises the narrowest word width. Further signal processing can be performed on 64-bit floating point data.

In the following, every data frame is subdivided into numerous ROIs per prostate slice using the sliding window technique in order to attain spatially distributed tissue characterization images. The ROIs used in this approach consist of 128 sample points in the transducers' axial direction and 16 scan lines in the lateral direction. Their axial and lateral overlap is 75 and 50%, respectively. As the transducer that was used during this work has sector geometry with an angle of 224°, the actual area that is encircled by the ROIs changes over depth. Each ROI comprises an area of approximately 1.5 mm × 2.0 mm in diameter at a typical focal depth of 20 mm. The average lesion that can be detected by the system, thus, covers approximately 3.0 mm^2. To be precise, the spatial resolution of the system consists of 1.5 mm^2 directly at the transducer surface, and of 10.5 mm^2 at the deepest penetration depth, which is rarely needed when imaging human prostates. A whole data frame consists of 1,680 ROIs, but as the prostate typically does not extend over the whole imaging plane, average prostate data frames consisted of up to 1,000 ROIs with a mean value of 680 ROIs per data frame. For attenuation measurements, adjacent ROIs are combined for each single attenuation estimation, as the ROI sizes mentioned are too small to support reliable attenuation estimation.[53]

Subsequently, all ROIs are transformed into frequency domain using fast Fourier transform on every echo line after windowing using a Hamming window of the ROI's length to avoid spectral leakage.[77] This step is exceptionally omitted for the calculation of autoregressive model parameters, as described in section "System Identification Parameters: AR Model."

The RF data are compensated for system and depth-dependent effects using the system's point spread function (PSF) over depth as an inverse filter within the system's effective bandwidth.[78] By using this approach, it is possible to compensate partly for the system's effects due to focusing and for the electromechanical characteristics of the transducer.[54] An error is induced, as the system's point spread function is constructed by interpolating echo sequences from a wire phantom in degassed water recorded at different distances of the transducer.[79] By using a glass plate instead of a wire phantom, the amplitude of the reflected signal can easily overdrive the imaging system's input stage. For this reason, a wire phantom was used to keep the echo amplitude within a feasible range for the calibration procedure. Instead of only recording the echo data of a wire at the focus position, several recordings have been made at different depth positions of the wire, as the spectral characteristics of the reflected signal can differ over depth.[51]

During the last stage of the preprocessing procedure, the echo data are compensated for local attenuation. As the local attenuation is not only estimated for reasons of attenuation compensation, but also to be used as a parameter describing the local tissue characteristics, this concept is described in detail in the following section "Parameter Extraction." *The concept of estimating tissue attenuation using pulse echo systems has been widely used, although it has not been accepted by every scientist working in ultrasonic tissue characterization.*

Parameter Extraction

In the following subsections, different parameter or feature extraction procedures are discussed in detail. Eight different groups of parameters were used in the system developed by the author. A discussion and review comparing all parameter groups with each other closes the discussion on feature extraction.

The extracted parameters used in this approach are not claimed to be completely independent of the underlying ultrasound imaging equipment. The parameters used for classification are calculated from the frequency spectrum and from the time domain, partly before and partly after demodulation.[80] A block diagram of the parameter extraction procedure is given in the lower part of Fig. 16.2.

Information Model

Considering the information model shown in Fig. 16.3, the whole information that is apparent about the patient and the prostate may be divided into four domains, which, more or less, interfere with each other. In addition to spatially distributed information in form of spectral and textural parameters, so-called clinical information may be included in a classification system. A typical clinical variable is the amount of PSA within the patient's blood, but clinical variables may also include the age and race of the patient[81, 82] and *even the ori-*

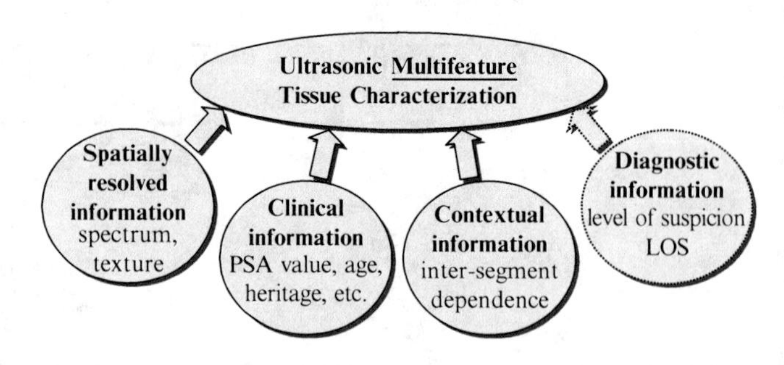

FIG. 16.3. Information model for multifeature tissue characterization systems. Four different information domains can be integrated into computer-aided classification systems. The system discussed in this chapter makes use of spatially resolved information, clinical information, and contextual information. Additional diagnostic information is not integrated due to its dependency on the physician

gin or the disease history of the patient might yield additional information that can be evaluated by ultrasonic tissue characterization systems.[83] Clinical variables have been analyzed by different groups.[84] As a drawback, clinical variables are no longer spatially distributed, as they are not extracted from single ROIs but belong to one patient at a time and, thus, need a huge database to lead to reliable results.

Contextual information can also be described as intersegment dependence. *Contextual features contain information derived from ROIs surrounding the ROI being analyzed.*[85] Considering a ROI, which is to be analyzed and which is surrounded by a certain amount of other ROIs belonging to a certain class, the probability of the ROI being analyzed belonging to the same class as the majority of the surrounding ROIs is higher than the probability of it belonging to another class. Under this assumption, the size of the optimal and most significant neighborhood can be calculated during the training procedure.

The fourth information domain, which is not used in this approach but which is also discussed as it is used by other groups, consists of additional diagnostic information, which has been gathered by physicians during their examinations of the patient. In approaches of other groups working in the field of ultrasonic tissue characterization for prostate diagnostics, the so-called LOS is used as an additional feature in neural network classification.[44, 46, 47] As this domain contains information dependent on the skills of the conducting physician, features originating from this domain should be used with great caution in order to maintain independence of the system. When integrating parameters such as the LOS into an ultrasonic tissue characterization system, the system will lose its independence from other diagnostic modalities and from the operator himself. *The system developed by the author of this chapter is aimed at being independent of other diagnostic systems, thus, yielding a new diagnostic modality, which can be used in addition to conventional diagnostic modalities by the conducting physician.*

Spectrum Parameters

Three different ways to analyze the spectral characteristics of the backscattered echo signal are discussed in this chapter. The first approach consists of conventional Fourier transform-based spectrum analysis. To be precise, only the magnitude of the Fourier spectrum is analyzed in the first approach, while the phase of the complex echo signals is ignored. This approach, which is widely used by the tissue characterizing community, is described in this subsection. The second approach, which is presented in section "System Identification Parameters: AR Model," uses autoregressive model-based spectrum estimation methods, thus, bypassing the windowing process needed when applying conventional Fourier-based spectrum analysis. This approach is often used, to keep ROI sizes as small as possible. The third method, which is described in detail in section "Generalized Spectrum Parameters," is based on the estimation of the generalized spectrum, and, therefore, utilizes information coded in the phase of the complex echo signal.

Following the first approach, spectrum parameters are typically calculated after applying a gating window to the TGC-compensated RF echo data of each ROI, computing the Fourier transform and converting the resultant power spectrum to dB.[77] Spectral results of each scan line are averaged to form an estimate of the average power spectrum within each ROI.[86, 87] A linear regression line is fitted to the averaged power spectrum to extract descriptive features. The regression line is fitted within the effective bandwidth of the system. The typical procedure is shown in Fig. 16.4. Although the linear fit is completely defined by two parameters, usually three parameters, the axis intercept, the slope, and the midband value, of the linear fit are evaluated.

The primary set of spectrum parameters evaluated by the author consists of five measures of backscatter calculated for the signal bandwidth: axis intercept, slope, midband value, square deviation, and normalized square deviation of the linear regression spectrum fit.[43, 52, 67, 88–90] Backscatter parameters can be compensated for attenuation effects, e.g., using the multinarrow band method.[49, 73, 91–93]

It has been shown by Thijssen et al.[93] and Oosterveld et al.[73] that excluding all ROIs with overflows, underflows, or severe inhomogeneities is important for the calculation of attenuation parameters. Under these circumstances, the estimation of the frequency-dependent attenuation coefficient leads to unreliable results. ROIs containing these properties should be discarded before calculation. After estimating the attenuation for all possible ROIs, the missing attenuation values for ROIs containing overflows, underflows, or severe inhomogeneities

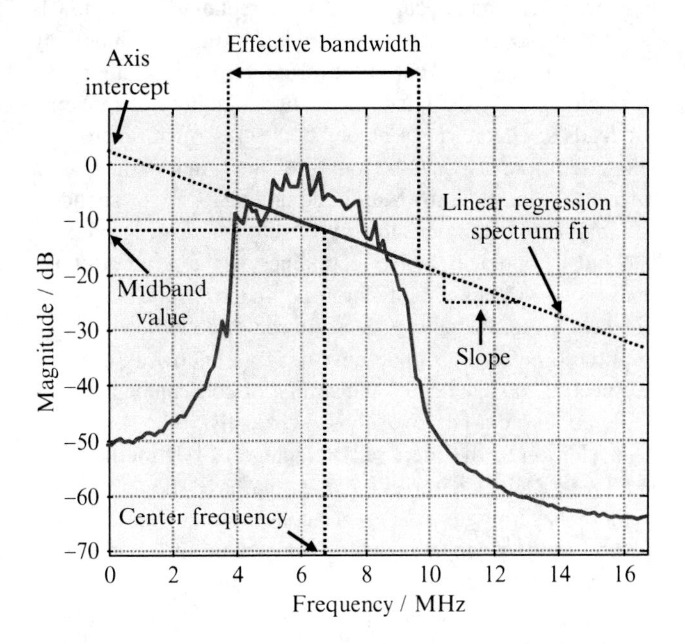

FIG. 16.4. Diagram of a typical RF echo spectrum. The linear regression spectrum fit within the effective bandwidth is used to calculate axis intercept, slope, and midband value. The deviation between the estimated spectrum and the linear spectrum fit can additionally be used as a tissue-characterizing feature

can be constructed by averaging the attenuation estimates of the surrounding ROIs. This step can be made to obtain complete parameter maps without missing entries, which is essential for the following processing steps.

A statistical framework for ultrasound spectral parameter imaging has been proposed by Huisman and Thijssen [74] and Lizzi et al.[69–71, 75] Further information on the underlying statistics can be found in these publications. Applications on different organs are presented in a short overview by Feleppa et al. in Ref. [94].

System Identification Parameters: AR Model

Since finding even small lesions within the prostate should be one objective of ultrasonic tissue characterization, the spatial resolution of the malignancy maps plays an important role. Admittedly, there is a discrepancy between the accuracy of the feature estimations and the underlying size of the ROIs. *On the one hand, as many data as possible are needed for an accurate parameter estimation, which demands large size ROIs; on the other hand, the resolution of the malignancy maps is required to be as high as possible to achieve fine resolved tumor areas and to keep the smallest detectable lesion size as small as possible.*[95, 96] Autoregressive (AR) methods are said to be able to cope with this discrepancy better than conventional Fourier-based methods.[97]

In many approaches, conventional Fourier transform is used to convert the underlying echo signals into frequency domain and to calculate the power spectral density from which the features are extracted. When using Fourier transform, the underlying time series have to be windowed to cope with spectral leakage, which may occur when only a rectangular window is used for the sliding window technique. During the windowing process, a certain amount of "information" is lost due to the masking effect of the window function. The loss of information leads to a decreased accuracy of the classification process. This effect increases as the length of the window decreases. Due to this loss of information, some groups recommend to use analyzing techniques that bypass the windowing process. The most popular of these techniques is the autoregressive analysis or system identification approach.[96, 98] When using AR techniques, the power spectrum can directly be estimated from the time series without involving a windowing process. No spectral leakage occurs and similar effects can be avoided, if the model order has been chosen correctly.[99, 100]

In addition to the proposed advantage of AR methods for small size ROIs, Chaturvedi and Insana have shown that AR methods have an advantage over conventional Fourier-based spectral analysis when analyzing noisy data. In[101] both methods were compared for different signal-to-noise ratios. and AR methods performed significantly better than Fourier methods for datasets involving low SNR.

Several methods for the estimation of the autoregressive coefficients are used today. However, Burg's algorithm has been found to be an efficient method when dealing with applications in ultrasonic tissue characterization.[100]

Six autoregressive spectral parameters are usually calculated from the spectrum and from the linear regression spectrum fit: axis intercept, slope, midband value, square deviation of the spectrum fit from the estimated spectrum, maximum value, and minimum value of the estimated spectrum.

Wear et al. have shown that the relative advantage of AR-based methods over conventional FFT-based methods increases with decreasing gate length.[100] However, it has to be mentioned that in the approach of Wear et al., FFT-based results were calculated without windowing the time series before Fourier transform, which cannot be recommended with respect to spectral leakage. Due to this fact, the results of Wear et al. cannot be taken as the final recommendation for applying ultrasonic tissue characterization based on spectrum analysis. Detailed results of the AR-based feature extraction approach described in this chapter can be found in Refs. [102] and [103].

Generalized Spectrum Parameters

Both the approaches described sections "Spectrum Parameters" and "System Identification Parameters: AR Model," one based on conventional Fourier transform, the other based on autoregressive models, have one property in common: they both only incorporate the magnitude of the frequency spectrum. The phase of the underlying echo signal, which might contain additional information about the underlying tissue, is not analyzed in these approaches. *In contrast to conventional spectral parameters, which are usually extracted after calculating the squared magnitude of the tissue response,* [45, 69–71]*parameters that are based on the generalized spectrum(GS)take into account the phase.*[104–106] The generalized spectrum is also referred to as spectral autocorrelation (SAC) function.

Parameters extracted from the generalized spectrum have been used in the field of breast tissue characterization by Donohue et al.,[104, 107] in the field of liver diagnostics by Vargese and Donohue,[106, 108] and in the field of prostate diagnostics by Scheipers et al.[1]

For an RF signal segment in time and its spectral component, the generalized spectrum is defined over the so-called bifrequency plane by vector multiplication (outer product) of the complex spectral component with its complex conjugate. The vector multiplication results in a matrix with real values (zero phase) along the main diagonal and with complex values in the off diagonal elements. While the main diagonal consists of the magnitude of the Fourier spectrum, the off-diagonal magnitude components depend on the degree of coherence between different frequency components from different regions of the Fourier spectrum and on the original spectrum magnitudes. According to these assumptions, the coherence of the backscattered echo signal, which is said to be an indicator for different tissue types, can be analyzed by the generalized spectrum.

To extract a reduced set of parameters from the generalized spectrum, a collapsed average (CA) is applied over the bifrequency plane.[104] A typical estimation of a collapsed average is shown in Fig. 16.5.

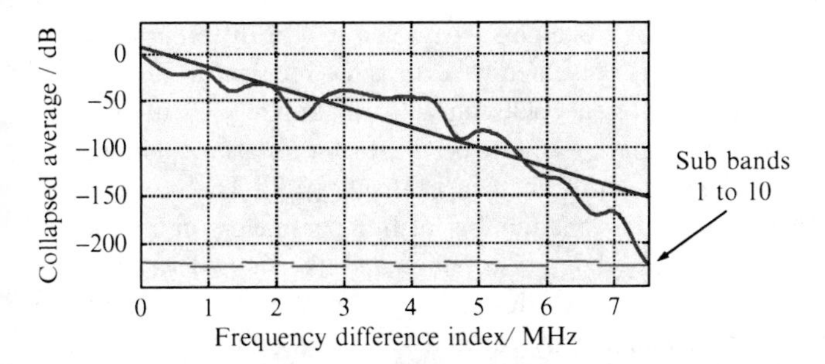

FIG. 16.5. Collapsed average (*red*) as estimated from a typical ROI. The linear regression fit (*blue*) as well as the markings of the ten sub-bands (*green*) are added to the graph. The axis intercept, the slope, the midband fit, and the energy within the sub-bands can be extracted as tissue characterization parameters

Magnitude normalization of the generalized spectrum may be useful.[104] Magnitude normalization scales the magnitudes of the elements of the generalized spectrum to unity, thus, only keeping the original phase differences. The sum of off-diagonal components over a single diagonal is a vector sum where each element has a unit magnitude. Thus, the coherence (consistent phase differences) of the spectral pairs over the ROI determines the final magnitude of the generalized spectrum estimate. Donohue et al. mention that this kind of normalization may be useful to get rid of system-induced artifacts, which, according to Donohue et al., mostly consist of magnitude effects and seldom affect the phase.[104] Magnitude normalization can be avoided, if normalization for the system's point spread function is applied instead.[1]

Donohue et al. suggest using a smoothing procedure on the data points, which consists of calculating an initial least square fit estimate and then sorting out 50% of the points with the greatest error before calculating the final least square fit to the remaining points. This procedure is intended to limit the effects of peaks and nulls due to periodic structures, if present. If the signal is averaged over several lines of each ROI, and at the same time, small enough ROIs have been chosen to keep the inner correlation high, the estimated expected values will lead to smooth estimations of collapsed averages without further smoothing procedures.[1]

Generalized spectrum parameters were directly extracted from the collapsed average. After applying a least squares fit to the collapsed average, which can be seen in Fig. 16.5, the axis intercept, the slope, and the midband value, which is the same as the area under the collapsed average, are extracted.[1] In addition, the maximum of the collapsed average can be used as a feature. Regions containing strong isolated scatterers or boundaries with sharp changes in density yield high values for the area under the collapsed average. Specular echoes directly affect the slope and intercept values, too. The slope indicates the rate at which coherence is lost as a function of frequency difference, and the intercept value relates to both the area under the collapsed average and the slope. Important features of the collapsed average for detecting and estimating regularly spaced or periodic scatterers are the areas under the collapsed average separated into several sub-bands. The collapsed average curve is linearly divided into ten sub-bands within the transducer bandwidth because different-sized structures, e.g., spacings, layers, scatterer pairs, correspond to different regions under the curve.

First-Order Texture Parameters

Texture parameters consist of first- and second-order (i.e., co-occurrence) parameters. *First-order texture parameters do not take into account the spatial relationship between adjacent pixels or sample points.* Second-order texture parameters allow the evaluation of spatial relations between adjacent sample points. *For complex structured signals, such as ultrasound echo data, the use of spatial information seems to be unavoidable.* Some features of typical ultrasound B-mode images of the prostate that are used by physicians or sonographers during diagnostics can easily be evaluated by first-order texture parameters: hyperdense or darker areas within the B-mode image are sometimes an indicator for prostate cancer. When taking this into consideration, the simple mean or minimum value of a ROI, a first-order parameter, should contain discriminating power.

Two different groups of first-order texture parameters are encountered in tissue characterization. The first group, which is described in this subsection, consists of numerous measures, which are directly statistically motivated. The second group consists of measures that are calculated by estimating numerical fits of different orders to the histogram of the backscattered echo signal. As this second group has found popularity with many groups working on ultrasonic tissue characterization[109–117] and is at the same time rather complex, this group is discussed in section "Backscatter Distribution Parameters," separately from the first group discussed in this subsection.

Texture parameters can be calculated directly from video or image data or after detecting the envelope of RF echo, e.g., using Hilbert transform to calculate the analytic signal, shifting the complex analytic signal into base band, and taking the squared magnitude. Typical first-order texture parameters that consist of different estimates of intensity are: maximum value, minimum value, mean value, standard deviation, contrast, which is the same as the variance when dealing with first-order parameters, skewness, kurtosis, signal-to-noise ratio, ratio of squares, entropy, and the full width at half maximum of the gray level histogram.

Backscatter Distribution Parameters

In addition to conventional first-order texture parameters, features based on probability distribution models, which are fitted to the estimated histogram of the backscattered signal's intensities, can be estimated and used for ultrasonic tissue characterization. An exemplary fitting procedure is shown in Fig. 16.6.

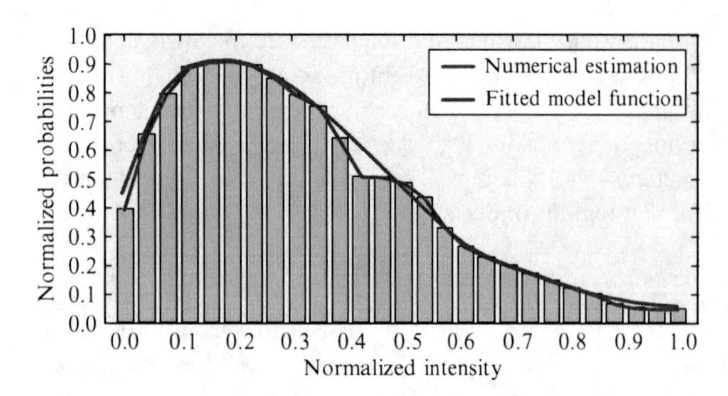

FIG. 16.6. A typical histogram of echo intensities (*gray*). Echo intensities are estimated for each ROI (*read*). Different parametric model functions (*blue*) are fitted to the estimated intensity distribution using least square fits. The model parameters are used as tissue describing features

Tissue parameters extracted from curve fittings of backscatter distribution models belong to the class of first-order texture parameters, as they do not take into account the spatial distribution of the intensities within the ROIs. *Models of ultrasound backscatter, especially of the echo envelope of the demodulated radiofrequency signal, can provide clinically useful information about the regularity and density of scatterers* (small structures in tissues, such as cells) *and, thus, can be useful in medical diagnostics.*

Statistics of speckle patterns in ultrasound backscatter were first described in general by Wagner at al.[80] Backscatter distribution estimates have recently been used for tissue characterization in general by Dutt et al., [118] Georgiou et al.,[112] Shankar,[119, 120] Prager et al.[116] and Dumane et al.[121] In the field of applied tissue characterization, first approaches in breast cancer diagnostics have been published by Shankar et al.[117, 122, 123] and Dumane et al. [109]. In addition, backscatter distribution estimates have been used in combination with parameters from different fields of tissue characterization for breast diagnostics.[111] In addition to breast cancer diagnostics, ultrasound backscatter distributions have been used for diagnostics of muscle tissue of the back after surgery by Pesavento et al.,[115] for cardiac imaging by Hao et al.,[113] and for prostate cancer diagnostics by Scheipers.[1] An overview of different distribution models is presented by Dutt and Greenleaf in Ref. [110].

Several different backscatter distribution models of different model order have formerly been used for ultrasonic tissue characterization for prostate cancer diagnostics.[1] The model order is determined by the number of free parameters in the model. At first, the Rayleigh distribution and its simple derivative, the Rice distribution, are discussed. As both the Rayleigh and the Rice distribution only account for certain types of ultrasound backscatter behavior, the more complex K distribution is evaluated in the next step. The K distribution is discussed in its basic form and in its generalized expansion. Both models have been designed to cope with irregular forms of backscatter, which is discussed in the subsections concerning these distribution models. The subsection on backscatter distribution models closes with two additional models based on the Nakagami distribution. A diagram of possible scatterer distributions is presented

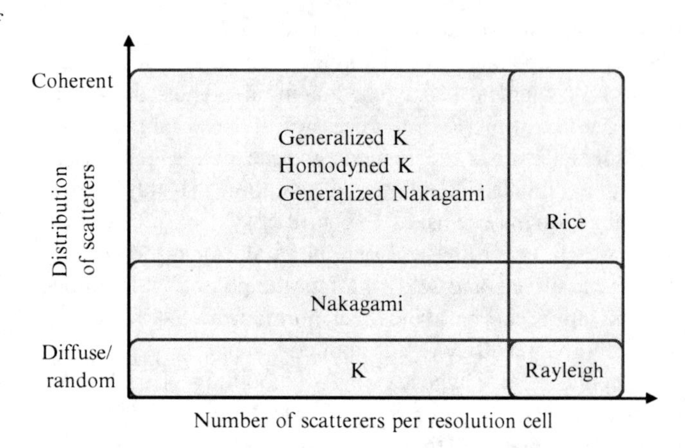

FIG. 16.7. Diagram of possible scatterer distributions. The Rayleigh distribution is only applicable to large numbers of scatterers per resolution cell and random distributed scatterers. The Rice distribution can also be used if there is a coherent part in the signal. The K distribution can model signals where the number of scatterers per resolution cell is small. The whole range of scatterer distributions can be covered by the generalized or homodyned K distributions

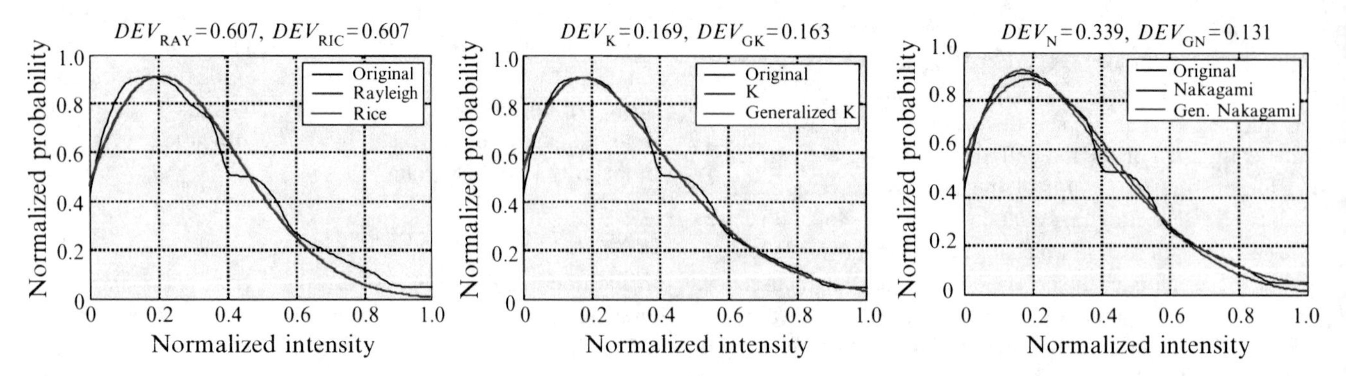

FIG. 16.8. Fitting process of typical ultrasound backscatter distribution models. The differences between the Rayleigh and the Rice distribution and between the K and the generalized K distribution are marginal; thus, they are hardly visible in the plots. The differences between the Nakagami distribution and the generalized Nakagami distribution are more significant. Axes have been normalized. The mean square errors of the fits are given in the title

in Fig. 16.7. A visualization of the six models fitted to a typical prostate dataset is presented in Fig. 16.8.

Parameters that describe the distribution model or parameters derived from them are used as features for tissue characterization. In addition to these features, the deviation of the estimated histogram from the best model fit, e.g., mean square error, can be used as a descriptive feature for tissue characterization. In addition to curve-fitting procedures, approaches based on the estimation of the moments of the distributions are used in some approaches.[120, 123] Approaches based on moment estimations are unavoidable for mathematically complex distributions such as the homodyned *K* distribution, which contains an infinite series.[110] In the approach described here, conventional curve-fitting algorithms based on unconstrained nonlinear optimization procedures[124] are used to estimate the distribution parameters. The model functions are usually fitted after demodulating the RF echo data, but before compression.

Rayleigh Distribution

The echo signal from a scattering medium such as biological tissue can be modeled as the sum of individual backscattered signals from a number of scattering points within the medium. The amplitudes of the individual backscattered signals are assumed to be randomly distributed due to random backscatter coefficients of each individual scatterer. In addition to the amplitudes, the phases are also considered to be randomly distributed due to the random locations of the individual scatterers.

In ultrasound imaging, the echo signal has a statistical nature arising out of interference signals from a large number of randomly distributed scatterers. If the number of scatterers per resolution cell is large, the size of the scatterers is small in comparison with the wavelength, and the distribution of the scatterers is random, the resulting speckle pattern is called "fully developed."[80] In such cases, the only useful information that can be extracted from the echo signal is the mean backscattered energy.

The Rayleigh distribution model suits ideal ultrasound backscatter conditions, but in typical applications of medical ultrasound, the backscattered signal cannot be assumed to be Rayleigh distributed. In many cases, at least one of the following conditions leads to the necessity for so-called post-Rayleigh distributions:

- The number of scatterers per resolution cell might not be large enough
- The effective scatterer size or scatterer cross-subsection might be large in comparison with the wavelength (which actually is implied in the first condition)
- The scatterers might not be located randomly (due to periodicity, structure, clusterings, or specular reflectors)

The violation of at least one of these conditions leads to extended backscatter models that are described on the following pages.

Rice Distribution

The Rice distribution model,[125] which is also referred to as the Rician or the Ricean distribution model, is an extension of the Rayleigh distribution model that adds a "coherent" signal to the backscattered signal that underlies the Rayleigh distribution and, thus, extends the usage of the model. The Rice distribution is completely defined by two parameters.

In contrast to the Rayleigh distribution, the Rice distribution can be used to model unresolved structures such as periodicity in the spatial scatterer distribution. The question, whether this advantage of the Rice distribution yields increased classification results in comparison to the Rayleigh distribution, is examined during the usual classification experiments. Nonuniformities in the spatial scatterer distribution such as clusterings in scatterers or regions with smaller effective numbers of scatterers cannot be modeled by the Rice distribution.

K Distribution

In contrast to the Rice distribution, the *K* distribution can be used to model nonuniformities in the spatial scatterer distribution such as clusterings in scatterers or regions with smaller effective numbers of scatterers.[112, 123, 126]

Neither the Rice distribution, nor the *K* distribution can model a combination of both ultrasound backscatter phenomena, coherent scatterers or a reduced number of scatterers per resolution cell.

Generalized *K* Distribution

The Rice distribution is a generalization of the Rayleigh distribution and allows the modeling of structural and periodic components in the echo signal. The *K* distribution, however, is a generalization of the Rayleigh distribution that allows the modeling of clusterings of scatterers or a reduced effective number of scatterers within the medium. A combination of the Rice distribution and the *K* distribution could model the whole range of speckle statistics that occur in ultrasound imaging by combining the advantages of both approaches. Two approaches are used: the generalized *K* distribution and the homodyned *K* distribution.[114] While the homodyned *K* distribution contains an infinite series and, thus, is computationally adverse, the generalized *K* distribution can be evaluated without greater effort.[127] In the definition of the generalized *K* distribution, the scaling of the *K* distribution is expanded using an additional factor, which integrates the coherent part of the backscattered ultrasound signal.

Nakagami Distribution

Another approach for modeling the backscattered signal, the Nakagami distribution, has been extensively investigated by Shankar et al.[117, 119, 120] and Dumane et al.[109, 121] The Nakagami distribution is an extended form of the Rayleigh distribution and follows a different definition to cope with non-Rayleigh conditions of ultrasound backscatter. The Nakagami distribution is especially aimed at handling a reduced number of scatterers per resolution cell, but can also model coherent scatterers to a certain degree.

As the Nakagami distribution cannot cope with coherent scattering conditions, an extended form, the generalized Nakagami distribution, has been introduced.

Generalized Nakagami Distribution

A generalized form of the Nakagami distribution, which is intended to cope better with coherent scattering, has been proposed by Shankar.[120] The Nakagami distribution is transformed into the generalized Nakagami distribution by introducing an additional shape adjustment parameter.

A visualization of the six model functions fitted to a typical prostate dataset is given in Fig. 16.8. These plots only show one exemplary case, but they demonstrate the typical behavior of the model functions and the fitting procedure. The estimated mean square deviation for the evaluated functions is given in the title of each plot.

The differences between the Rayleigh and the Rice distribution and between the K and the generalized K distribution are marginal; thus, they are hardly visible in the plots. The differences between the Nakagami distribution and the generalized Nakagami distribution are more significant and can be seen clearly in the plots. *For prostate cancer diagnostics, the Nakagami distribution model was shown to outperform the other presented distribution models.*[1]

Second-Order Texture Parameters

In contrast to first-order texture parameters, second-order texture parameters are based on spatial relations between pixel or sample point gray levels and, therefore, can describe spatial distributions of information in data. Second-order texture parameters have been used extensively in the field of tissue characterization, especially for liver[128, 129] and breast cancer diagnostics.[130]

Spatial structures within the data are evaluated by computing co-occurrence matrices of the underlying ROIs. Co-occurrence matrices are also referred to as spatial gray tone dependence matrices. The use of co-occurrence matrices for the evaluation of spatial structures has been proposed by Haralick,[131] Valckx and Thijssen,[132] and Valckx et al.[133]

Elements of co-occurrence matrices are calculated by evaluating the spatial distribution of intensities within an image, a dataset, or a ROI. In a co-occurrence matrix of a defined size, the entries of the matrix represent the probability or relative frequency of the co-occurrence of two quantized intensity level of a pair of pixels or samples under a given distance and orientation angle. For applications in image processing, typically orientation angles of 0°, 45°, 90° and 135° are calculated when using neighborhoods of eight. Sometimes neighborhoods of four are used as well. With respect to the kind of neighborhood, a so-called full co-occurrence matrix can be constructed by element-wise addition of co-occurrence matrices of all relevant orientation angles. Furthermore, the combination, i.e., the sum of two co-occurrence matrices calculated for opposing directions, always yields a symmetric matrix.

When using a sector-based ultrasound scanner, as usually applied during transrectal ultrasound, co-occurrence matrices should only be calculated in axial direction because of the nonlinear geometry of the scan area. When a sector-based geometry is used, the lateral resolution changes rapidly with depth, thus making the calculation of comparable tissue parameters difficult. This characteristic is quantitatively visualized in Fig. 16.9.

Even when an ultrasound probe with linear geometry is used, the calculation of symmetric gray tone spatial dependence matrices combining all directions may be uncertain because of focusing and diffraction effects. It has to be admitted that diffraction and focusing effects influence the axial resolution over depth, even when the data have been compensated for these effects by filtering with the inverse transfer function of the system. Therefore, even texture parameters that are only calculated in the axial direction may exhibit depth dependency, but on a smaller scale than texture parameters calculated in the lateral direction.

Various parameters from common co-occurrence matrices can be calculated in the spatial domain from demodulated data or from image data for different distances, i.e., step sizes between pixels.[34] The following second-order texture parameters are usually evaluated: angular second moment is a measure of the local homogeneity of the data and represents the energy within the co-occurrence matrix. In other approaches, the variance of the co-occurrence matrix, which only differs by a linear factor, is used instead. Contrast is a measure of the amount of local variations present in the data and, thus, can directly characterize edges and specular structures. Correla-

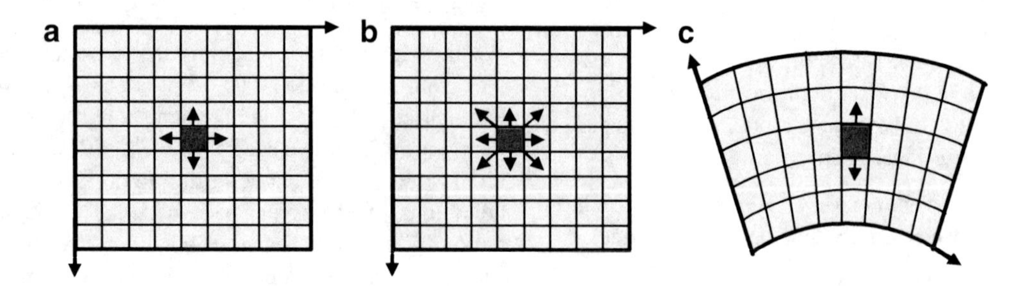

Fig. 16.9. Calculation of co-occurrence matrices. (**a**) A neighborhood of four is shown. (**b**) Shows a neighborhood of eight. Both approaches are typically used in the field of image processing. (**c**) The typical geometry of an ultrasound sector scanner is shown. Due to this geometry, only axial intensity distributions should be evaluated

tion is a measure of local linear dependencies and can be useful to characterize local periodic texture patterns. Dimension is a weighted measure of the local information content. Entropy is often used to characterize diffuse echoes and other highly disordered texture patterns. Inverse difference moment is related to the dimension measure, but does not use a weighting term. Kappa stresses the relationships between equal intensities and, therefore, can characterize specular reflections. Peak density is a simple measure of homogeneity relations within the ROI and can evaluate harmonics as well as other periodicities. All parameters should be estimated in axial direction only and should be averaged over echo lines.[1]

A problem of this parameter group is the dependence of some co-occurrence parameters on the linear attenuation of the system. Correlation and inverse difference moment are depth variant parameters. It is possible to compensate for the depth dependency by normalizing the data as proposed in Ref. [131] or by normalizing each ROI locally. All other co-occurrence parameters evaluated in this approach are independent of depth. Texture parameters, which are based on intensity data, are highly dependent on the scaling of the underlying data. It is recommended to use RF echo data of the ultrasound imaging system for the parameter calculation and, thus, allow scaling of the intensity maps for the extraction of texture parameters as required. Approaches of other groups use ultrasound B-mode video images for tissue characterization and, thus, cannot choose the scaling freely. It is preferable to give more weight to the low-amplitude patterns relative to large amplitude spike. This method is referred to as amplitude compression. Different nonlinear scaling methods are proposed in the literature,[104] but often simply taking the logarithm of the intensity values has proven to lead to reliable results, as in the work underlying this chapter.

Morphological Parameters

All parameter groups discussed in the previous subsections are based on features extracted from radiofrequency or image data. Thus, these parameters describe the characteristics of the underlying tissue of each single ROI of the ultrasound dataset by means of texture, attenuation, and spectral nature. The parameters described in this subsection are based on the morphology of the organ, i.e., the prostate. *Parameters extracted from information about the morphological nature of an organ can make up a completely complementary group of features which shows little correlation with parameters extracted from RF or video data.*[1, 134]

Under certain circumstances, some tissue parameters discussed in the preceding subsections might lead to unreliable results. For example, *attenuation measurements can fail if calculated behind calcifications due to the fact that the largest part of the signal energy is reflected by the calcification.* Only a small amount of energy is left behind the calcification, which does not support reliable attenuation estimation. While attenuation estimations yield reliable results in the absence of calcifications, some co-occurrence parameters that are independent of the mean intensity can still yield satisfying results under adverse circumstances such as calcifications. Because calcifications, in most cases, are found in the lower subsection of the prostate, this observation led to the inclusion of morphological descriptors.[1] *Morphological descriptors, if integrated in a nonlinear classifier, can allow classification system to choose different parameter combinations for different positions within the prostate.* For example, parameters extracted from attenuation estimations are chosen by the system when dealing with near-field ROIs, texture parameters based on co-occurrence matrices are used for deep positions within the prostate.

Eight so-called morphological descriptors have been proposed. The calculation of these morphological descriptors is illustrated in Fig. 16.10. As the first parameter, the axial distance of the ROIs from the center of the ultrasound probe can be evaluated. The sagittal position and the lateral position of the ROIs within the prostate with respect to a Cartesian grid are evaluated using two interpretations. On the one hand, the lateral position ranging from −1 on the left-hand side to +1 on the right-hand side can be evaluated. On the other hand, an additional interpretation normalized on the center of the prostate and, thus, ranging from +1 on the left-hand side to 0 in the center position and again to +1 on the right-hand side can also be evaluated. The second interpretation is normalized on the center of the prostate because it is intended to prevent the system from differentiating between the left-hand and the right-hand subsection of the prostate. The lateral position of the ROIs in reference to the scan beam is coded in three different parameters. The first measure contains the position of the ROIs ranging from −1 on the left-hand side to +1 on the right-hand side of the prostate. The second measure is again normalized on the center of the prostate slice, thus ranging from +1 on the left-hand side to 0 in the center position and again to +1 on the right-hand side of the organ. This normalization is performed again in order to prevent the system from

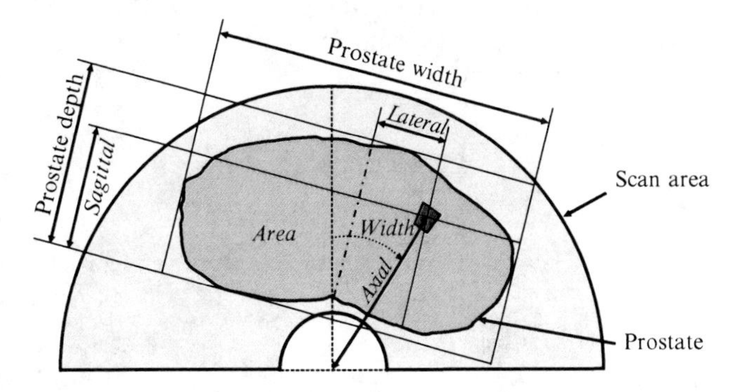

FIG. 16.10. Sketch of a typical prostate with some morphological measures attached. The distances Organ depth and Organ width are used to normalize the morphological descriptors *Sagittal*, *Axial*, *Lateral*, and *Width*. The area of the prostate slice is evaluated as an additional parameter

differentiating between the left and the right subsection of the prostate. The third parameter, which is called "integrated width," contains an estimation which is calculated by measuring the width over the whole prostate slice at the current position of the ROI, thus only yielding one value per sagittal position. The last of the eight morphological features stands for the area of the prostate slice at the examined position, thus only yielding one value per prostate slice.

All parameters except area and the integrated width estimate should be normalized on the size of each individual prostate slice to yield values between 0 and +1 or −1 and +1, respectively. This normalization is performed in order to keep these parameters independent of individual prostate slice sizes.

As approximately 70–80% of all prostate carcinoma are found in the peripheral zone of the prostate, which extends at the lower bound of the organ, the parameters triggering on the sagittal position of the ROI can be expected to yield high classification results during single parameter classification experiments. The lateral measures are expected to provide additional discriminating power, as cancer only spreads from the inside of the organ in very few cases. However, classification rates of lateral measures are expected to lie below the rates of the sagittal measures.

Clinical Features

In addition to classical tissue parameters and morphological features, clinical features make up a third group of parameter, which can be used for tissue characterization. *Clinical features typically consist of all variables which concern the life and condition of a patient and which can be recorded in a numerical form.* Typical examples of clinical features are the age of the patient and the amount of PSA in the patient's blood. Other personal variables, such as the race or heritage of the patient and special diets or medication, can also be considered as clinical features. If known, the disease history can be very valuable. *Clinical features are usually highly independent of the other parameter groups because of their completely different nature.* This independence can lead to increased classification rates if clinical variables are used together with conventional tissue parameters and morphological parameters in a single classification procedure.

In the system underlying this chapter, the age of the patient in years at the day of the transrectal ultrasound examination was recorded and stored as a parameter. In addition to the patient's age, the conventionally acquired amount of PSA in the patient's blood [4, 135] was stored as a parameter. Extended PSA measures such as free PSA value [10, 135, 136] or the PSA speed [4, 6] can also be included.

Additionally, the physician's results of the DRE were recorded for every patient and stored as a parameter.[28, 137] These values are only of interest during first interpretations of the data and for comparing the results of the different types of diagnostics. The results of DRE are highly dependent on the conducting physician's skills and, thus, are not recommended for integration in computer-aided diagnostic systems, which are intended to remain independent of the operator.

Several works have been carried out on the combination of clinical variables in order to produce precise diagnostics. An overview of neural networks classification for urology is given by Wei in Ref. [138]. In a general approach, the clinical features of 1,787 patients were evaluated and high classification accuracies were reported.[139] Most previous approaches only combined parameters from the so-called clinical feature group. Feleppa et al. report the successful combination of spectral parameters and clinical features using a neural network.[44, 46, 47]

All previously described parameters yield one value for each ROI or at least one parameter per prostate slice. The clinical features discussed in this subsection only yield one value per patient. *When working on small patient databases, the integration of clinical parameters into the system can easily cause problems.* Taking the central limits theorem into consideration, the amount of information might be too small to support a reliable training procedure. *Clinical parameters should only be used, when the patient database consists of a relative larger patient contingent, e.g., a few hundred.*

Discussion of Parameter Groups

A correlation matrix shown in Table 16.1 was calculated for all parameter groups. The correlation matrix is calculated as a simple measure of the linear correlation coefficient between the different parameter groups. If the correlation coefficient between two or more parameter groups is high, the "information" stored in these features is regarded to be similar; thus,

TABLE 16.1. Correlation matrix over all groups of parameters.

Parameter group	Spectr.	AR	GS	Text. 1	Distri.	Text. 2	Morph.	Clinic.
Spectral	1.00	0.23	0.16	0.17	0.09	0.16	0.38	0.03
AR model	0.23	1.00	0.35	0.33	0.15	0.39	0.06	0.03
Generalized spectrum	0.16	0.35	1.00	0.71	0.68	0.34	0.06	0.03
Texture first order	0.17	0.33	0.71	1.00	0.80	0.52	0.07	0.01
Distribution model	0.09	0.15	0.68	0.80	1.00	0.40	0.04	0.02
Texture second order	0.16	0.39	0.34	0.52	0.40	1.00	0.05	0.02
Morphological	0.38	0.06	0.06	0.07	0.04	0.05	1.00	0.01
Clinical	0.03	0.03	0.03	0.01	0.02	0.02	0.01	1.00

only one of the high correlated features should be kept for further classification tasks.

The combination of different features originating from different groups of parameters can increase the final classification rates of computer-aided diagnostic systems. When the correlation coefficients in Table 16.1 are taken into consideration, it is apparent that the correlation between the two first-order texture parameters groups ("Texture first order" and "Distribution model") is high in comparison to the other correlation coefficients. The correlation between conventional first-order texture parameters and features extracted from backscatter distribution models is 0.80. This leads to the assumption that an additional *integration of backscatter distribution model parameters in addition to conventional first-order texture parameters will probably not lead to a significant increase in classification rate.*

The correlation coefficients between first- and second-order texture parameters are in acceptable ranges between 0.40 and 0.52, which gives rise to the assumption that different tissue characteristics are evaluated by these groups of parameters, as has already been proposed in the appropriate subsections. The correlation coefficients between morphological and clinical features and nearly all other parameter groups are low when compared to other correlation coefficients. This leads to the assumption that the integration of morphological and clinical features, in addition to conventional tissue characterizing parameters, will increase classification rates. *Very low correlation coefficients* ranging between 0.01 and 0.03 *are found in all combinations of parameters involving the clinical parameter group. This motivates the integration of the PSA value, the age of the patient, and other clinical values into the classification system.*

Similar correlation coefficients are found in nearly all combinations involving the morphological parameter group, which give rise to correlation coefficients between 0.01 and 0.07, except for the spectral parameter group, which achieves 0.38.

The parameter group based on generalized spectrum parameters shows correlation coefficients of 0.68 and 0.71 when evaluated against first-order texture parameters. This would not have been expected for these combinations. An interesting observation is the fact that all three frequency domain-based parameter groups, spectral parameters, autoregression parameters, and generalized spectrum parameters, yield relatively low correlation coefficients.

Classification

After the data acquisition and preprocessing as the first step in ultrasonic tissue characterization and the parameter extraction as the second step, the classification procedure makes up the third step. *In general, there are different classification methods in use today, but due to the mathematical characteristics of the underlying parameters, only a subset of these methods is adequate for ultrasonic tissue characterization systems.* The whole range of classification methods can be divided into two groups: numerical and parametrical classifiers.

Numerical classifiers typically store numerous known cases in a large database and consult this so-called knowledge base when looking for a specific diagnosis on a new case. As information about known cases is usually stored in numerical form, these classifiers are called "numerical." A known diagnosis found in the database, which shows similar features as the new case, is then accepted as diagnosis for the new case. Numerical classifiers, also known as nonparametric classifiers, are computationally inefficient because not only the whole database has to be stored inside the system, but also the whole database has to be searched for entries, which match each single new case. Typically, the databases are downsampled to a practical size to increase both storage space and the required computational power, while accepting a loss in accuracy. The searching procedure, also referred to as table-lookup method, may include interpolating algorithms to increase accuracy. Typical numerical classifiers are nearest neighbor or k-nearest neighbor classifiers. The description "nearest neighbor" originates from the procedure of looking for "neighbors" of the actual case in the feature space. For the example of computer-aided diagnostic systems, the "neighbors" stand for known diagnoses for known cases described by similar parameters as the actual case.

In contrast to numerical classifiers, parametrical classifiers analyze the underlying data and estimate model functions, which model the behavior and the interdependency of the underlying parameter vectors. Instead of storing the whole set of known cases, parametrical classifiers outline the numerical properties of the features. Simple parametrical classifiers such as the minimum distance classifier, the Bayesian classifier, and the maximum likelihood classifier are only able to model linear relationships between features. *If nonlinear relationships between evaluated features are expected, as typically is in ultrasonic tissue characterization, higher-order parametrical classifiers such as neural networks and fuzzy inference systems are the methods of choice.* Fuzzy inference systems and artificial neural networks have proven to be successful in handling the nonlinear behavior of tissue parameters.[1, 53, 68, 140]

One property, which all higher-order classifiers have in common, is the need for training. Typically, the amount of available data is divided into training datasets and validation datasets to yield representative classification results during the design procedure of the classifier by evaluating the system with data that were formerly unknown to the system during training. More details about this concept called crossvalidation are given in section "Crossvalidation." A rough overview of classifier design is given in Fig. 16.11. The training procedure and especially the crossvalidation method, which describes the division of the whole dataset into training and validation datasets, are discussed in detail in section "Crossvalidation."

The classification procedure used in the system developed by the author consists of several stages, which are described in

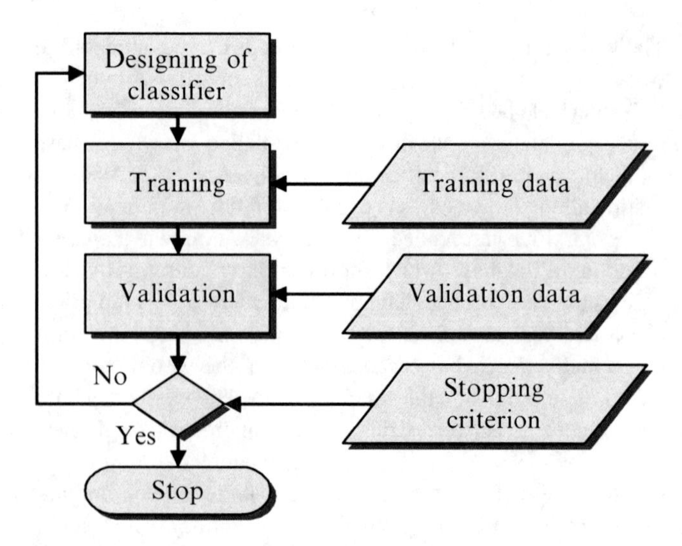

FIG. 16.11. Basic principle of classifier design, which consists of two main stages: training and validation. When neural networks or fuzzy inference systems are considered, the classifier is iteratively optimized until a criterion is met. When considering simple classifiers, such as numerical or minimum distance classifiers, no iterative steps are taken

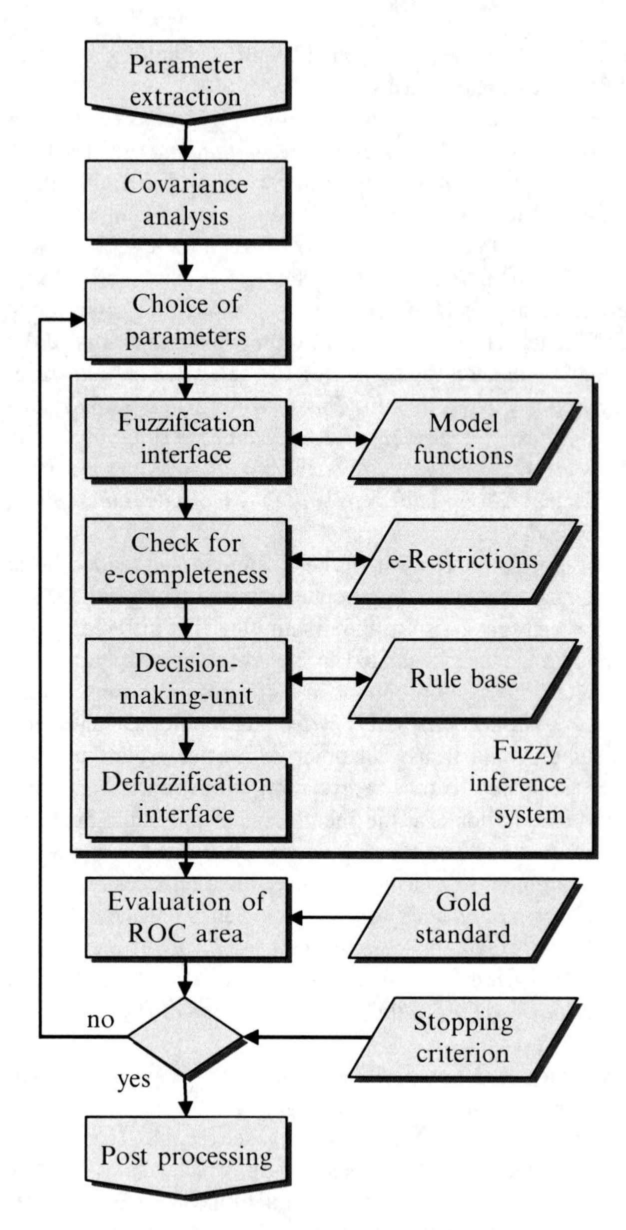

FIG. 16.12. Block diagram of training procedure. During this procedure, the different tissue characterization parameters are analyzed, the rule base of the fuzzy inference system is determined and the optimal combination of parameters is selected

detail in the following subsections. An introductory overview of the classification procedure is given in the block diagram shown in Fig. 16.12, which visualizes the training procedure of the system. The classification procedure applied during the training stage differs from the classification procedure implemented for the final evaluation and application of the system. The latter procedure, thus, is described separately in section "Evaluation Stage."

When using higher-order classifiers, several pitfalls have to be dealt with. *If the model order of the classifier is too high, the model may overfit the training data, which can lead to poor classification results during crossvalidation.* The consequential application of crossvalidation methods during training can only cope with this problem to a certain degree.

Fuzzy Inference Systems

The adaptive network-based fuzzy inference systems proposed in this chapter are designed to classify and separate the ROIs into two classes. The first class, or target group, consists of all negative or benign ROIs. The second target group consists of all positive or malignant ROIs. On the underlying data, two FIS are used in parallel: one FIS is trained to find all hypoechoic and hyperechoic positive ROIs, while the other FIS is designed to detect all isoechoic positive ROIs. Thus, overall three target groups are implemented in the system, as the positive target group is divided into two positive subgroups.

The fundamentals of fuzzy logic and of the idea behind fuzzy models can be found in detail in the publications of Zadeh [62, 63] and Mendel [65] and in several textbooks by various authors. An overview of network-based fuzzy systems is given by Jang in Ref. [141]. The mathematical background, especially the learning or training process of the FIS, is described in detail by Jang in Ref. [64]. Due to the complexity of fuzzy inference, only a rough overview and a few important details can be given here. The interested reader is motivated to get further details from the cited literature.

Fuzzy inference systems use so-called membership functions to fit the underlying parameter probability distributions in the multidimensional parameter domain concerning each target group. Typically, Gaussian membership functions are used when working on normally distributed data. As mentioned in section "Parameter Extraction," not all parameter vectors implemented in this work can be considered to be normally distributed.[69–71] This means that the use of Gaussian membership functions may be considered unsafe in a statistical way, but the use of fuzzy inference systems in combination with Gaussian membership functions has been proven to lead to reliable results, even if the underlying data are not completely normally distributed. In a typical fuzzy inference system, each processed feature is not only modeled by one single membership function, but by several independent functions. The number of membership functions per parameter is determined during the classification procedure and is part of the design process. To model each feature using several membership functions instead of only one model function each makes it possible to cope with a wider range of possible distributions within the data:

- Multiple clusters within the input data space can be modeled using several Gaussian membership functions per parameter
- Non-Gaussian distributed clusters within the input data space can be modeled using several Gaussian membership functions per parameter in superposition

A set of membership functions is combined according to so-called rules. The combination of membership functions into rules is shown later in Fig. 16.15. An increasing number of membership functions yields a decreasing classification error when considering the fit of the model functions to the training dataset alone. When considering crossvalidation methods (see section "Crossvalidation"), an increasing number of membership functions might result in decreasing generalization. Therefore, *the correct choice of the number of membership functions is very essential for the design of robust fuzzy inference systems.*

The fuzzy inference systems used on the underlying data are based on Sugeno-type systems[142] with up to 15 Gaussian model functions per parameter. A Sugeno-type system has been chosen because this type of fuzzy inference system is computationally efficient and easily permits the use of propagation algorithms. The exemplary block diagram of a typical first-order Sugeno-type fuzzy inference system is presented in Fig. 16.13. In this example, three different input parameters are evaluated by two membership functions each, thus, resulting in two rules. The results of both rules are combined to form an output value.

The whole feature space is defined by a certain rules, which each consist of a model function for each parameter. Several membership functions belonging to a typical classification problem are shown in Fig. 16.14. In this example, the membership functions of two rules combining six parameters are given.

As can be seen in Fig. 16.14, two clusters yielding high probabilities for the target group are found in the six-dimensional feature space spanned by the six input parameters. Both clusters are modeled using Gaussian membership functions of different widths and different center positions.

After the membership functions have been estimated during the training procedure, the system can be used to evaluate the validation dataset. All measured input parameters of a fuzzy inference system are weighted by the membership functions as shown in Fig. 16.15. This step is called fuzzyfication, as the crisp values of the input parameters are transformed into fuzzy values by weighting the crisp input values with the formerly determined membership functions. The estimated degree of membership is then processed by the rules. Often, simply the

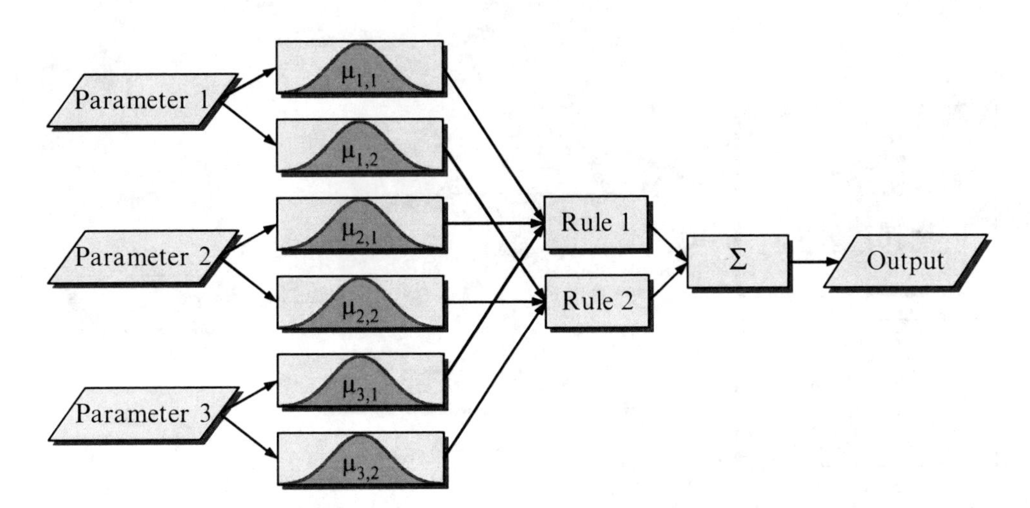

FIG. 16.13. Block diagram of a typical Sugeno-type fuzzy inference system. Three different input parameters are evaluated by two membership functions each, thus, resulting in two rules. The estimated degrees of membership are evaluated by the rules. The results of both rules are combined to form an output value

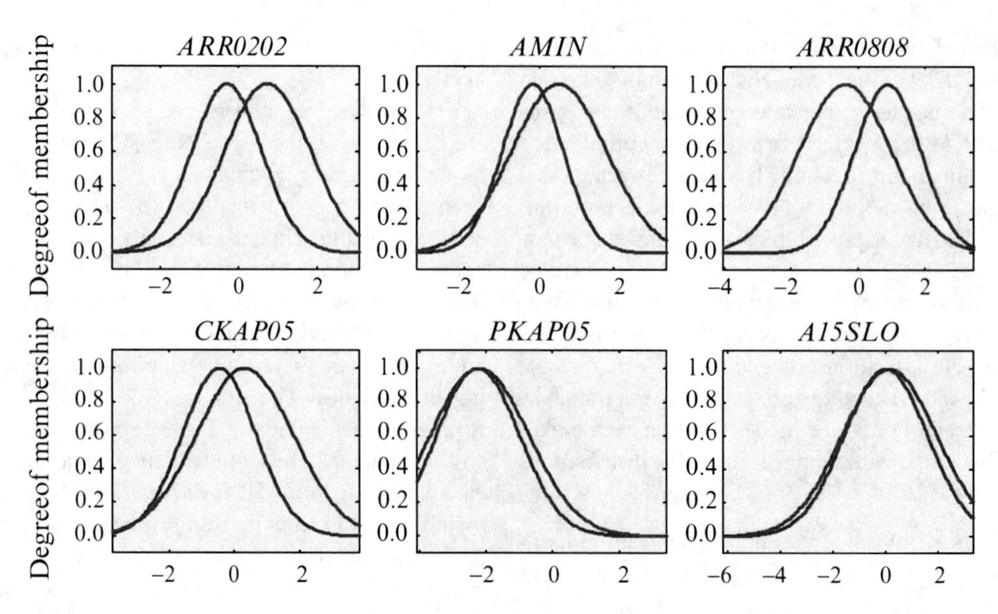

FIG. 16.14. Twelve membership functions, as determined for six different tissue characterization parameters. The functions are plotted over the normalized output ranges of the parameters. Two rules have been found by the classification system to best characterize the underlying data. All membership functions belonging to the first rule are drawn in *red*. All membership functions belonging to the second rule are drawn in *blue*

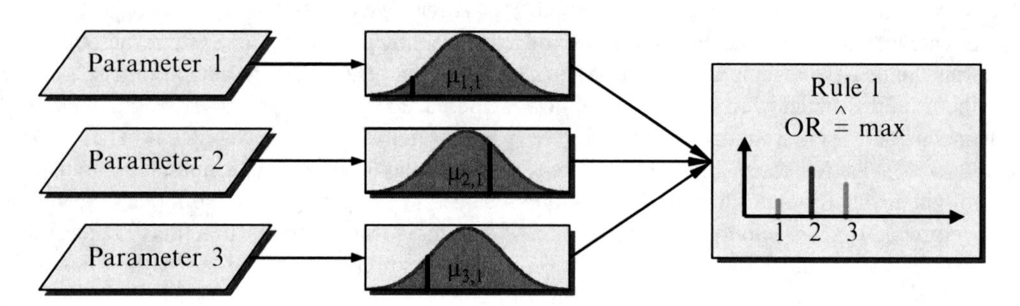

FIG. 16.15. Fuzzyfication procedure and application of fuzzy rules. All input parameters of a fuzzy inference system are weighted by the membership functions as depicted in thefigure. This is called the fuzzyfication procedure. The estimated degree of membership is then processed by the rules. Often, simply the maximum value is used as the output, which is called the "winner takes all" strategy

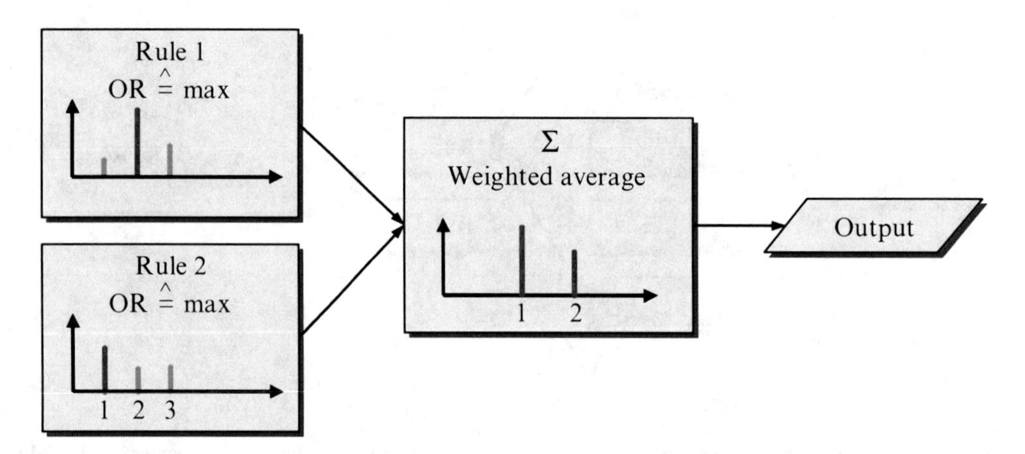

FIG. 16.16. Defuzzyfication stage of a typical fuzzy inference system. The output values of all rules are combined during the so-called defuzzyfication stage. Often, simply the weighted average is used as output value of the fuzzy inference system

maximum value is used as the output value as shown in the figure. In this example, only the first of the two rules involved in the fuzzy inference process is shown for reasons of simplicity. Here, parameter 2 achieves the highest membership value; thus, this value is forwarded to the next stage.

During the next stage, as shown in Fig. 16.16, the output of all rules belonging to a fuzzy inference system is combined. This procedure is called the defuzzyfication stage. In this example, simply the weighted average is used as the output value of the fuzzy inference system. Complex procedures, such as taking the center of gravity of the rules, have been proven useful in many applications and, therefore, may be used as well in ultrasonic tissue characterization. Sometimes, the output values are scaled using arbitrary output functions. If involved, these output functions are also considered to be part of the fuzzy inference system. If using an output threshold-independent performance measure for evaluating the classification system, such as the area under the ROC curve, scaling of the output does not alter classification results and, thus, can be ignored.

As mentioned earlier, the number of rules is adaptively chosen by the system. Subtractive clustering, which is an extension of the mountain clustering method, is often used as the initial step in the supervised learning procedure to find natural clusters in the data space. During this step, the center position of the Gaussians in the feature space is determined. Subtractive clustering is a realization of the "scatter partitioning" method described by Jang.[141] A hybrid adaptive training algorithm based on backpropagation and least square error estimation with adaptive step sizes is used to train the system.[64, 143] The use of adaptive step sizes during backpropagation increases training speed, especially if the initialization of the rules is far from optimal. The initial setting of the membership functions is found using the clustering procedures mentioned. Nevertheless, training speed is increased by using adaptive step sizes. Batch learning is applied to set the width parameters and to refine the center position of the Gaussians.

During the training procedure, the best combination of parameters and the appropriate membership functions are stored in a rule base, which is used during the evaluation procedure described later in section "Evaluation Stage." This rule base forms the knowledge base of the fuzzy inference system. *Radial basis neural networks are mathematically similar to network-based fuzzy inference systems and can be implemented to behave in the same way as network-based fuzzy inference systems if required.*[144] *In comparison to more complex neural network designs like the multilayer perceptron, fuzzy inference systems and radial basis neural networks have the important advantage of being more transparent or easier to see through.* Although the underlying data will not always be normally distributed, normally distributed data should be considered as the model or best case when designing a classification system to be used in ultrasonic tissue characterization. Therefore, *using classification systems that apply a combination of Gaussians to model the underlying data should be considered first.*

Crossvalidation

Methods for estimating the accuracy of diagnostic tests and, thus, for comparing different classifiers require independence of the test results in the samples. For this reason, fivefold crossvalidation methods have been used for the selection and combination of parameters for the tissue characterization system underlying this chapter. *Crossvalidation methods are known to yield an almost unbiased prediction error, although it must be accepted that the results can be highly variable.*[145] Fivefold crossvalidation is a method well known in the field of pattern recognition and classification, which consists of dividing the whole amount of data into five subsets of approximately the same size, training the classifier with four of the subsets, and testing the trained classifier with the fifth remaining subset. Training and testing procedures are repeated five times with all possible permutations of the data subsets.

Consequently, no data that are involved in the training should be used for evaluation. Only datasets that were not used during the training procedure are used during evaluation. The same amounts from both target groups, positive and negative, are used during the training procedure. During the evaluation procedure, the remaining data are used. The division into five equally sized subsets is based on experiences with similar datasets[1, 67, 68] and represents a compromise between the achieved accuracy of the classification results and acceptable computation time.

To provide an overall classification result for the classifier, the mean value and the standard deviation of the classifier can be calculated over all five results. While the mean value is a good estimation for the overall performance of a classifier, the standard deviation or variance indicates the stability. In the field of pattern recognition and classification, the estimation of the standard deviation over small cases such as five is typically accepted.

In approaches where there are multiple cases from the same patient, the estimation and inference of the accuracy of the diagnostic test must account for intracluster correlation. *To account for intracluster correlation, crossvalidation methods should be used on datasets, which are constructed considering a division of the number of patients, not the amount of ROIs.*[146] Small differences in the sizes of the subsets can be accepted. When using crossvalidation methods and not keeping in mind that possible intracluster correlation exists, the classification results will be unreliable because they are too positively weighted. Thus, a strict differentiation between patients has to be maintained during the evaluation of classification systems.

Once the design of the classifiers is finished, leave-one-out classification methods over patients can be performed for the final classification results, in order to achieve results that provide the highest possible accuracy, not considering computational costs. Leave-one-out crossvalidation should also be performed over patients and not over abstract datasets to avoid intracluster correlation. When considering this system developed by the author, the original database consisted of data originating from 100 patients. Thus, leave-one-out crossvalidation is performed by training the classifier with the data of 99 patients and classifying the data of the remaining patient with the resulting classification system. Again, both measures, the mean classification performance and the standard deviation, should be estimated. For leave-one-out crossvalidation, the estimation of the standard deviation can be considered being completely unbiased. Leave-one-out crossvalidation is also referred to as complete crossvalidation or total crossvalidation, as it is performed on the smallest sizes of crossvalidation data subsets possible.

Using crossvalidation methods during training only leads to representative performance measures if performed on independent datasets. In addition, generalization of the classifier can easily be achieved if using crossvalidation methods during training and design of the classifier.

Selection of Parameters

As discussed in section "Parameter Extraction," several parameter groups have been evaluated by the author with regard to their classification power and practicability for ultrasonic tissue characterization for prostate cancer detection. The intention is to integrate different parameters originating from different parameter groups into multifeature classifiers. The selection of adequate parameters from the pool of different parameter groups is discussed in this subsection.

The block diagram of the training and parameter selection procedure is given in Fig. 16.12. The parameter selection procedure starts by calculating the classification power of each single feature. In order to use a decision-based criterion[147] instead of an approximation-based criterion (e.g., mean square error), the classification power is expressed as the area under the ROC curve.[148] Details on the estimation of ROC curves are given in section.[149, 150]

Once the area under the ROC curve has been calculated for every single parameter, the parameter with the largest area is chosen as the first feature of choice. During the next step, this parameter is evaluated in combination with all other remaining parameters. The parameters belonging to the pair with the largest area under the ROC curve are chosen as the parameters of choice for the next iteration. This procedure is repeated until the area under the ROC curve stalls or even decreases as the total number of parameters increases.

As this stepwise selection procedure is rather time consuming, a step reduction procedure has been proposed by Sugeno.[142] When the approach of Sugeno is followed, the current parameters of choice are only evaluated in combination with new parameters that performed better during the last iteration step, as the best combination of parameters two iteration steps ago. In most cases, this reduction has been proven useful as the best combination of parameters was found with a reduced number of evaluations. With regard to computational costs, this step reduction approach remarkably reduces computation time. No exact reduction factors are given here due to the variability in different datasets. An exemplary scheme, which involves the Sugeno reduction method, is demonstrated in Fig. 16.17.

It has to be admitted that this reduced selection procedure is not the optimal method as regards the accuracy of the best parameter estimation. The optimal set of parameters can only be estimated if every possible combination of parameters is evaluated and compared with all other possible combinations. However, as the optimal method is too time consuming to be practical, the near-optimal method proposed here is considered a very good choice for applications in ultrasonic tissue characterization.

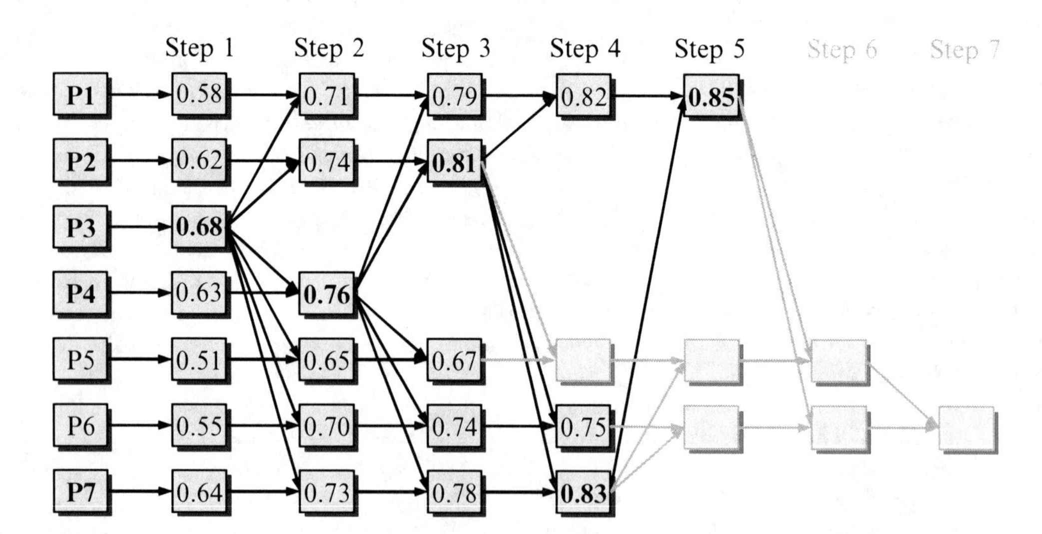

Fig. 16.17. Stepwise selection of parameters. The parameter selection is performed according to the exemplary scheme shown. Parameters are discarded during the selection procedure according to the Sugeno reduction method (P5 and P6), which is implemented to reduce the number of calculations needed to reach the optimal parameter combination. Skipped calculation steps are shown in *gray*

Figure 16.18 displays the results of a parameter combination process. The mean area under the ROC curve is shown together with error bars. Eight parameters have been combined successfully using a fuzzy inference system. An increase in the area under the ROC curve is observed throughout the combination process. The example shown is typical for parameter combination procedures using fuzzy inference.

Postprocessing

When considering a single ROI that is going to be analyzed, it is proposed that the probability of this ROI belonging to a particular target group is high if the ROI to be analyzed is surrounded by ROIs, which also belong to this particular target group. This assumption leads to the integration of so-called contextual information, which describes the properties of a ROI considering its context or surrounding environment within the organ.

A typical postprocessing stage is depicted in Fig. 16.19. The output of the first stage, the fuzzy inference system, is filtered and thresholded, which produces increased classification results and malignancy maps that are easier to interpret.

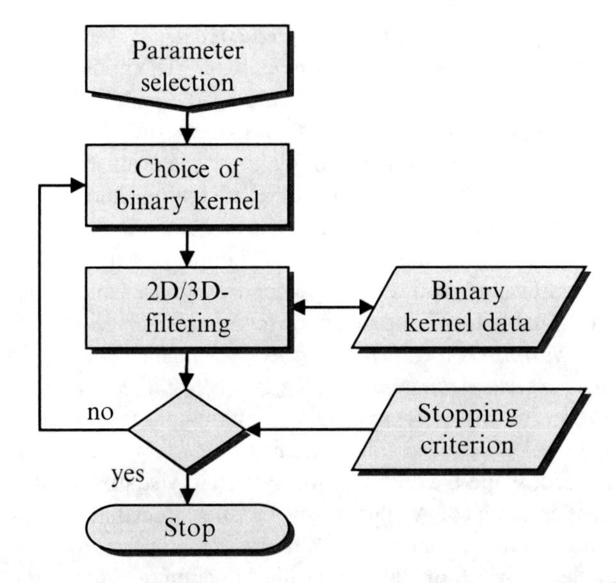

Fig. 16.19. Postprocessing stage. This stage evaluates contextual information by analyzing the environment or context of the ROIs in two or three dimensions using 2D or 3D filter kernels

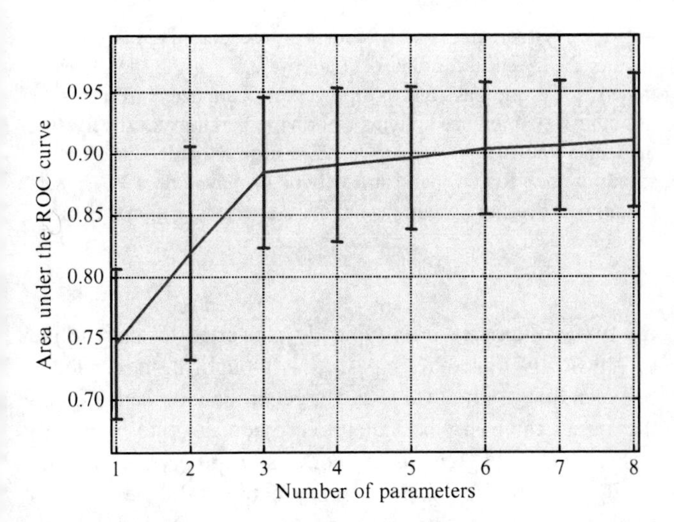

Fig. 16.18. Results of a typical parameter combination process. The mean area under the ROC curve (*red*) is shown together with error bars (*blue*). Eight parameters have been combined using a fuzzy inference system

This so-called morphological analysis combines clusters in the output maps of the fuzzy inference systems to mark areas of similar tissue characteristics. The clustering procedure is implemented by the two-dimensional filtering of the output maps with symmetric binary kernels of a systematically determined size and subsequently thresholding the obtained maps by formerly determined filter thresholds. As this procedure does not only include the filtering of malignancy maps but also includes thresholding using specific filter thresholds, this procedure exceeds simple low pass filtering procedures but represents a nonlinear operation on the data. Typical filter kernels that can be applied during contextual post processing are shown in Fig. 16.20.

During the training procedure, *the optimal kernel sizes and filter thresholds can be determined by systematically varying*

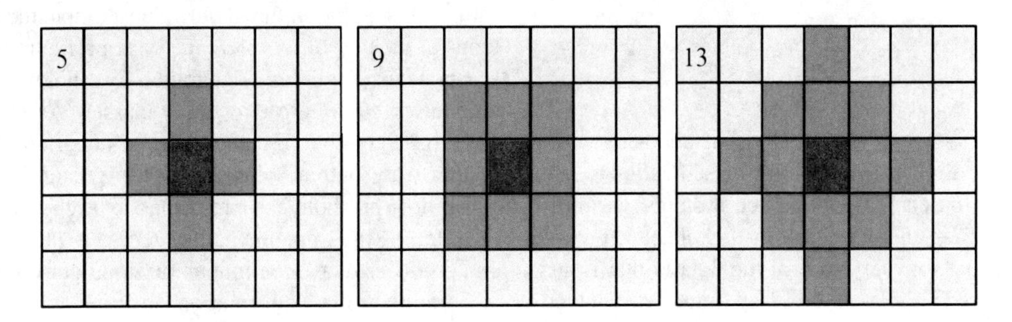

Fig. 16.20. Typical symmetrical and binary 2D filter kernels of sizes 5, 9, and 13. The ROI which is being analyzed (*red*) is evaluated in correlation with the surrounding ROIs (*orange*). The optimal size of the filter kernel and the optimal cut-off threshold should be determined during the training stage

kernel sizes and filter thresholds and comparing the classification results to find optimal combinations. The optimal kernel sizes and filter thresholds should be determined for the whole range of separation thresholds, thus, still allowing a free choice of separation threshold during the evaluation procedure. During the training procedure, the optimal kernel sizes and filter thresholds can be stored in a database for use during the evaluation procedure. In addition to improving the classification rates, this postprocessing step makes malignancy maps more readable for the physician or sonographer.

The postprocessing step increases the influence of compact formed regions, which are rather typical for prostate tumors. However, during the clustering step, the output resolution of the system is reduced. The presentation of larger lesions is enhanced, while the ability of the system to visualize smaller lesions is reduced. As this postprocessing procedure can be considered problematic in certain cases, the operator should be able to switch off this stage during patient examinations. However, as has been experienced during our clinical studies, fuzzy inference systems tend to underestimate the malignant area, thus, motivating the use of morphological postprocessing routines.[1]

Evaluation Stage

All system design parameters, such as those describing the membership functions of the fuzzy inference systems and the filter kernels and separation thresholds of the morphological postprocessing stage, which were previously estimated during training, are now finally used to classify the underlying ultrasound data. The appropriate evaluation procedure is shown in Fig. 16.21. As the composition of the evaluation stage shows many parallels to the actual training procedure, no additional discussion is needed concerning the appertaining block diagram.

The results of the two fuzzy inference systems are combined after morphological postprocessing to build a so-called combined malignancy map, which consists of a conventional B-mode image of the organ in which areas of high cancer probability are marked. Typically, these areas are colored in red to show the malignancy. The combination or fusion of the output of the two fuzzy inference systems is made by simply superimposing (disjunction) the single binary output maps of the two systems.

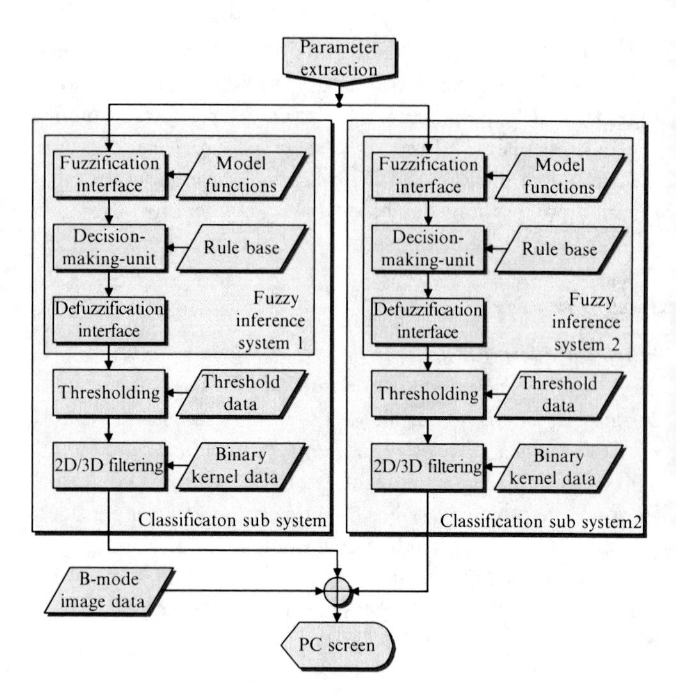

Fig. 16.21. Block diagram of evaluation procedure. During this procedure, the given ultrasound data are evaluated using the predetermined fuzzy rule base and postprocessing parameters. The results of both fuzzy inference systems working in parallel and supervising their own knowledge base are fused to form a single classification value for each ROI, which can easily be displayed on a PC screen. Usually an overlay of malignancy maps over conventional B-mode images is used

Visualization

The fourth and last stage in ultrasonic tissue characterization consists of the visual presentation of the classification results. Adaptive network-based fuzzy inference systems, as implemented by the author and discussed in this chapter, provide a fuzzy output value for every ROI of the dataset that is analyzed and classified. This so-called fuzzy output value stands for a certain probability of the ROI being negative or positive, respectively. As this fuzzy output value is not a crisp number directly indicating absolute probabilities or sensitivities, the fuzzy output value is typically converted to an absolute or physically motivated measure. Although the dependency between fuzzy output value and target probability is nonlinear, the output can easily be scaled to provide absolute probabilities. A block diagram of the conversion procedure is given in Fig. 16.22. Typically, the fuzzy output values are scaled to absolute probabilities belonging to a certain target group. The scaling of the output values into sensitivity or specificity values is commonly used as well.

For the fusion of the output maps of both fuzzy inference systems, the specificities of both classification systems are matched in order to provide comparable sensitivity values for estimated separation threshold values. Often, the fuzzy output maps of the two fuzzy inference systems are transformed into binary maps applying a separation threshold to separate the amount of cases into two target classes. As can be seen in Fig. 16.22, the binarization is carried out after the conversion of the fuzzy output values into crisp sensitivity values. The separation threshold can be selected to be chosen freely by the operator, as the implemented system is a quantitative system and produces quasi-continuous fuzzy output vectors.

Certainly, some "information" is discarded during the binarization step, but the output of the system becomes easier to interpret and, thus, more readable for the physician or sonographer. *The aim of the system is to provide the operator with*

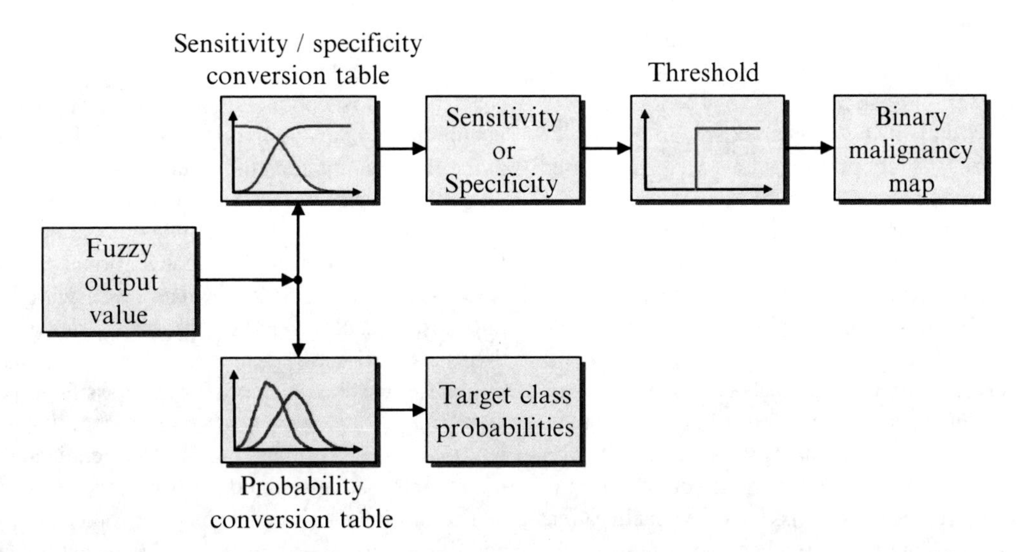

FIG. 16.22. Visualization procedure of an ultrasonic tissue characterization system. The block diagram shows the fourth and final step in ultrasonic tissue characterization. The output values of the fuzzy inference systems are converted and scaled to provide representative diagnostic images. Binary malignancy maps are used for the clinical study underlying this work

the information to probe further in a certain region within the prostate which yields an estimated high probability for cancer. Numerically scaled probabilities can be difficult to interpret, even when using sophisticated visualization schemes involving selected color maps. The malignancy map can be presented to the physician on a PC screen and, thus, can supplement the existing methods of diagnostics. Malignancy maps can easily be printed or archived, which is an important step in biopsy planning.[151]

In addition to two-dimensional presentations of prostate slices, volumetric modalities have been developed to open up new fields of diagnostics. The segmentation of the organ itself is an important diagnostic modality, as the shape of the organ can change due to diseases such as prostate cancer.[85, 152] In the later stages of prostate cancer, the shape of the organ can change because of excessive tumor growth. Furthermore, the mere volume of the prostate, which is highly correlated with benign prostate hyperplasia, is an important diagnostic parameter in urology.[152] In addition to diagnostic aims, volumetric representations of malignancies can help during therapy planning and during treatment itself. Looking into the future, the targeting of radiation therapy doses, when considering external beam radiotherapy, afterloading techniques or Brachytherapy, will be easier to plan. Thermal therapies may be easier to conduct when using volumetric representations of organ and tumor borders.

Results

During the clinical study on the detection of prostate carcinoma underlying most of the development of the tissue characterization system presented in this chapter, radiofrequency ultrasound data from 100 patients were acquired and processed. On the day of the examination, the youngest patient was 48 years old, the eldest 79 years. Both the mean and the median age of the patients were 64 years. All patients in this study underwent prostatectomy. Prostate slices with histological diagnosis following prostatectomy act as the gold standard and "teacher data." Histological analysis is usually accepted as the gold standard; nevertheless, it is subject to error.[153]

The concentration of the PSA in the patient's blood was recorded together with possible medication and hormonal data. The results of the clinical examinations, involving DRE and conventional B-mode transrectal ultrasound, have been recorded two allow crossvalidation.

As shown in Table 16.2, the PSA values of the patients were in the range of 1–93 ng ml^{-1} with a mean value of 12.8 ng ml^{-1} and a median value of 8.5 ng ml^{-1}. 17 patients had a PSA value greater than 20 ng ml^{-1}, which is a fairly certain indicator of the presence of prostate cancer. 21 patients had a PSA value between 10 and 20 ng ml^{-1}, which still stands for a certain probability of prostate cancer. The greatest amount of patients, in total 49, had a PSA value between 4 and 10

TABLE 16.2. PSA values encountered in the clinical study.

PSA value	Number of patients
PSA ≤ 4 ng ml^{-1}	9
4 ng ml^{-1} < PSA ≤ 10 ng ml^{-1}	49
10 ng ml^{-1} < PSA ≤ 20 ng ml^{-1}	21
20 ng ml^{-1} < PSA	17
Not recorded	4
Sum	100

ng ml^{-1}, an amount that makes a conclusion rather unreliable. Nine patients had a PSA value below 4 ng ml^{-1}. No PSA values were recorded for four patients.

Looking at the results of the clinical examinations, which are shown in Table 16.3, about 44 patients were diagnosed T3, 41 patients were diagnosed T2, and 11 patients received a diagnosis of T1. One patient was diagnosed T4. In three cases, no carcinoma could be diagnosed. Gleason scores are not evaluated in this study, because they have only been recorded for a few patients and, thus, cannot be discussed in a representative manner.

The RF datasets have been divided as described in section "Data Acquisition and Preprocessing," resulting in a sum of 129,967 benign and 40,517 malignant ROIs. An exact overview is presented in Table 16.4. After prostatectomy, a minimum of three prostate slices was dissected for each patient while maintaining the angle of the slices according to the angle of the ultrasound transducer during the data acquisition. Prostate tissues have been stained and marked on the prostate slices with hematoxylin and eosin. Malignant areas have been encircled on the glass plates by the pathologists after the preparation of the slices using microscopic examination of the specimen. The contours have been transferred to the workstation by experienced physicians, thus, enabling a definite assignment of dataset ROIs to tissue classes. For transferring the contours to the workstation, the B-mode images of all recorded datasets of one patient are displayed on the workstation screen. The physician chooses the datasets that fit the prostate slices best and transfers the contour to the workstation, interactively encircling the prostate and cancerous areas with the mouse. Only datasets that exactly match the prostate slices are kept for further processing. This results in approximately two or three validated datasets per patient.

The tumors have been divided into two different classes. The first class (PS) consists of all tumors that were visible in the conventional B-mode image. In total this class consists of 27,608 ROIs. Hypoechoic tumors have also been included in this class as hyperechoic tumors. The second class (PU) consists of all isoechoic tumors, which are tumors that are not visible in the conventional B-mode.[2, 154] These tumors appear in the B-mode image in the same way as healthy tissue. Overall, 12,909 ROIs belong to this class. When considering these amounts, it can easily be concluded that about one-third of all tumors cannot be seen with conventional B-mode imaging. Nevertheless, this result correlates well with former studies on transrectal ultrasound imaging.[2, 30] Prior work has shown that the partitioning of the entire amount of malignant ROIs into these two classes improves the classification results quite significantly.[52] However, a separation of the first class PS into two subclasses that consist of isoechoic and hyperechoic tumors, respectively, could further improve the system.

The third class (N) consists of all other kinds of tissue. In addition to normal tissue ROIs, ROIs that consist of benign prostate hyperplasia also belong to this class. It has to be mentioned that all other kinds of "unusual" tissue, e.g., stones, etc., belong to the class N, too. In total, class N comprises 129,967 ROIs.

The manual transfer of prostate and tumor contours from histological prostate slices to the workstation screen is a procedure that is very sensitive to errors. The physician or sonographer has to work properly and precisely to keep transfer errors as low as possible during the training procedure. The transferring procedure can be conducted reasonably well for tumors that are more or less visible in the conventional B-mode image, but requires great skills from the physician in the case of isoechoic tumors, thus, only allowing the physician to use typical landmarks such as the prostate border, stones, and the urethra/seminal duct for navigation. During the preparation, the prostate slices are often deformed, making a proper correlation even more complicated. From the current point of view, an automatic transfer procedure, based on acquiring images of the histological prostate slices using a scanner and digital image processing, does not seem to be able to satisfy the required demands. For this reason, the transfer procedure was conducted manually by two physicians.

Two fuzzy inference systems were trained in succession using the histological findings as "teacher data." Details of the training process and the fuzzy inference systems involved in this work are discussed in section "Methods." The first fuzzy inference system was trained to distinguish the class PS, which consists of hypoechoic and hyperechoic tumors, from class N, which consists of "normal" tissue in the sense of tumor detection. The second system was used to distinguish between the class PU, which consists of isoechoic tumors, and the class N.

Table 16.3. Results of clinical examination.

Results of examination	Number of patients
None	3
T1	11
T2	41
T3	44
T4	1
Sum	100

Table 16.4. Overview of regions of interest acquired during the clinical study.

Class	Acronym	Number of ROIs
Noncancerous tissue	N	129,967
Hyperechoic and hypoechoic tumors	PS	27,608
Isoechoic tumors	PU	12,909
Sum		170,484

Results of Tissue Characterization

Each of the two fuzzy inference systems involved in the classification process provides a fuzzy output value for each ROI of the ultrasound dataset. The fuzzy output value is a measure of the estimated probability of the ROI being malignant or benign. The frequencies of occurrence of a classification of the benign and malignant ROIs for different normalized output values are shown in Fig. 16.23 for FIS 1 and in Fig. 16.24 for FIS 2, respectively.

These curves will also be used for the conversion between fuzzy output values and crisp values when the absolute probabilities of class membership are requested. Typically, the output values are expected to be normally distributed. As can be seen from the figures, only three of the four curves exhibit normal behavior. The complex shape of the positive curve of FIS 1 is unexpected but, as the system provides reliable results, the distribution of the output values is considered to be of minor importance. As several tissue parameters involved in the classification process exhibit non-Gaussian behavior, the not-normally shaped distribution of the fuzzy output values can be explained as originating from the distributions of the underlying tissue parameters.

ROC curves are calculated by continuously varying the separation threshold.[146, 149, 150] The ROC curves for the two systems are shown in Fig. 16.25. The area under the ROC curve is 0.86 for the first system and 0.84 for the second system, respectively. The capability of the system has been determined using the leave-one-out classification method over patients, which means that the system has been trained on 99 patients to classify the remaining 100th patient.[145] After 100 single calculations, the results are averaged to form the final classification results. The standard deviations of the repeated classification tests are 0.01 for the first system and 0.02 for the second system, respectively. Calculating sensitivities and specificities for the example point of sensitivity = specificity, a.k.a. equal error rate, leads to a classification rate of 0.75.

The results of the eight different tissue characterization parameter groups are given in Table 16.5. Analyzing the results of the single parameter groups, the conventional spectral parameters based on Fourier transform processing of the underlying RF echo data allow by far the best discrimination between malignant and benign ROIs. Followed by the results of second-order texture parameters and by the morphological group, conventional spectral parameters clearly outperform AR model parameters and parameters based on the generalized spectrum. Clinical parameters did not perform significantly

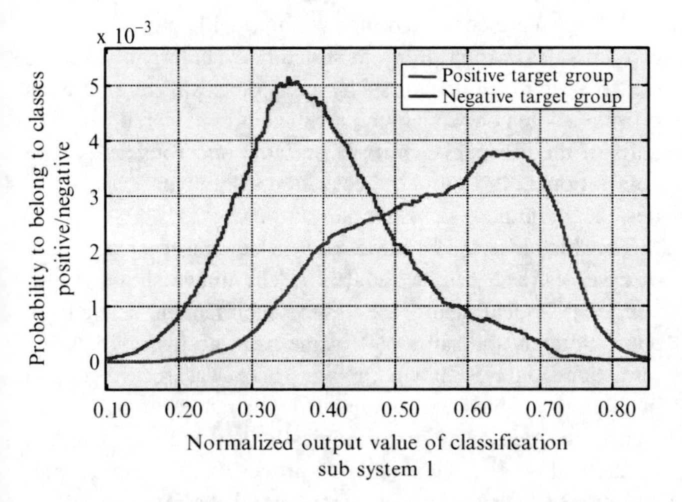

Fig. 16.23. Probabilities of the output values of classification system 1 (hyperechoic and hypoechoic tumors against normal tissue) belonging to a certain target group. The Gaussian shape of the negative class is apparent, while the positive class exhibits a not-normally distributed shape

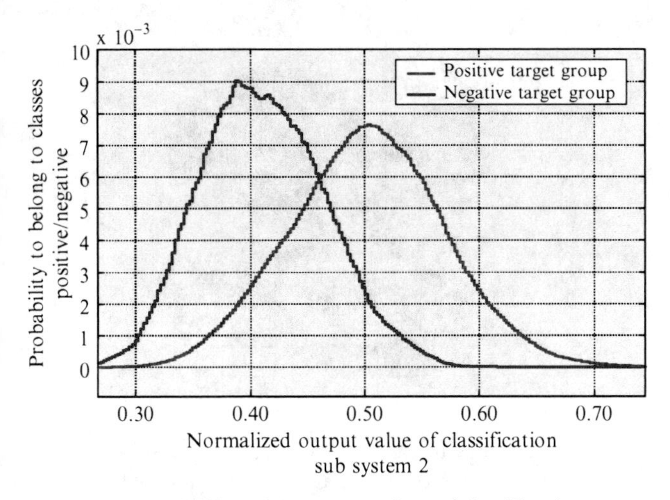

Fig. 16.24. Probabilities of the output values of classification system 2 (isoechoic tumors against normal tissue) belonging to a certain target group. The Gaussian shape is apparent for both classes

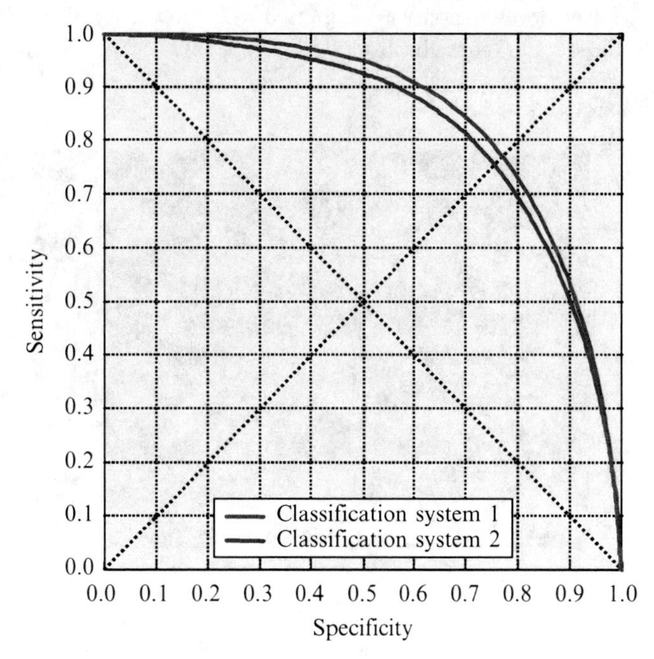

Fig. 16.25. ROC curves of the two classification systems. The mean area under is ROC curve is 0.86 with a standard deviation of 0.01 for the first system (*red*), and 0.84 with a standard deviation of 0.02 for the second system (*blue*), respectively

TABLE 16.5. Classification results of single parameter groups.

	System 1		System 2	
Parameter group	ROC area	Standard dev.	ROC area	Standard dev.
Spectral	0.77	0.01	0.64	0.03
AR model	0.64	0.05	0.58	0.02
Generalized spectrum	0.64	0.03	0.57	0.02
Texture first order	0.68	0.02	0.60	0.05
Distribution model	0.63	0.01	0.55	0.05
Texture second order	0.72	0.02	0.62	0.04
Morphological	0.72	0.01	0.64	0.04
Clinical	0.54	0.02	0.52	0.06

when analyzed alone, but it has to be remembered that the correlation between the clinical parameter group and all other groups was low, thus, still motivating the integration of clinical parameters into a nonlinear classification system.

Classification results of system 2 are in general inferior in comparison to the classification results of system 1. However, a similar relationship between the different parameter groups can also be observed here.

Case A

The first patient, whose case is discussed in detail, here called case A, was 57 years old on the day of the examination. The PSA value found in the blood specimen taken on the day of the examination was high at 29 ng ml^{-1}. He was diagnosed T2 with a Gleason score of three. This diagnosis was made after DRE, PSA value analysis, and conventional transrectal ultrasound examination.

A cancerous region was diagnosed in the lower right lobe of the organ. When the B-mode image shown in Fig. 16.26 is investigated, an abnormal hypoechoic area can be detected in the lower right area. When the left and right lower parts of the organ are compared, no symmetrical behavior is found as both sides exhibit different structures. The organ border is clearly seen in the image as a hyperechoic seam encircling the prostate. When only the B-mode image is considered, all other parts of the prostate seem to be free of cancerous areas. The conventional ultrasound image does not show any abnormalities except in the lower right part of the organ.

The histological findings after a radical prostatectomy of case A are shown in Fig. 16.27. The image shows a conventional optical scan of a tissue specimen dissected from approximately the same part of the prostate from which the ultrasound dataset shown in Fig. 16.26 was recorded. The prostate tissue has been stained using hematoxylin and eosin. Cancerous areas were microscopically detected and encircled by the pathologist. The histology proves that the tumor actually spread over the whole lower part of the prostate. In the conventional B-mode image shown in Fig. 16.26, only the right part of the tumor was visible and, thus, could be diagnosed as malignant.

Experienced physicians transferred the contours encircled on the histological specimen shown in Fig. 16.27 to the tissue

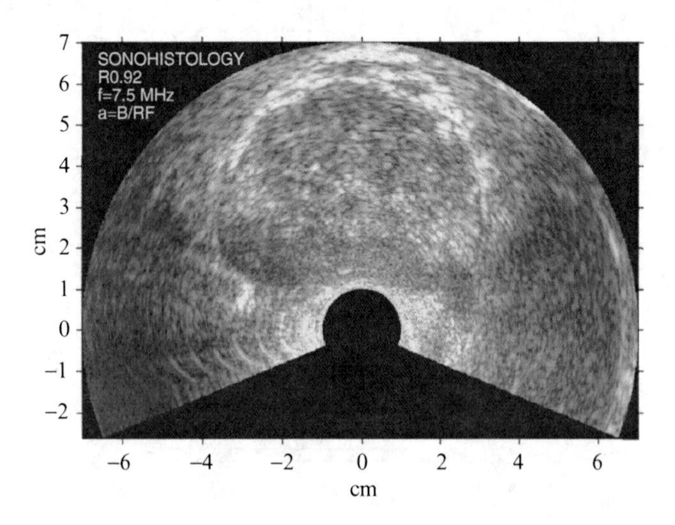

FIG. 16.26. Conventional B-mode image of case A. An abnormal hypoechoic region is visible in the lower right area of the prostate. When the left and the right lobes of the organ are compared, the lower part does not look symmetrical but exhibits different structures on both sides

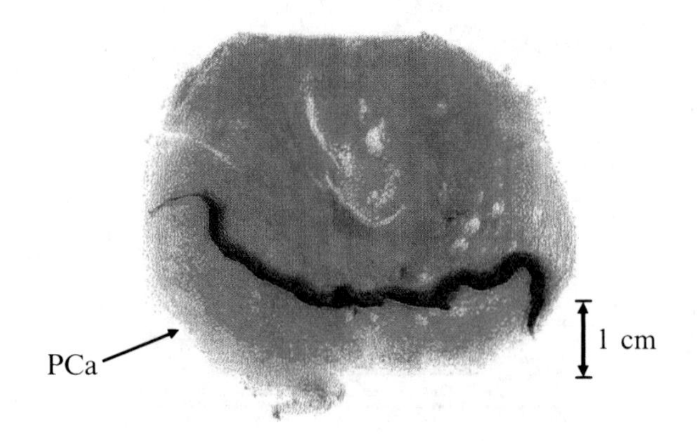

FIG. 16.27. Histology of case A. The image was scanned optically from a prostate slice fixed on a glass plate. The prostate tissue has been stained using hematoxylin and eosin. A cancerous area (PCa), here encircled by the pathologist, was detected spreading over the lower part of the organ

characterization workstation for the evaluation of the classification system. Several histological specimens dissected from different parts of the organ were matched with several ultrasound datasets recorded at different positions of the organ. The shape of the organ and typical landmarks such as urethra, prostate stones, and the seminal duct were used for matching and navigation. The contours of a prostate slice of case A, as transferred to the computer, are shown in Fig. 16.28. The whole organ is encircled in green while cancerous areas are encircled in red.

The output of the classification system for case A is shown as a malignancy map in Fig. 16.29. Not only the right-hand part of the tumor is correctly classified, but also a distinct part on the left-hand side of the organ was correctly classified as cancerous, though this part appears as isoechoic tissue in the conventional B-mode ultrasound image.

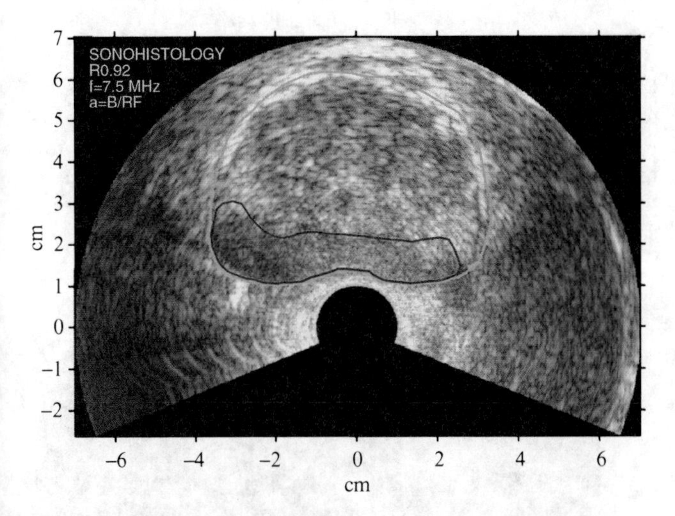

Fig. 16.28. Contour plot of prostate slice of case A. Experienced physicians transferred the contours encircled on the histological specimen shown in Fig. 16.27 to the tissue characterization workstation for the evaluation of the classification system. The whole organ is encircled in *green*, cancerous areas are encircled in *red*

Case B

The second patient, whose case is discussed in detail, here called case B, was 64 years old on the day of the examination. The PSA value found in the blood specimen taken on the day of the examination was slightly elevated at 6 ng ml^{-1}. The patient was diagnosed T2 with a Gleason score of two. The diagnosis was made after DRE, PSA value analysis, and conventional transrectal ultrasound.

A cancerous region was diagnosed in the lower left part of the organ. When the B-mode image shown in Fig. 16.30 is investigated, a hypoechoic area can be detected in the lower left area. When comparing left and right lower parts of the organ, no symmetrical behavior is found. Again, the organ border is clearly seen in the image as a hyperechoic seam encircling the prostate. The prostate itself appears less echoic than the surrounding tissue. When only the B-mode image is considered, all other parts of the prostate seem to be free of cancerous areas, though the tissue of the organ is more irregular than the tissue in case A. The conventional ultrasound B-mode image does not exhibit any abnormalities except the irregularity of the whole organ and the compact region in the lower right part of the organ.

The histological findings after prostatectomy of case B are shown Fig. 16.31. The image shows a conventional optical scan of a tissue specimen dissected from approximately the same part of the prostate from which the ultrasound dataset shown in Fig. 16.30 was recorded. The histology proves that

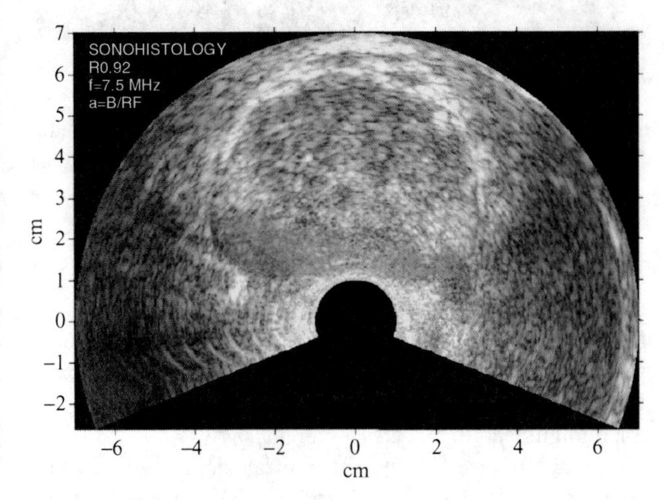

Fig. 16.29. Malignancy map of case A. The final classification results of the classification system are shown. Areas of the prostate exhibiting high cancer probability are marked in *red*. Not only the right part of the tumor was highlighted by the classification system but nearly the whole extension of the cancerous region was detected

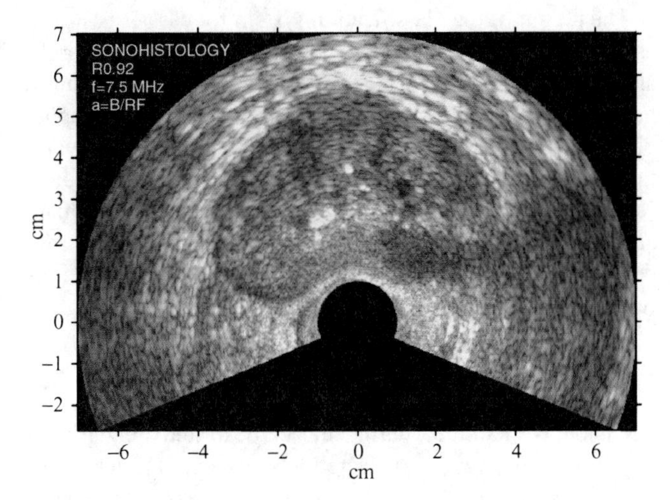

Fig. 16.30. Conventional B-mode image of case B. A compact hypoechoic region is visible in the lower left area of the prostate. When the left and the right lobes of the organ are compared, it seems that the lower part of the organ is not symmetrical. A slight shadow is visible behind the hypoechoic region

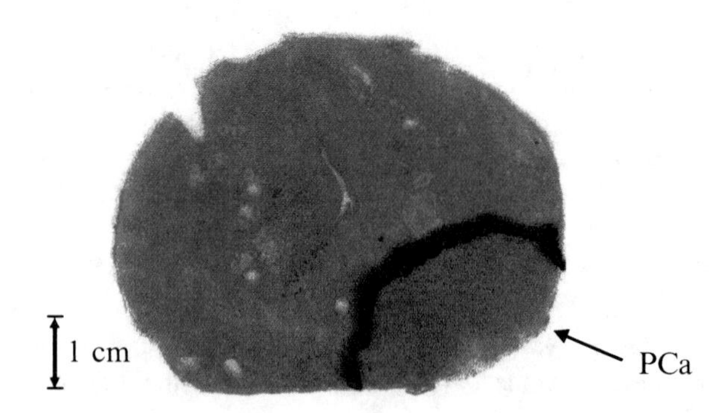

FIG. 16.31. Histology of case B. The image was scanned optically from a prostate slice fixed on a glass plate. The prostate tissue has been stained using hematoxylin and eosin. A cancerous area, here encircled by the pathologist, was detected in the lower right part of the organ

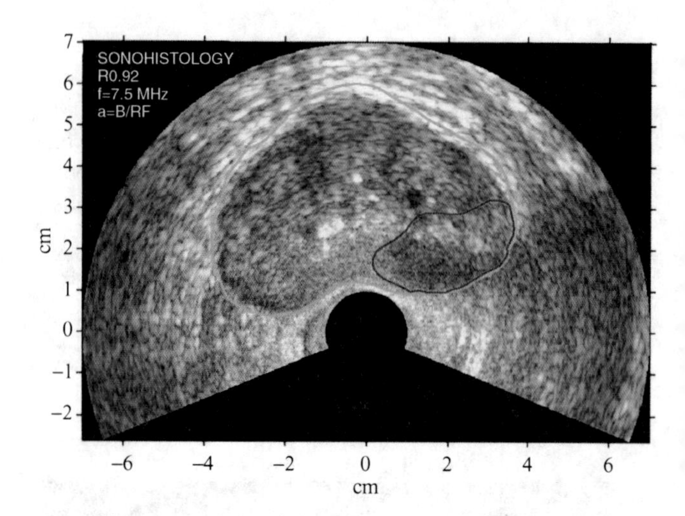

FIG. 16.32. Contour plot of prostate slice of case B. Using the histological findings shown in Fig. 16.31 experienced physicians transferred the contours encircled on the histological specimen to the tissue characterization workstation for the evaluation of the classification system. The whole organ is encircled in *green*, cancerous areas are encircled in *red*

the tumor actually extends over the compact region in the lower left part of the prostate and, thus, is much bigger than actually diagnosed using conventional ultrasound B-mode and DRE. In the conventional B-mode image only the lower right part of the tumor was visible and, thus, could be diagnosed as malignant.

Using the histological findings shown in Fig. 16.31, experienced physicians transferred the contours encircled on the histological specimen to the tissue characterization workstation for the evaluation of the classification system. Several histological specimens dissected from different parts of the organ were matched with several ultrasound datasets recorded at different positions of the organ. The shape of the organ and typical landmarks such as prostate stones and the seminal duct are used for matching and navigation. The contours of the prostate slice of case B, as transferred to the tissue characterization workstation, are shown in Fig. 16.32. The whole organ is encircled in green while cancerous areas are encircled in red.

The output of the classification system for case B is shown as a malignancy map in Fig. 16.33. Areas of high cancer probability are marked in red. Not only the lower part of the tumor has correctly been classified, but also the extension to the upper part of the organ was correctly classified as cancerous. Nearly the whole area of the cancerous part of the organ was detected. In addition to two-dimensional representations of malignant areas, volumetric representations can be constructed by rendering classification results. Typical volumetric presentations of case B's prostate are shown in Fig. 16.34.

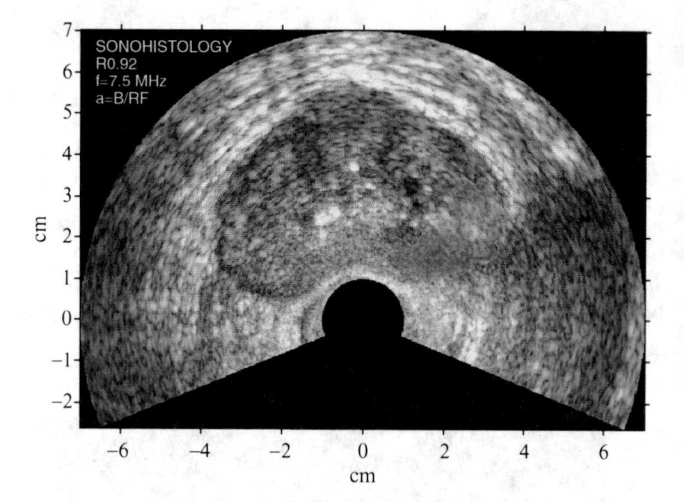

FIG. 16.33. Malignancy map of case B. Areas of the prostate exhibiting high cancer probability are marked in *red*. Not only the lower part of the tumor has been highlighted by the classification system, but nearly the complete extension of the cancerous region was detected

Discussion

All patients examined during the clinical study underlying this work underwent prostatectomy. However, long-term process checkups of patients who underwent prostatectomy have shown that about 40% were prone to biochemical relapse, which is indicated by a consecutive rising PSA value.[28] Most likely, these patients did not profit from excision. These results demand superior diagnostic staging and planning before the actual surgery. Only an exact analysis of preoperative tumor characteristics can lead to a decrease in relapse.[28] Sophisticated ultrasonic tissue characterization systems can provide the physician with an improved analysis of prostate tissue, which might lead to a decrease in relapse.

In addition to conventional prostatectomy and external beam radiation therapy, which still are the preferred methods for high-risk patients in many countries,[155] alternative methods like Brachytherapy are on the rise.[156] Because Brachytherapy is aimed at the low-risk patient, where the tumor is located in one side of the prostate only and the prostate capsule is still

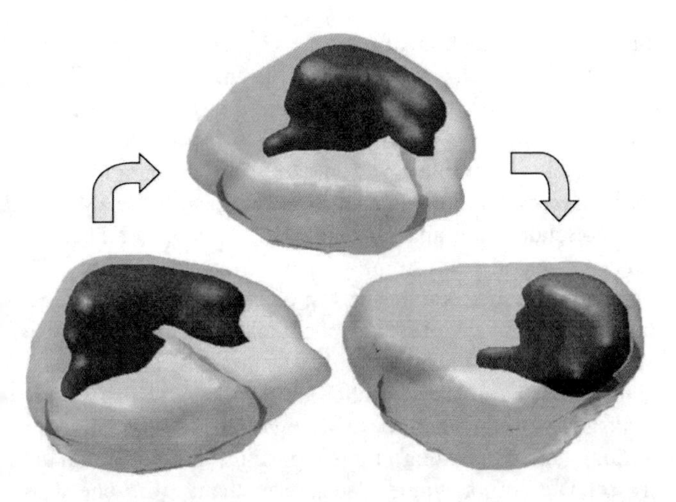

FIG. 16.34. Volumetric representations of prostate carcinoma and organ boundaries as seen from different viewing angles. The carcinoma is visualized in *opaque red*, while the whole organ is shown in *transparent yellow*. Rendered volumes can be rotated to any angle to aid in therapy planning and diagnostics

intact,[157,158] especially volumetric reconstructions of the whole organ, based on ultrasonic tissue characterization including malignant areas within the prostate, will result in improved planning for the application of Brachytherapy.

Another radiation-based method, the afterloading technique, is based on a combination of a temporarily implanted iridium load and percutaneous irradiation. This method may also be used for high-risk patients.[158] The dose of both modalities, the implanted iridium load and the percutaneous irradiation, has to be planned properly in order to irradiate the whole malignant area while sparing unaffected tissue. Because of the high accuracy demands of the method, volumetric representations of the prostate and cancerous areas might successfully supplement the afterloading technique.

Cryoablation[159] and high-intensity focused ultrasound (HIFU),[160] two nonionizing methods, are used minimally invasive. Even combinations of irradiating and nonionizing methods are used today, for example, thermo-radiotherapy that consists of a combined usage of interstitial hyperthermia and conformal radiation therapy.[161] Again, these therapies might benefit from ultrasonic tissue characterization in two ways: firstly, volumetric reconstructions may aid in planning therapy. Secondly, tissue characterization methods may be used to characterize the treated tissue and to monitor the treatment procedure. For tumors, which are not considered, to be curable, hormonal therapy is the therapy of choice.[162] Hormonal therapy is also used to shrink tumors before treatment by surgery or radiotherapy. Ultrasonic tissue characterization may help to monitor the therapy process. Especially volumetric representations of tumors can be used to calculate tumor shrinkage due to hormonal influence.

Chemotherapy[163] is the method of choice in special cases, usually when all other modalities, even hormone therapy, are not successful. Although no clinical studies have been conducted on this matter so far, ultrasonic tissue characterization may be used to monitor the changes in tissue due to chemotherapy. Improved medication and the improved adjustment of medication during therapy might be possible in the future.

Focus on Brachytherapy

Permanent-implant Brachytherapy is a technique that is becoming more and more popular for the treatment of the early-stage prostate carcinoma. Since the radioactive sources are implanted directly within the tumor, Brachytherapy provides a very effective way of delivering a full radioactive dose to the diseased area while sparing radiation exposure to normal tissue.[48,164] Typically, between 40 and 100 seeds are placed within the prostate. The major limitation today is the effective planning and placement of the seeds within the malignant region of the prostate. Several works dealing with software solutions for the placement problem have been published. An overview is given in Ref. [164]. As the tumor region is seldom recognized with a high grade of accuracy when using conventional diagnostics, seeds are typically implanted within the whole prostate, in order not to save any malignant regions. When this method is considered, it is apparent that a high overall dose has to be applied to the patient to treat all malignant regions while keeping the false negative rate of untreated malignant regions as low as possible. The approach described in this work may lead to better planning modalities for Brachytherapy using tissue characterization-based volumetric reconstructions of prostate regions. As has been shown in this work, the classification system is able to detect cancerous regions within the prostate with a high grade of accuracy. Using volumetric reconstructions, the cancerous regions can be modeled in three dimensions. The tumor model can be used as input for conventional Brachytherapy planning software, which calculates the radioactive dosage and its appropriate seed positions.[164] Improved planning modalities for radioactive seed implantations will result in better results of Brachytherapy. The patient's overall exposure to radiation will be kept as low as possible while increasing the irradiation at malignant areas.

Conclusion

Ultrasonic tissue characterization for prostate cancer diagnostics is a revolutionary approach toward precise cancer diagnostics. A sophisticated system for ultrasonic tissue characterization based on multifeature processing and nonlinear classifiers has been proposed and discussed as an exemplary case. Systems for ultrasonic tissue characterization usually comprise four main processing stages: data acquisition and preprocessing, parameter extraction, classification, and visualization, all which have been discussed in detail. Numerous ways of extracting tissue describing parameters originating from different parameter groups have been described in the literature. The most popular of these groups have been discussed. In the exemplary system proposed in this chapter, several of these parameters are combined to produce spatially resolved malignancy maps using a multifeature approach based on fuzzy reasoning. The classification engine of the proposed system consists of two network-based fuzzy inference systems working in parallel. In addition to 2D malignancy maps, the output of the tissue characterization systems can be rendered to yield volume reconstructions of the prostate and of carcinoma within the prostate.

It has been shown that *ultrasonic multifeature tissue characterization is able to detect the prostate carcinoma with a high grade of accuracy. This means that ultrasonic tissue characterization systems can supplement the existing methods of prostate diagnostics to improve the early detection of prostate cancer and to achieve an increased reliability in diagnostics.*

The ROC curve area of the proposed system is 0.86 for the first subsystem, which was trained to distinguish between hyperechoic and hypoechoic tumors and normal tissue, and 0.84 for the second subsystem, which was trained to distinguish between isoechoic tumors and normal tissue. The standard deviations are 0.01 for the first subsystem and 0.02 for the second subsystem, respectively. Tumors that are not visible in the conventional B-mode image can be located. The planning of biopsies may be improved, unnecessary biopsies may be avoided and performed biopsies may be guided with increased reliability. In comparison to the work of Feleppa et al.[45–47, 57] and Balaji et al.,[48] who include the so-called LOS of the physician as an additional parameter in their classification system, only conventional parameters are used in the proposed approach. However, a high grade of accuracy could still be achieved without losing the independence from the conducting physician.

The problem of conventional B-mode ultrasound imaging for the detection of prostate cancer is the interobserver variability, which is the dependence of diagnostic results on the abilities of the conducting physician or sonographer. A highly trained physician or sonographer may be able to detect the majority of tumors, while a novice physician or sonographer may oversee small tumors or tumors with isoechoic properties, which, therefore, cannot be seen in conventional B-mode imaging. *An ultrasonic tissue characterization system can automate the process of finding suspicious regions and hence help to reduce the wide gap in ultrasound imaging diagnostic results between expert and novice physicians and sonographers. As ultrasonic tissue characterization systems even evaluate characteristics of the ultrasound echo signal that cannot be seen in the conventional B-mode image, the approach may also be of great help to the expert*

Acknowledgments The author would like to thank everyone who was involved in the development of the tissue characterization system discussed in this chapter, especially Dr. Georg Schmitz, who started the project on tissue characterization for the early detection of prostate cancer many years ago, Dr. Andreas Lorenz, who pushed the integration of Fuzzy inference systems into the classification engine, Dr. Helmut Ermert, who made everything possible from the technical side, all physicians involved in acquiring the data over the years, especially Dr. Hans-Jörg Sommerfeld, Dr. Miguel Garcia-Schürmann, and Dr. Katharina König, Dr. Theodor Senge who made everything possible from the clinical side, Dr. Stathis Philippou who was in charge of the histological examinations of the prostate specimen and therefore for the gold standard, and last but not least, the KMR (Kompetenzzentrum Medizintechink Ruhr), the DFG (Deutsche Forschungsgesellschaft), and the BMBF (Bundesministerium für Bildung und Forschung) for supporting and financing the project.The author would also like to thank everyone who took a key position in adapting the tissue characterization system for the application on other organs, especially Dr. Christian Perrey for the experiments on coronary plaques involving intravascular ultrasound, Stefan Siebers for the experiments on monitoring thermal ablation therapy of liver tumors and on staging of deep venous thrombosis, Christian Hansen for the experiments on monitoring metabolism effects in the liver, Dr. Frank Gottwald, Dr. Alessandro Bozzato, Dr. Johannes Zenk, and Dr. Heinrich Iro for the study on the classification of tumors of the parotid gland, and again to Stefan Siebers and Dr. Helmut Ermert for pushing this very promising study into another round.

References

1. Scheipers U, Sonohistology – Methods and Systems for Ultrasonic Tissue Characterization based on a Multifeature Approach and Fuzzy Inference Systems (Logos: Berlin, 2005).
2. Scardino PT, Early Detection of Prostate Cancer, The Urologic Clinics of North America 1998, 16(4):635–656.
3. Clements R, The Role of Transrectal Ultrasound in Diagnosing Prostate Cancer, Current Urology Reports 2002, 3(3):194–200.
4. Schmid HP, Prikler L, Sturgeon CM, Semjonow A, Diagnosis of Prostate Cancer – The Clinical Use of Prostate Specific Antigen, EAU Update Series 2003, 1:3–8.
5. Catalona WJ, Richie JP, Ahmann FR, et al.. Comparison of Digital Rectal Examination and Serum Prostate Specific Antigen in the Early Detection of Prostate Cancer: Results of a Multicenter Clinical Trial of 6,630 Men, Journal of Urology 1994, 151: 1283–1290.
6. Barry MJ, Prostate-Specific-Antigen Testing for Early Diagnosis of Prostate Cancer, The New England Journal of Medicine 2003, 344(18):1373–1377.
7. Scardino PT, The Prevention of Prostate Cancer – The Dilemma Continues, The New England Journal of Medicine 2003, 349(3):295–297.
8. Renty P, d'Hauwers K, van Camp C, Verheyden B, Gentens P, Wyndaele JJ, Value of Transrectal Prostatic Echography, Prostate-Specific Antigen and Rectal Examination in the Diagnosis of Prostate Cancer. Relationship with the Result of Prostatic Biopsies, Acta Urologica Belgica 1996, 64(3):7–12.

9. Bangma CH, Rietbergen JB, Schroder FH, Prostate-Specific Antigen as a Screening Test. The Netherlands Experience, The Urologic Clinics of North America 1997, 24(2):307–314.
10. Bangma CH, Screening for Prostate Cancer, Urologe A 2000, 39:334–340.
11. Luboldt HJ, Rübben H, PSA-Based Early Detection of Prostate Cancer, Urologe A 2000, 39:20–26.
12. Luboldt HJ, Hüsing J, Altwein JE, et al.. Early Detection of Prostate Cancer in German Urological Practice by Digital Rectal Examination and Prostate-Specific Antigen, Urologe A 2000, 39:20–26.
13. Schröder FH, Kranse R, Verification Bias and the Prostate-Specific Antigen Test – Is there a Case for a Lower Threshold for Biopsy?, The New England Journal of Medicine 2003, 349(4):393–395.
14. Marchant J, Screening Trials Focus on Prostate Cancer, Diagnostic Imaging Europe 2002, 2002:21–24.
15. Schmitz G, Advances in Endoscopical Ultrasound of the Prostate, Frequenz 2001, 55:25–30.
16. Ophir J, Céspedes I, Ponnekanti H, Yazdi Y, Li X, Elastography: A Quantitative Method for Imaging the Elasticity of Biological Tissues, Ultrasonic Imaging 1991, 13:111–134.
17. Lorenz A, Sommerfeld HJ, Garcia-Schürmann M, Philippou S, Senge T, Ermert H, Diagnosis of Prostate Carcinoma using Multicompression Strain Imaging: Data Acquisition and First In Vivo Results, Proceedings Ultrasonics Symposium 1998, 1761–1764.
18. Lorenz A, Sommerfeld HJ, Garcia-Schürmann M, Philippou S, Senge T, Ermert H, A New System for the Acquisition of Ultrasonic Multicompression Strain Images of the Human Prostate In Vivo, Transactions on Ultrasonics, Ferroelectrics and Frequency Control 1999, 46(5):1147–1154.
19. Lorenz A, Zwei neue Verfahren zur Früherkennung von Prostatatumoren mit diagnostischem Ultraschall, (Shaker: Germany, 1999).
20. Pesavento A, Perrey C, Krueger M, Ermert H, A Time-Efficient and Accurate Strain Estimation Concept for Ultrasonic Elastography Using Iterative Phase Zero Estimation, Transactions on Ultrasonics, Ferroelectrics and Frequency Control 1999, 46(5):1057–1066.
21. Lorenz A, Pesavento A, Scheipers U, et al., Ultrasonic Tissue Characterization – Assessment of Prostate Tissue Malignancy In Vivo Using a Conventional Classifier Based Tissue Classification Approach and Elastographic Imaging, Proceedings Ultrasonics Symposium 2000, 1845–1848.
22. Pesavento A, Lorenz A, Real Time Strain Imaging and in-vivo Applications in Prostate Cancer, Proceedings Ultrasonics Symposium 2001, 2:1647–1652.
23. Sommerfeld HJ, Garcia-Schürmann M, Schewe J, et al. Prostatakarzinomdiagnostik durch Ultraschall-Elastographie – Vorstellung eines neuartigen Verfahrens und erste klinische Ergebnisse, Urologe A 2003, 42:941–945.
24. König K, Scheipers U, Pesavento A, Lorenz A, Ermert H, Senge T, Initial Experiences with Real-Time Elastography Guided Biopsies of the Prostate, Journal of Urology 2005, 174:115–117.
25. Jager GJ, Severens JL, Thornbury JR, de la Rosette JJMCH, Ruijs SHJ, Barentsz JO, Prostate Cancer Staging: Should MR Imaging Be Used? – A Decision Analytic Approach, Radiology 2000, 215:445–451.
26. Engelhard K, Hollenbach HP, Riedl C, Ott G, Hausmann J, Risse W, Magnetresonanztomographie bei Prostataerkrankungen, Electromedica 2001, 69(1):38–43.
27. Macilquham MD, Gong J, Lavoipierre AM, MR Widens Options for Prostate Imaging, Diagnostic Imaging Europe 2003, 2003:37–45.
28. Graefen M, Hammerer P, Noldus J, et al. Prognostic Markers for Prostate Cancer, Urologe A 2000, 39:14–21.
29. Roy C, Buy X, Lang H, Ultrasound Contrast Alters Prostate Protocol, Diagnostic Imaging Europe 2003, 2003:29–33.
30. Sedelaar JPM, Vijverberg PLM, De Reijke TM, et al. Transrectal Ultrasound in the Diagnosis of Prostate Cancer: State of the Art and Perspectives, European Urology 2001, 40:275–284.
31. Sedelaa JPM, Leenders GJLH, Hulsbergen-van de Kaa CA, et-al.., Microvessel Density: Correlation between Contrast Ultrasonography and Histology of Prostate Cancer, European Urology 2001, 40:285–293.
32. Sedelaa JPM, Goossen TEB, Wijkstra H, de la Rosette JJMCH, Reproducibility of Contrast-Enhanced Transrectal Ultrasound of the Prostate, Ultrasound in Medicine & Biology 2001, 27(5): 595–602.
33. Potdevin TC, Moskalik AP, Fowlkes JB, Bude RO, Carson PL, Doppler Quantitative Measures by Region to Discriminate Prostate Cancer, Ultrasound in Medicine & Biology 2001, 27(9):1305–1310.
34. Basset O, Sun Z, Mestas JL, Gimenez G, Texture Analysis of Ultrasonic Images of the Prostate by Means of Cooccurrence Matrices, Ultrasonic Imaging 1993, 15:218–237.
35. Huynen AL, Giesen RJB, De La Rosette JJMCH, Aarnink RG, Debruyne FMJ, Wijkstra H, Analysis of Ultrasonographic Prostate Images for the Detection of Prostatic Carcinoma: the Automated Urologic Diagnostic Expert System, Ultrasound in Medicine & Biology 1994, 20(1):1–10.
36. Giesen RJB, Huynen AL, Aarnink RG, et-al.., Computer Analysis of Transrectal Ultrasound Images of the Prostate for the Detection of Carcinoma: A Prospective Study in Radical Prostatectomy Specimens, Journal of Urology 1995, 154:1397–1400.
37. Loch T, Leuschner I, Genberg C, et-al.., Artificial Neural Network Analysis (ANNA) of Prostatic Transrectal Ultrasound, The Prostate 1999, 39:198–204.
38. Loch T, Leuschner I, Genberg C, et al. Weiterentwicklung des transrektalen Ultraschalls, Der Urologe A 2000, 4:341–347.
39. Jenderka KV, Gärtner T, Zacharias M, Heynemann H, Cobet U, System Independent Tissue Typing of Human Testis and Prostate, Proceedings Ultrasonics Symposium 1999, 2:1377–1380.
40. Jenderka KV, Gärtner T, Cobet U, Zacharias M, Heynemann H, Tissue Characterization by Imaging the Local Frequency Dependent Relative Backscatter Coefficient, Ultrasonic Imaging and Signal Processing, Proceedings of SPIE 2000, 3982:270–277.
41. Feleppa EJ, Kalisz A, Sokil-Melgar JB, et al. Typing of Prostate Tissue by Ultrasonic Spectrum Analysis, Transactions on Ultrasonics, Ferroelectrics and Frequency Control 1996, 43(4):609–619.
42. Feleppa EJ, Liu T, Kalisz A, et al. Ultrasonic Spectral-Parameter Imaging of the Prostate, International Journal of Imaging Systems & Technology 1997, 8(1):11–25.
43. Feleppa EJ, Fair WR, Liu T, et al. Two-Dimensional and Three-Dimensional Tissue-Type Imaging of the Prostate Based on Ultrasonic Spectrum Analysis and Neural-Network Classification, Medical Imaging, SPIE 2000, 1(27):152–160.
44. Feleppa EJ, Ketterling JA, Kalisz A, et al. Advanced Ultrasonic Tissue-Typing and Imaging Based on Radio-Frequency Spectrum Analysis and Neural-Network Classification for Guidance

of Therapy and Biopsy Procedures, Proceedings of CARS 2001, 333–337.
45. Feleppa EJ, Ennis RD, Schiff PB, et al. Spectrum-Analysis and Neural-Networks for Imaging to Detect and Treat Prostate Cancer, Ultrasonic Imaging 2001, 23:135–146.
46. Feleppa EJ, Porter CR, Ketterling JA, et al. Recent Developments in Tissue-Type Imaging (TTI) for Planning and Monitoring Treatment of Prostate Cancer, Ultrasonic Imaging 2004, 26:71–84.
47. Feleppa EJ, Porter CR, Ketterling JA, Dasgupta S, Ramachandran S, Sparks D, Recent advances in ultrasonic tissue-type imaging of the prostate: improving detection and evaluation, Acoustical Imaging, M.P. Andre (Ed.) (Springer: Dordrecht, 2007) vol. 28, pp. 331–339.
48. Balaji KC, Fair WR, Feleppa EJ, et al. Role of Advanced 2 and 3-Dimensional Ultrasound For Detecting Prostate Cancer, Journal of Urology 2002, 168:2422–2425.
49. Schmitz G, Ermert H, Senge T, Tissue Characterization of the Prostate Using Kohonen-Maps, Proceedings of Ultrasonics Symposium 1994, 2:1487–1490.
50. Lorenz A, Zwei neue Verfahren zur Früherkennung von Prostatatumoren mit diagnostischem Ultraschall (Shaker: Germany, 1999).
51. Schmitz G, Ein Verfahren zur Ultraschall-Gewebscharakterisierung der Prostata (VDI: Berlin, 1995).
52. Lorenz A, Blüm M, Ermert H, Senge T, Comparison of Different Neuro-Fuzzy Classification Systems for the Detection of Prostate Cancer in Ultrasonic Images, Proceedings Ultrasonics Symposium, 1997, 2:1201–1204.
53. Schmitz G, Ermert H, Senge T, Tissue Characterization and Imaging of the Prostate Using Radio Frequency Ultrasonic Signals, Transactions on Ultrasonics, Ferroelectrics and Frequency Control 1999, 46:126–138.
54. Thijssen JM, Spectroscopy and Image Texture Analysis, Ultrasound in Medical Biology 2000, 26(1):S41–S44.
55. Delorme S, Zuna I, Ad multos annos, Ultraschall in der Medizin 2000, 21:230–232.
56. Schmitz G, Ermert H, Senge T, Ultraschall-Gewebecharakterisierung der Prostata mit Kohonen-Maps, Biomedizinische Technik 1994, 39:36–37.
57. Feleppa EJJ, Diller Kalisz A, Rosado AL, Ultrasonic Tissue Typing of Prostate Tissue, Proceedings Ultrasonics Symposium 1994, 1483–1486.
58. Feleppa EJ, Fair WR, Liu T, et al. Improved Prostate Biopsy Guidance Using Ultrasonic Tissue-Typing Images, Proceedings Ultrasonics Symposium 1996, 1163–1166.
59. Scheipers U, Lorenz A, Pesavento A, et al. Ultrasonic Multifeature Tissue Characterization for the Early Detection of Prostate Cancer, Proceedings International Ultrasonics Symposium 2001, 1265–1268.
60. Scheipers U, Ermert H, Lorenz A, et al. Neuro-Fuzzy Inference System for Ultrasonic Multifeature Tissue Characterization for Prostate Diagnostics, Proceedings International Ultrasonics Symposium 2002, 1347–1350.
61. Kadah YM, Farag AA, Zurada JM, Badawi AM, Youssef ABM, Classification Algorithms for Quantitative Tissue Characterization of Diffuse Liver Disease from Ultrasound Images, Transactions of Medical Imaging 1996, 15(4):466–478.
62. Zadeh LA, Outline of a New Approach to the Analysis of Complex Systems and Decision Processes, Transactions of System, Man, and Cybernetics 1973, 3(1):28–44.
63. Zadeh LA, Knowledge Representation in Fuzzy Logic, Trans Knowledge Data Engineering 1989, 1:89–100.
64. Jang JSR, ANFIS: Adaptive Network-Based Fuzzy Inference Systems, Transactions of System, Man, and Cybernetics 1993, 23(3):665–685.
65. Mendel JM, Fuzzy Logic Systems for Engineering: A Tutorial, Proceedings of the IEEE 1995, 83(9):345–377.
66. Furuhashi T, Fusion of Fuzzy/Neuro/Evolutionary Computing for Knowledge Acquisition, Proceedings of the IEEE 2001, 89(9):1266–1274.
67. Scheipers U, Ermert H, Sommerfeld HJ, et al. Ultrasonic Tissue Characterization for Prostate Diagnostics: Spectral Parameters vs. Texture Parameters, Biomedizinische Technik 2003, 48(5):122–129.
68. Scheipers U, Ermert H, Sommerfeld HJ, Garcia-Schürmann M, Senge T, Philippou S, Ultrasonic Multifeature Tissue Characterization for Prostate Diagnostics, Ultrasound in Medicine & Biology 2003, 29(8):1137–1149.
69. Lizzi FL, Astor M, Feleppa EJ, Shao M, Kalisz A, Statistical Framework for Ultrasonic Spectral Parameter Imaging, Ultrasound in Medicine & Biology 1997, 23(9):1371–1382.
70. Lizzi FL, Feleppa EJ, Astor M, Kalisz A, Statistics of Ultrasonic Spectral Parameters and Liver Examinations, Transactions on Ultrasonics, Ferroelectrics and Frequency Control 1997, 44(4):935–942.
71. Lizzi FL, Alam SK, Mikaelian S, Lee P, Feleppa EJ, On the statistics of ultrasonic spectral parameters, Ultrasound in Medicine & Biology 2006, 32(11):1671–1685.
72. Blackmore S, Intelligent Sensing and Self-Organizing Fuzzy-Logic Techniques Used in Agricultural Automation, Asae/Csae Meeting 1994, 931048, Silsoe College, Cranfield University.
73. Oosterveld BJ, Thijssen JM, Hartman PC, Romijn RL, Rosenbusch GJE, Ultrasound Attenuation and Texture Analysis of Diffuse Liver Disease: Methods and Preliminary Results, Physics in Medicine & Biology 1991, 36:1039–1064.
74. Huisman HJ, Thijssen JM, Precision and Accuracy of Acoustospectrographic Parameters, Ultrasound in Medicine & Biology 1996, 22(7):855–871.
75. Lizzi FL, Greenebaum M, Feleppa EJ, Elbaum M, Theoretical Framework for Spectrum Analysis in Ultrasonic Tissue Characterization, Journal of the Acoustical Society of America 1983, 73(4):1366–1373.
76. Oelze ML, O'Brien Jr. WD, Frequency-Dependent Attenuation-Compensation Functions for Ultrasonic Signals Backscattered from Random Media, Journal of Acoustical Society of America 2002, 11(5):2308–1319.
77. Wear KA, A Gaussian Framework for Modeling Effects of Frequency-Dependent Attenuation, Frequency-Dependent Scattering, and Gating, Transactions on Ultrasonics, Ferroelectrics and Frequency Control 2002, 49(11):1572–1582.
78. Liu CN, Fatemi M, Waag RC, Digital Processing for Improvement of Ultrasonic Abdominal Images, Transactions on Medical Imaging 1983, 2(2):66–75.
79. Angelsen BAJ, Ultrasound Imaging (Emantec AS: Trondheim, Norway, 2000).
80. Wagner RF, Smith SW, Sandrik JM, Lopez H, Statistics of Speckle in Ultrasound B-Scans, Transactions on Sonics Ultrasonics 1983, 30(3):156–163.
81. Centers for Disease Control and Prevention, Screening with the Prostate Specific Antigen Test – Texas, 1997, MMWR 2000, 49(36):818–820.

82. Centers for Disease Control and Prevention, Recent Trends in Mortality Rates for Four Major Cancers, by Sex and Race/Ethnicity – United States, 1990–1998, MMWR 2002, 51:49–53.
83. Khan J, Wei JS, Ringner M, et al. Classification and Diagnostic Prediction of Cancers Using Gene Expression Profiling and Artificial Neural Networks, Nature Medicine 2001, 7(6):673–679.
84. Parkes C, Wald NJ, Murphy P, et al. Prospective Observational Study to Asses Value of Prostate Specific Antigen as Screening Test for Prostate Cancer, BMJ 1995, 311(7016):1340–1343.
85. Prater JS, Richard WD, Segmenting Ultrasound Images of the Prostate Using Neural Networks, Ultrasonic Imaging 1992, 14:159–185.
86. Lang M, Ermert H, Heuser L, In Vivo Study of On-Line Liver Tissue Classification Based on Envelope Power Spectrum Analysis, Ultrasonic Imaging 1994, 16:77–86.
87. Thijssen JM, Ultrasonic Tissue Characterization and Echographic Imaging, Physics in Medicine and Biology 1989, 34(11):1667–1674.
88. Scheipers U, Lorenz A, Pesavento A, et al. Ultraschall-Gewebecharakterisierung für die Prostatadiagnostik, Biomedizinische Technik 2001, 46(1):72–73.
89. Scheipers U, Ermert H, Lorenz A, et al. Ultraschall-Gewebecharakterisierung für die Früherkennung von Prostatatumoren, Ultraschall in der Medizin 2001, 22(1):43.
90. Scheipers U, Ermert H, Lorenz A, et al. Ultrasonic Multifeature Tissue Characterization for Prostate Diagnostics, Proceedings in Acoustics, DAGA 2002, 28:689–690.
91. Cloostermans MJTM, Thijssen JM, A Beam Corrected Estimation of the Frequency Dependent Attenuation of Biological Tissues from Backscattered Ultrasound, Ultrasonic Imaging 1983, 5(2):136–147.
92. Cloostermans MJTM, Verhoef WA, Thijssen JM, Generalized Description and Tracking Estimation of the Frequency Dependent Attenuation of Ultrasound in Biological Tissue, Ultrasonic Imaging 1985, 7(1):133–141.
93. Thijssen JM, Oosterveld BJ, Hartman PC, Rosenbusch GJ, Correlations between Acoustic and Texture Parameters from RF and B-mode Liver Echograms, Ultrasound in Medicine & Biology 1993, 19(1):13–20.
94. Feleppa EJ, Liu T, Lizzi FL, et al. Three-Dimensional Ultrasonic Parametric and Tissue-Property Imaging for Tissue Evaluation, Treatment Planning, Therapy Guidance, and Efficacy Assessment, Medical Imaging SPIE 2000, 1(27):68–76.
95. Wear KA, Wagner RF, Insana MF, Hall TJ, Application of Autoregressive Spectral Analysis to Cepstral Estimation of Mean Scatterer Spacing, Transactions on Ultrasonics, Ferroelectrics and Frequency Control 1993, 40(1):50–58.
96. Gorce JM, Friboulet D, Dydenko I, D'hooge J, Bijnens BH, Magnin IE, Processing Radio Frequency Ultrasound Images: A Robust Method for Local Spectral Features Estimation by a Spatially Constrained Parametric Approach, Transactions on Ultrasonics, Ferroelectrics and Frequency Control 2002, 49(12):1704–1719.
97. Nair A, Obuchowski N, Kuban BD, Vince DG, Classification of Atherosclerotic Plaque Composition by Spectral Analysis of Intravascular Ultrasound Data, Proceedings Ultrasonics Symposium 2001, 2001:1569–1572.
98. Böhme JF, Stochastische Signale (B.G. Teubner: Stuttgart, 1993).
99. Wear KA, Wagner RF, Garra BS, High Resolution Ultrasonic Backscatter Coefficient Estimation Based on Autoregressive Spectral Estimation Using Burg's Algorithm, Transactions on Medical Imaging 1994, 13(3):500–507.
100. Wear KA, Wagner RF, Garra BS, A Comparison of Autoregressive Spectral Estimation Algorithms and Order Determination Methods in Ultrasonic Tissue Characterization, Transactions on Ultrasonics, Ferroelectrics and Frequency Control 2995, 42(4):709–716.
101. Chaturvedi P, Insana MF, Autoregressive Spectral Estimation in Ultrasonic Scatterer Size Imaging, Ultrasonic Imaging 1996, 18:10–24.
102. Scheipers U, König K, Sommerfeld H, et al. Ultrasonic Tissue Characterization for the Classification of Prostate Tissue, Proceedings WCU 2003, 2003:637–640.
103. Scheipers U, König K, Sommerfeld HJ, et al. Diagnostics of Prostate Cancer based on Ultrasonic Multifeature Tissue Characterization, Proceedings Ultrasonics Symposium 2004, 2004:2153–2156.
104. Donohue KD, Huang L, Burks T, Forsberg F, Piccoli CW, Tissue Classification with Generalized Spectrum Parameters, Ultrasound in Medicine & Biology 2001, 27(11):1505–1514.
105. Huang L, Donohue KD, Genis V, Forsberg F, Duct Detection and Wall Spacing Estimation in Breast Tissue, Ultrasonic Imaging 2000, 22(3):137–152.
106. Varghese T, Donohue KD, Estimating Mean Scatterer Spacing with the Frequency-Smoothed Spectral Autocorrelation Function, Transactions on Ultrasonics, Ferroelectrics and Frequency Control 1995, 42(3):451–463.
107. Donohue KD, Forsberg F, Piccoli CW, Goldberg BB, Analysis and Classification of Tissue with Scatterer Structure Templates, Transactions on Ultrasonics, Ferroelectrics and Frequency Control 1999, 46(2):300–310.
108. Varghese T, Donohue KD, Characterization of Tissue Microstructure Scatterer Distribution with Spectral Correlation, Ultrasonic Imaging 1993, 15(3):238–254.
109. Dumane VA, Shankar PM, Piccoli CW, et al. Classification of Ultrasonic B Mode Images of the Breast Using Frequency Diversity and Nakagami Statistics, Transactions on Ultrasonics, Ferroelectrics and Frequency Control 2002, 49(5):664–668.
110. Dutt V, Greenleaf JF, Ultrasound Echo Envelope Analysis Using a Homodyned K Distribution Signal Model, Ultrasonic Imaging 1994, 16:265–287.
111. Gefen S, Tretiak OJ, Piccoli CW, et al. ROC Analysis of Ultrasound Tissue Characterization Classifiers for Breast Cancer Diagnosis, Classification of Ultrasonic B Mode Images of the Breast Using Frequency Diversity and Nakagami Statistics 2003, 22(2):170–177.
112. Georgiou G, Cohen FS, Statistical Characterization of Diffuse Scattering in Ultrasound Images, Classification of Ultrasonic B Mode Images of the Breast Using Frequency Diversity and Nakagami Statistics 1998, 45(1):57–64.
113. Hao X, Bruce CJ, Pislaru C, Greenleaf JF, Characterization of Reperfused Myocardium from High-Frequency Intracardiac Ultrasound Imaging Using Homodyned K Distribution, Classification of Ultrasonic B Mode Images of the Breast Using Frequency Diversity and Nakagami Statistics 2002, 49(11):1530–1542.
114. Jakeman E, Tough RJA, Generalized K Distribution: A Statistical Model for Weak Scattering, Journal of the Optical Society of America 1987, A(9):1764–1772.

115. Pesavento A, Ermert H, Broll-Zeitvogel E, Grifka J, High Resolution Imaging of Generalized K-Distribution Parameters using Maximum Likelihood Estimation for Ultrasonic Diagnosis of Muscle After Back Surgery, Proceedings Ultrasonics Symposium 1998, 2:1353–1356.
116. Prager RW, Gee AH, Treece GM, Berman L, Decompression and Speckle Detection for Ultrasound Images Using the Homodyned K-Distribution, Technical Report CUED/F-INFENG/TR 397 2000, University of Cambridge, Department of Engineering.
117. Shankar PM, Dumane VA, Reid JM, et al. Classification of Ultrasonic B-mode Images of Breast Masses Using Nakagami Distribution, Transactions on Ultrasonics, Ferroelectrics and Frequency Control 2001, 48(2):569–580.
118. Shankar PM, A Compound Scattering PDF for the Ultrasonic Echo Envelope and Its Relationship to K and Nakagami Distributions, Transactions on Ultrasonics, Ferroelectrics and Frequency Control 2003, 50(3):339–343.
119. Shankar PM, A General Statistical Model for Ultrasonic Backscattering from Tissues, Transactions on Ultrasonics, Ferroelectrics and Frequency Control 2000, 47(3):727–736.
120. Shankar PM, Ultrasonic Tissue Characterization Using a generalized Nakagami Model, Transactions on Ultrasonics, Ferroelectrics and Frequency Control 2001, 48(6):1716–1720.
121. Dumane VA, Shankar PM, Use of Frequency Diversity and Nakagami Statistics in Ultrasonic Tissue Characterization, Transactions on Ultrasonics, Ferroelectrics and Frequency Control 2001, 48(4):1139–1146.
122. Shankar PM, Molthen R, Narayanan VM, et al. Studies on the Use of Non-Rayleigh Statistics for Ultrasonic Tissue Characterization, Ultrasound in Medicine & Biology 1996, 22(7):873–882.
123. Shankar PM, Dumane VA, Reid JM, et al. Use of the K-Distribution for Classification of Breast Masses, Ultrasound in Medicine & Biology 2000, 26(9):1503–1510.
124. Lagarias JC, Reeds JA, Wright MH, Wright PE, Convergence Properties of the Nelder-Mead Simplex Method in Low Dimensions, SIAM Journal of Optimization 1998, 9(1):112–147.
125. Sijbers J, den Dekker AJ, Scheunders P, Van Dyck D, Maximum-Likelihood Estimation of Rician Distribution Parameters, Transactions on Medical Imaging 1998, 17(3):357–361.
126. Wachowiak MP, Smolikova R, Zurada JM, Elmaghraby AS, Estimation of K Distribution Parameters using Neural Networks, Transactions on Biomedical Engineering 2002, 49(6):617–620.
127. Prager RW, Gee AH, Treece GM, Berman L, Speckle Detection in Ultrasound Images Using First Order Statistics, Technical Report CUED/F-INFENG/TR 415 2001, University of Cambridge, Department of Engineering.
128. Bleck JS, Ranft U, Gebel M, et al. Random Field Models in the Textural Analysis of Ultrasonic Images of the Liver, Transactions on Medical Imaging 1996, 15(6):796–801.
129. Coolen J, Engelbrecht MR, Thijssen JM, Quantitative Analysis of Ultrasonic B-mode Images, Ultrasonic Imaging 1999, 21(3):157–172.
130. Lefebvre F, Meunier M, Thibault F, Laugier P, Berger G, Computerized Ultrasound B-Scan Characterization of Breast Nodules, Ultrasound in Medicine & Biology 2000, 26(9):1421–1428.
131. Haralick RM, Shanmugam K, Dinstein I, Textural Features for Image Classification, Transactions of System, Man, and Cybernetics 1973, 3(6):768–780.
132. Valckx FMJ, Thijssen JM, Characterization of Echographic Image Texture by Cooccurrence Matrix Parameters, Ultrasound in Medicine & Biology 1997, 23(4):559–571.
133. Valckx FMJ, Thijssen JM, van Geemen AJ, Rotteveel JJ, Mullaart R, Calibrated Parametric Medical Ultrasound Imaging, Ultrasonic Imaging 2000, 22:57–72.
134. Alam SK, Lizzi FL, Feleppa EJ, Liu T, Kalisz A, Ultrasonic Multifeature Analysis Procedures for Breast Lesion Classification, SPIE Medical Imaging 2000, 3982:196–201.
135. Wolf JM, Borchers H, Boeckmann W, Habib FK, Jakse G, Increased Differentiation Between Prostate Cancer and Benign Prostatic Hyperplasia Through Measurement of the Percentage of Free Prostate-Specific Antigen, Urologe A 1997, 36:255–258.
136. Polascik TJ, Oesterling JE, Partin AW, Prostate Specific Antigen: A Decade of Discovery – What We Have Learned and Where We Are Going, Journal of Urology 1999, 162:193–306.
137. Nelson WG, De Marzo AM, Isaacs WB, Prostate Cancer, The New England Journal of Medicine 2003, 349(4):366–381.
138. Wei JT, Zhang Z, Barnhill SD, Madyastha KR, Zhang H, Oesterling JE, Understanding Artificial Neural Networks and Exploring Their Potential Applications for the Practicing Urologist, Urology 1998, 52:161–172.
139. Snow PB, Smith DS, Catalona WJ, Artificial Neural Networks in the Diagnosis and Prognosis of Prostate Cancer: A Pilot Study, Journal of Urology 1994, 152:1923–1926.
140. Bishop CM, Neural Networks for Pattern Recognition (Oxford University Press: Oxford, UK, 1995).
141. Jang JSR, Sun CT, Neuro Fuzzy Modeling and Control, Proceedings of the IEEE 1995, 83(3):378–406.
142. Sugeno M, Yasukawa T, A Fuzzy-Logic-Based Approach to Qualitative Modeling, Transactions on Fuzzy Systems 1993, 1(1):7–31.
143. Jang JSR, Fuzzy Modeling Using Generalized Neural Networks and Kalman Filter Algorithm, Proceedings of Ninth National Conference on Artificial Intelligence 1991:762–767.
144. Hoang TA, Nguyen DT, Optimal Learning for Patterns Classification in RBF Networks, Electronic Letters 2002, 38(20):1188–1190.
145. Efron B, Tibshirani R, Improvements on Cross-Validation: The .632+ Bootstrap Method, Journal American Statistical Associations 1997, 92:548–560.
146. Obuchowski NA, Nonparametric Analysis of Clustered ROC Curve Data, Biometrics 1997, 53:567–578.
147. Kung SY, Taur JS, Decision-Based Neural Networks with Signal/Image Classification Applications, Transactions on Neural Networks 1995, 6(1):170–181.
148. Kroschel K, Statistische Nachrichtentechnik (Springer: Berlin, 1996).
149. Scheipers U, Perrey C, Siebers S, Hansen C, Ermert H, A Tutorial on the Use of ROC Analysis for Computer-Aided Diagnostic Systems, Ultrasonic Imaging 2005, 27:181–198.
150. Scheipers U, A ROC Framework for Computer-Aided Detection Systems, in: C. H. Chen (Ed.), Ultrasonic and Advanced Methods for Nondestructive Testing and Material Characterization (World Scientific: London, 2007) 684 pp.
151. Djavan B, Ramzi M, Ghawidel K, Marberger M, Diagnosis of Prostate Cancer: The Clinical Use of Transrectal Ultrasound and Biopsy, EAU Update Series 2003, 1:9–15.
152. Aarnink RG, Giesen RJB, Huynen AL, De La Rosette JJMCH, Debruyne FMJ, Wijkstra H, A Practical Clinical Method for

Contour Determination in Ultrasonographic Prostate Images, Ultrasound in Medicine & Biology 1994, 20(8):705–717.
153. Hoppin JW, Kupinski MA, Kastis GA, Clarkson E, Barrett HH, Objective Comparison of Quantitative Imaging Modalities Without the Use of a Gold Standard, Transactions on Medical Imaging 2002, 21(5):441–449.
154. Ellis WJ, Brawer MK, The Significance of Isoechoic Prostatic Carcinoma, Journal of Urology 1994, 152:2304–2307.
155. Noldus J, Palisaar J, Huland H, Treatment of Prostate Cancer – The Clinical Use of Radical Prostatectomy, EAU Update Series 2003, 1:16–22.
156. Loening SA, Wirth M, Engelmann U, Alternative Therapien des lokalen Prostatakarzinoms, Urologe A 2001, 40:180.
157. Deger S, Böhmer D, Roigas J, Türk I, Budach V, Loening SA, Brachytherapie des lokalen Prostatakarzinoms, Urologe A 2001, 40:181–184.
158. Bolla M, Treatment of Localized or Locally Advanced Prostate Cancer: The Clinical Use of Radiotherapy, EAU Update Series 2003, 1:23–31.
159. Sommer F, Derakhshani P, Zumbé J, Engelmann U, Die Bedeutung der Kryotherapie beim lokalisierten Prostatakarzinom, Urologe A 2001, 40:185–190.
160. Thüroff S, Chaussy C, Therapie des lokalen Prostatakarzinoms mit hoch intensivem fokussiertem Ultraschall (HIFU), Urologe A 2001, 40:191–194.
161. Deger S, Böhmer D, Türk I, et-al.., Thermoradiotherapie mit interstitiellen Thermoseeds bei der Behandlung des lokalen Prostatakarzinoms, Urologe A 2001, 40:195–198.
162. Anderson J, Treatment of Prostate Cancer – The Role of Primary Hormonal Therapy, EAU Update Series 2003 1:32–39.
163. Heidenreich A, Schrader AJ, The Treatment of Hormone Refractory Prostate Cancer, EAU Update Series 2003 1:40–50.
164. Lee EK, Gallagher RJ, Silvern D, Wuu CS, Zaider M, Treatment Planning for Brachytherapy: An Integer Programming Model, two Computational Experiments with Permanent Prostate Implant Planning, Physics in Medicine and Biology 1999, 44:145–165.

Chapter 17
Augmented Reality for Computer-Assisted Image-Guided Minimally Invasive Urology

Osamu Ukimura and Inderbir S. Gill

Background

Surgery is considered to be a highly interactive process and significant surgical decisions need to be made during surgery. In this era of minimally invasive surgery, videoscopic procedures have increasingly made the surgeon distanced from the real surgical field, with diminishing tactile feedback. Imaging guidance is particularly crucial for such videoscopic minimally invasive surgery where the procedure is performed through small openings in the body, since the sensory information available to the surgeon is much more limited than in the open approach. Image-guided surgery has had significant growth in recent years and is becoming widely accepted by experts or professionals.[1–7] Conventional use of intraoperative imaging for surgical navigation, such as real-time ultrasound or open MRI, has critical issues including (1) operator dependency in interpretation of the image, (2) the need for ultrasound expertise, (3) the need of expensive equipment for open MRI, and (4) the limitation of its two-dimensional imaging feature. If using conventional 2D preoperative imaging alone, surgeons have generally needed extensive mental imagination to understand the 3D anatomy beyond the surgical view, by using tactile feedback or other available sensory information. On the other hand, intraoperative computer-assisted image guidance systems allow the surgeon to have detailed information available in the real surgical field during the surgical procedure, visualizing the 3D anatomy of the patient and also rendering the surgical instruments. The 3D patient information can be a preoperative imaging modality such as CT, MRI, or PET that requires a registration process onto the real anatomy during the procedure, or it can be a real-time imaging modality such as ultrasound or fluoroscopy that have the advantage of eliminating the registration process because of their real-time nature. The patient-specific surgical planning models can be made into 3D preoperative or intraoperative surgical planning models. Furthermore, integrating by digital information the interventional device and the 3D imaging, computer-assisted interventional treatment (such as in percutaneous or extracorporeal approaches) will significantly improve both the consistency of the intervention and the clinical follow-up data available for patient and statistical analysis to validate new therapeutic interventions. The goal of future computer-assisted image-guided surgery is not simply to replace the surgeon with a computer or robot, but to provide new valuable versatile tools that extend the surgeon's ability to achieve both oncological and functional outcomes of the surgery for the patient. The value of computer assistance can be measured in: (1) increased precision of the surgery, (2) reduced morbidity or error rates, (3) shortened operative times, and (4) a shortened learning curve for the novice.

Virtual reality has been used as a surgical simulator of the real world for training or planning.[8] The laparoscopic simulator is regarded as one of the recommended tools for training surgical residents, which might be enhanced by coupling it with a virtual reality simulation model. Augmented reality is the technology further advanced from virtual reality.[4,9–13] It is a powerful, new, intraoperative imaging technology allowing the merging of computer graphics and real surgical imagery into a single, coherent perception of the enhanced surgical world around the surgeon. This means that the image one sees on the endoscopic video screen comprises a real video image overlaid with a graphics image. This allows the surgeon directional interpretation of the 3D imaging information of the real endoscopic surgical field. The clinical application of augmented reality in the individual clinical setting will offer better realism, potentially not only improving precision in difficult surgery for the expert, but also decreasing the learning curve for the novice by minimizing adverse effects. Augmented reality technology potentially improves clinical outcomes, in a practical educational process.

Technical Aspects of Augmented Reality

Augmented reality was initially applied to neurosurgery, which has a relatively fixed small space, frames, and a bony reference, facilitating the registration of virtual and real images.[9,11] In clinical application of augmented reality technology, the challenge in laparoscopic surgery has included the deformation of the abdominal organs due to respiration, heartbeat, gas

O. Ukimura and I.S. Gill (eds.), *Contemporary Interventional Ultrasonography in Urology*,
DOI: 10.1007/978-1-84800-217-3_17,

insufflations, and surgical manipulation.[1,12] Key steps in the application of augmented reality involve the reconstruction of 3D surgical models from the imaging modality, registration of the image onto the real anatomy, and tracking the surgical instruments as well as tracking any motion of the targeted organs and surrounding anatomies. The system is designed to assist a surgeon in (1) performing a surgery with preoperative surgical planning models; (2) allowing intraoperative registration of preoperative surgical models onto the real surgical field, and (3) intraoperative use of the 3D surgical planning model integrated with the surgical instruments.

The preoperative surgical plan generally starts with 2D medical images, together with other available information about the patient, such as the pathology. For intraoperative use, a 3D surgical model can be developed from these preoperative images as well as intraoperatively acquired images. In the operating room, this information is registered onto the actual patient using an intraoperative position sensor system, which typically involves the use of a magnetic or optical 3D localization system, X-ray, or US images, or the use of a laser system. If necessary, the surgical plan can be updated intraoperatively with real-time imaging such as US, X-ray, or MRI.

The essential technology for augmented reality is the accuracy of the registration and tracking systems. The most common clinical applications for the registration and tracking system include (1) optical sensor systems, (2) electromagnetic sensor systems, or (2) a robot itself. (1) Optical tracking systems, using an infrared stereo camera and optical marker, are the most prevalent tracking systems used today for image-guided surgery. In general, optical tracking systems provide a simple tracking solution that achieves high accuracy, a fast sample rate to achieve a real-time nature, and relatively constant and isotropic measurement error for clinical practice. (2) Electromagnetic sensor systems have a field generator that produces one or more distinct magnetic fields, and a receiver with one or more sensor coils that picks up the signals. Unfortunately, electromagnetic sensor systems have the shortcoming that anything that distorts the generated field (such as metal in an operating gurney) will cause a decrease in accuracy. Key components of electromagnetic sensor systems include (1) the field generator to generate the magnetic fields, (2) the sensor to produce electrical signals in the presence of the induced magnetic fields, and (3) the system control unit to control the field generator, and to receive the sensor data and synchronizing it with the field generator output, performing calculations, and communicating with the host personal computer. (3) A robot can also prove to be a great localizational tool to provide digital information of the surgical instruments in the space. An accurately calibrated robot provides a very precise location within the calibrated workspace. A further method of tracking is the use of real-time medical imaging directly, for example, using fluoroscopy or ultrasound as well as, in the near future, using real-time CT fluoroscopy and MRI. Also in the future, a body-GPS (global positioning system) may be used for tracking the dynamic motion of the surgical target.

Augmented reality provides 3D anatomy to localize the tumor, adjacent organs, and vasculatures in order to determine the correct dissection planes. Potential advantages of the use of augmented reality in laparoscopic surgery include identifying ideal dissection planes or resection margins and the avoidance of any injury to invisible structures to improve the safety and efficacy of various percutaneous approaches or extracorporeal techniques such as radiofrequency ablation, cryosurgery, the cyber knife, or high-intensity focused ultrasound. Since the use of augmented reality will be simplified when automated image registration is developed for achieving the dynamic tracking of organ movement, we are currently working toward the use of a wireless body-GPS.

Initial Clinical Use of Augmented Reality in Urology: Cleveland Clinic Experience

In the Cleveland Clinic, we have first developed our system and software for augmented reality navigation to be compatible with laparoscopic urological procedures, from the original program of our coresearcher's augmented reality technique for breast-conservative cancer surgery in 1998.[13–15] We employed optical tracking systems, which have been the most prevalent tracking systems for image-guided surgery, as already mentioned (Fig. 17.1). The 3D anatomical information can be a preoperative high-resolution image such as CT or MRI for kidney surgery or a real-time imaging modality such as transrectal ultrasound (TRUS) (Figs. 17.2–17.8) or MRI (Fig. 17.9)

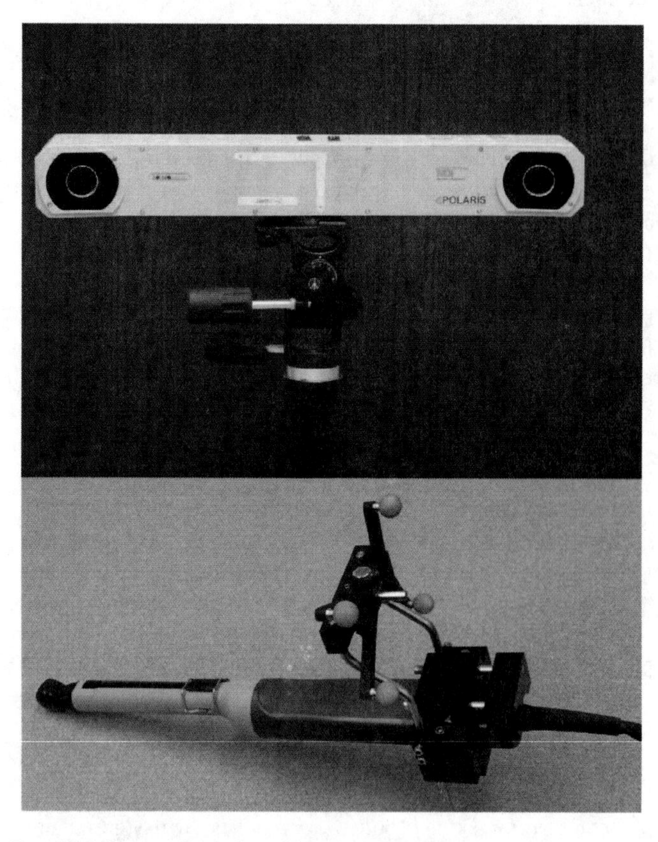

Fig. 17.1. Upper, Optical positions sensor with infrared optical camera, named by Polaris; Lower, Optical marker attached TRUS probe

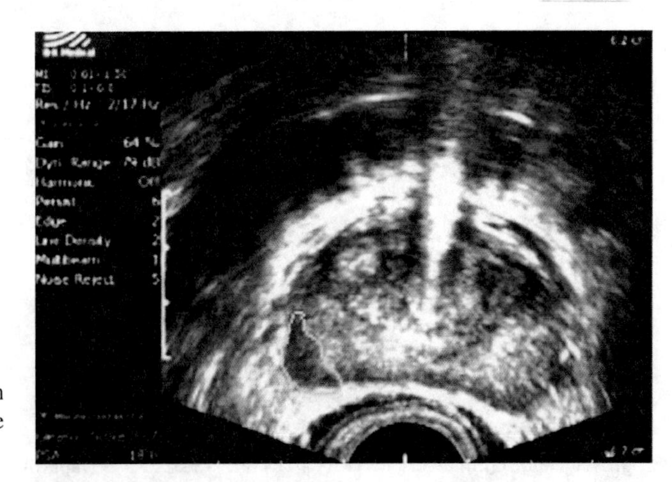

FIG. 17.2. Original intraoperatively acquired 2D TRUS picture with traced hypoechoic lesion (*yellow line*), which was proven by positive biopsy for cancer

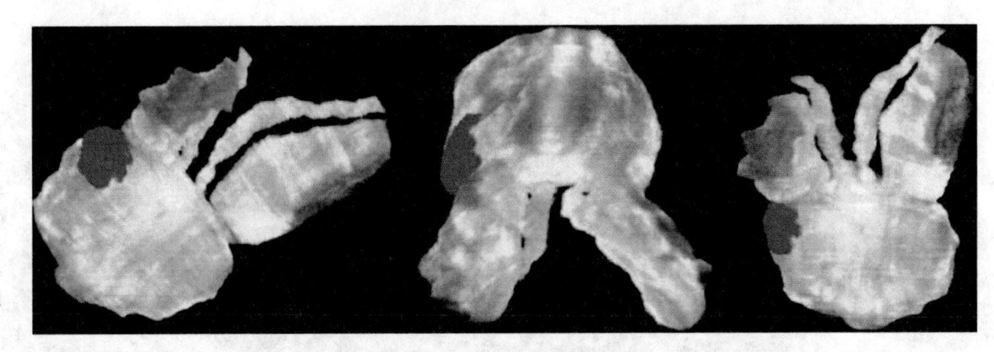

FIG. 17.3. Reconstructed 3D surgical model of the prostate and biopsy-proven cancer area (*blue*)

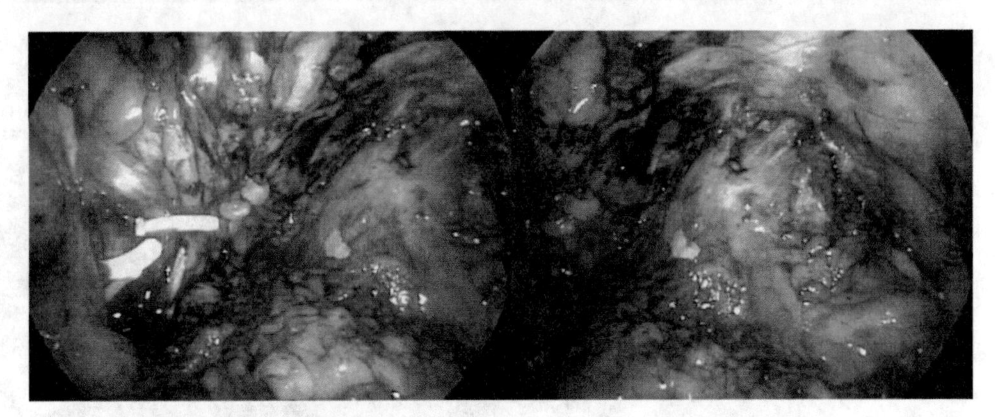

FIG. 17.4. Augmented reality visualization using the 3D TRUS image of biopsy confirmed cancer area (*rainbow colored*) onto the real-time laparoscopic view; augmented reality demonstrates the precisely superimposed 3D cancer area even when the directions of the endoscopic view were changed

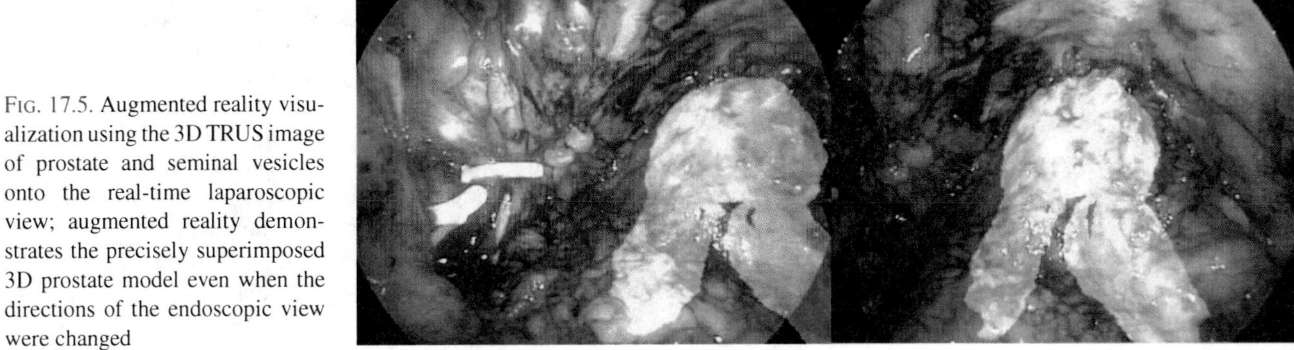

FIG. 17.5. Augmented reality visualization using the 3D TRUS image of prostate and seminal vesicles onto the real-time laparoscopic view; augmented reality demonstrates the precisely superimposed 3D prostate model even when the directions of the endoscopic view were changed

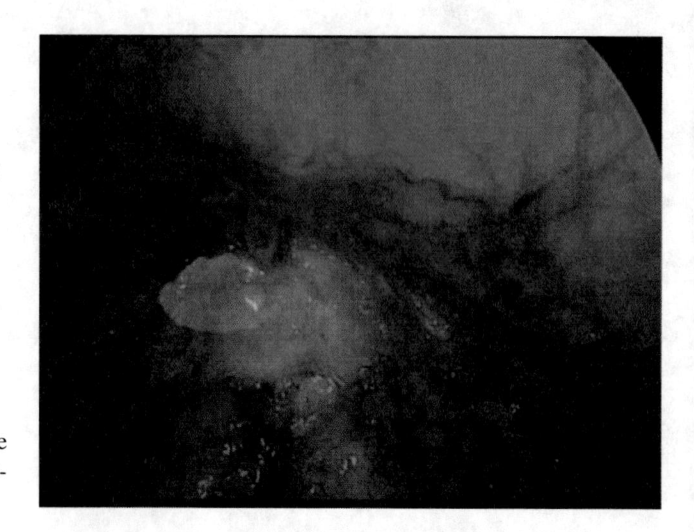

FIG. 17.7. Augmented reality visualization using the 3D TRUS image of prostate and seminal vesicles (Fig. 17.6) onto the real-time laparoscopic view

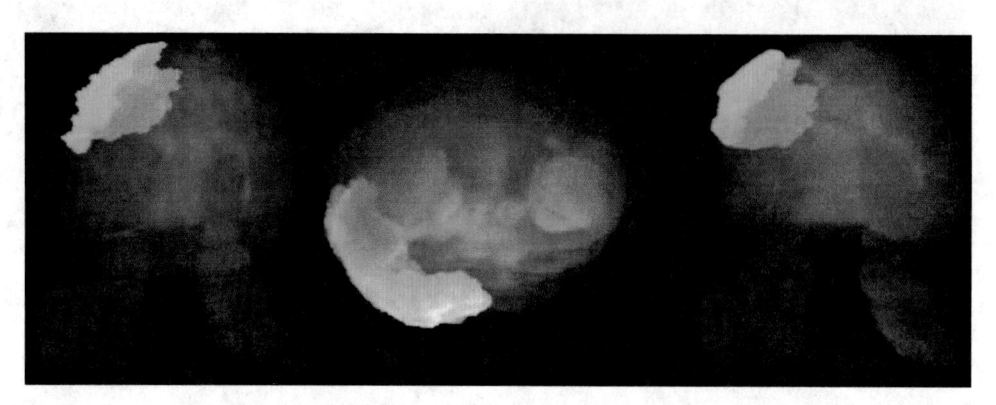

FIG. 17.6. Reconstructed 3D surgical model of the prostate (see-though *orange colored*) and biopsy-proven cancer area (*blue*)

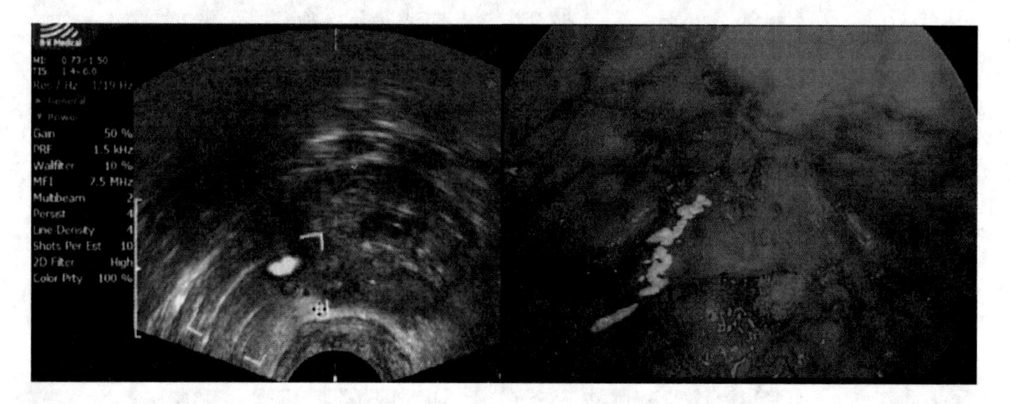

FIG. 17.8. *Left*: Original intraoperatively acquired 2D power Doppler TRUS picture, which was focused on the blood flow within the neurovascular bundle (NVB). *Right*: Augmented reality visualization using the reconstructed 3D TRUS model of the NVB, which was reconstructed from the series of the original pictures (shown in the *left* of figure) onto the real-time laparoscopic view

for prostate surgery. The ability to employ a 3D model from the intraoperatively acquired ultrasound image as well as the accuracy to register a preoperatively constructed 3D model by CT/MRI were our key steps, since the position and shape of the targeted organ might move and change according to the progress of the surgery.

In the summer of 2006, as our initial clinical series, we employed our augmented reality system in 25 laparoscopic cases: laparoscopic partial nephrectomy (LPN) ($n = 8$), laparoscopic radical nephrectomy (LRN) ($n = 2$), laparoscopic donor nephrectomy (LDN) ($n = 1$), laparoscopic radical prostatectomy (LRP) ($n = 13$), and laparoscopic radical cystopros-

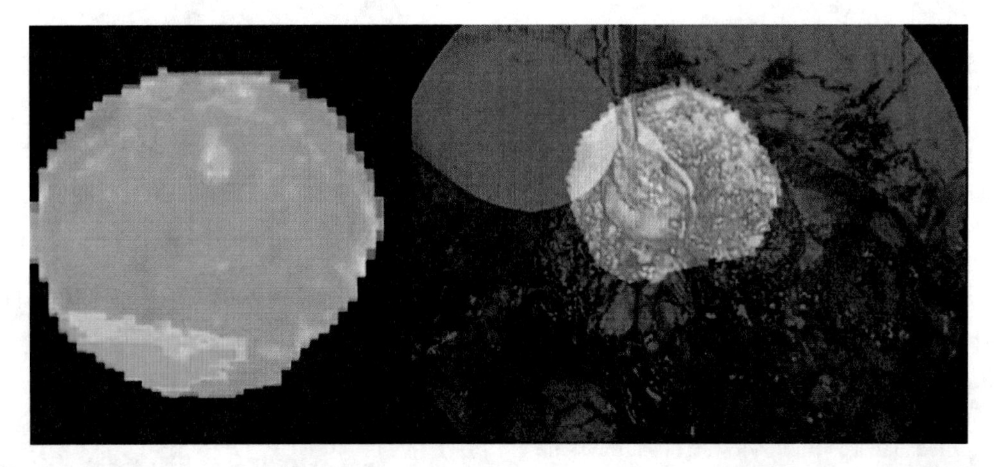

FIG. 17.9. *Left*: 3D surgical model of the prostate (*purple colored*) and biopsy-proven cancer area (*blue*), which was reconstructed from preoperative MRI image. *Right*: Augmented reality visualization using the reconstructed 3D MRI model (shown in the *left* of figure) onto the real-time laparoscopic view

tatectomy (LRC) (n = 1).[14,15] The system consists of surgical instruments (rigid laparoscope, laparoscopic surgical instruments) on which optical markers were attached, an infrared optical tracking sensor (Polaris, Northern Digital, Waterloo, Ontario, Canada), and a computerized workstation.

The practical process to perform image-guidance included (1) calibration of the instruments (TRUS probe, laparoscope, and surgical instruments), integrated with the optical position sensor system, (2) image acquisition and segmentation of the region of interest (such as a biopsy-proven hypoechoic cancer area), (3) 3D image reconstruction according to specific surgical planning in each case, (4) (when using preoperative CT or MRI), registration of 3D coordinates between real surgical fields and imaging data, and (5) superimposition of the 3D image onto the laparoscopic view.

In the tracking system of the intraoperative motion of the surgical instrument, on which 3–4 optical markers were attached, calibration of the instruments was performed one day before surgery, and then these instruments (including laparoscope, laparoscopic scissors, and pointer) were sterilized over night. Intraoperative ultrasound images of the surgical fields were obtained by a TRUS probe (Type 8818 or Type 8808, B-K medical, Copenhagen, Denmark) for the prostate (Fig.17.1), or an abdominal convex probe for the kidney, with an ultrasound machine (Pro-Focus, B-K medical, Copenhagen, Denmark). For calibration of the US probe, a specially shaped board was designed. A US image of the board, which was placed under water, was obtained, and then specified to determine 2D coordinates between the points imaged by US and the corresponding points on the board. An US image could be obtained intraoperatively at any time point during surgery, and immediately segmented for construction of 3D models of the tumor and surrounding structures to create a superimposed image. When using preoperative CT or MRI for the superimposed image, the CT or MRI image was obtained preoperatively, and all volume data were transferred into the workstation by a CD formatted by DICOM. 3D surgical planning models of CT or MRI were constructed one day before surgery and stored in the workstation.

For prostate surgery, intraoperative real-time TRUS was performed as reported previously.[5,6] The 3D motion of the ultrasound probes was followed with the aid of an optical tracking system which measured the position of the optical markers attached to the probes. The regions of interest containing the prostate and hypoechoic cancer lesion were defined manually on the stored 2D images using Virtual Place software (Medical Imaging Laboratory Inc., Tokyo, Japan) (Fig. 17.2). A surgical planning 3D model of the prostate and cancer area was created by the volume rendering method (Figs. 17.3 and 17.6). Since the US image is real time, and available at any time point during surgery, the constructed 3D geometry can be projected very precisely without a registration process (Figs. 17.4, 17.5, 17.7, and 17.8). This is achieved under the hypothesis that no movement of organs in the operative field occurred between acquisition and projection of the images. The prostate, biopsy-proven cancer area, and neurovascular bundles (NVB) were finally superimposed onto a real video image of the laparoscopic surgical field in accordance with the 3D coordinates (Figs. 17.4, 17.5, 17.7, and 17.8). To map the movements of the prostate at different surgical stages we ran the TRUS probe repeatedly to update the image.

In selected cases in which MRI could demonstrate the cancer area, 3D images of the MRI for the prostate were employed for the surgical planning model. In these cases, 3D models of the preoperative MRI images were reconstructed one day before, and superimposed with the technique of an image-to-image registration process, with overlapping of the 3D models of the preoperative MRI onto the 3D models of intraoperative US (Fig. 17.9).

Intraoperative US is most attractive for surgical navigation because US is real time and the 3D model can be updated at any time point during surgery. In our recent reports, the ability to acquire intraoperative TRUS images during nerve-sparing LRP has been proven to be useful for obtaining better surgical margins and erectile function recovery.[6,16] The most valuable information from intraoperative TRUS is to enable visualization of what is beyond what the surgeon can see directly, which includes the biopsy-proven cancer area and the neurovascular bundle. 3D images of the prostate anatomy and biopsy-proven cancer area were re-constructed from the intraoperative real-time TRUS. Augmented reality technology can superimpose a 3D US image of the blue-colored cancer area on the real surgical laparoscopic view. This allows the surgeon direct interpretation of the 3D relationship between the cancer and the NVB.

Conclusions

Real-time surgical navigation systems using augmented reality technology have been applied for various laparoscopic urologic procedures. Reconstructed 3D models included preoperative CT, MRI, and/or intraoperative ultrasound. Currently, intraoperative real-time ultrasound is the most attractive imaging modality and can be acquired at any time point during surgery to update the real-time surgical anatomy which can be changed from its preoperative status by respiration, heartbeat, and/or surgical manipulations.

References

1. Ackerman JD, Keller K, Fuches H: Real-time anatomical 3D image extraction for laparoscopic surgery. Stud Health Technol Inform. 81:18–22. 2001
2. Gill IS: Minimally invasive nephron-sparing surgery. Urol Clin N Am. 30:551–579. 2003
3. Gill IS, Matin SF, Desai MM, Kaouk JH, Steinberg A, Mascha E, Thornton J, Sherief MH, Strzempkowski B, Novick AC: Comparative analysis of laparoscopic vs. open partial nephrectomy for renal tumors in 200 patients. J Urol. 170:64. 2003
4. Marescaux J, Rubino F, Arenas M, Mutter D, Soler L: Augmented-reality-assisted laparoscopic adrenalectomy. JAMA. 292:2214–2215. 2004
5. Ukimura O, Gill IS, Desai MM, Steinberg AP, Kilciler M, Ng CS, Abreu SC, Spaliviero M, Ramani AP, Kaouk JH, Kawauchi A, Miki T: Real-time transrectal ultrasonography during laparoscopic radical prostatectomy. J Urol. 172:112–118. 2004
6. Ukimura O, Magi-Galluzzi C, Gill IS: Real-time transrectal ultrasound guidance during nerve-sparing laparoscopic radical prostatectomy: Impact on surgical margins. J Urol. 175:1304–1310. 2006
7. Hong J, Nakashima H, Konishi K, Ieiri S, Tanoue K, Nakamuta M, Hashizume M: Interventional navigation for abdominal therapy based on simultaneous use of MRI and ultrasound. Med Biol Eng Comput. 44:1127–34. 2006
8. Cameron BM, Robb RA: Virtual-reality-assisted interventional procedures. Clin Orthop Relat Res. 442:63–73. 2006
9. Iseki H, Masutani Y, Iwahara M, Tanikawa T, Muragaki Y, Taira T, Dohi T, Takakura K: Volumegraph (overlaid three-dimensional image-guided navigation). Clinical application of augmented reality in neurosurgery. Stereotact Funct Neurosurg. 68:18–24. 1997
10. Tang SL, Kwoh CK, Teo MY, Sing NW, Ling KV: Augmented reality systems for medical applications. IEEE Eng Med Biol Mag. 17:49–58. 1998
11. Kawamata T, Iseki H, Shibasaki T, Hori T: Endoscopic augmented reality navigation system for endonasal transsphenoidal surgery to treat pituitary tumors: technical note. Neurosurgery. 50:1393–1397. 2002
12. Shuhaiber JH: Augmented reality in surgery. Arch Surg. 139:170–174. 2004
13. Sato Y, Nakamoto M, Tamaki Y, Sasama T, Sakita I, Nakajima Y, Monden M, Tamura S: Image guidance of breast cancer surgery using 3-D ultrasound images and augmented reality visualization. IEEE Trans Med Imaging. 17:681–693. 1998
14. Ukimura O, Gill IS, Miki T: Recent achievements of laparoscopic ultrasonographic navigation: Initial experience of real-time TRUS-LRP and augmented reality in urology. Recent Adv Endourol. 10. 2008 (in press)
15. Ukimura O, Gill IS: Imaging assisted endoscopic surgery – Cleveland Clinic experience. J Endourol. 22(4): 803–810. 2008
16. Gill IS, Ukimura O: Thermal energy-free laparoscopic nerve-sparing radical prostatectomy: one-year potency outcomes. Urology. 70:309–314. 2007

Chapter 18
Robotic Percutaneous Interventions

Dan Stoianovici, Bogdan Vigaru, Doru Petrisor, and Pierre Mozer

Introduction

A robot is a mechanical device controlled by a computer. The first industrial robot was created by J. Engelberger and G. Deroe in 1961 and consisted of an articulated arm used in the automobile industry. The first robotic systems in the field of medicine began in the 1980s and were derived from industrial robots. However, the medical requirements for safety, sterility, and demanding constraints of the applications led to the development of specialized robots. In urology, robotics was introduced in 1989 by B. Davies at the Imperial College in London for transurethral resection of the prostate (TURP).[1]

Many classifications of robots can be found, and depending on the specifics of the applications these can be rather numerous.[2] A top-level classification in the medical field, however, may separate the systems based on the input that the system uses. The daVinci™ (Intuitive Surgical, Inc., CA), which is perhaps the most popular system today, is a *surgeon-driven* system, in which the robot is made to follow the input of the surgeon. The human operator directs the machine which does not have autonomous actions. The second type of robots is *image-guided*. These are connected to a medical imager (ultrasound, fluoroscopy, CT, MRI, etc.) and allow the physician to control the intervention under image feedback. Special algorithms are used to drive the robots in the space of the image (robot to image registration and navigation). With these and other image-guidance methods, the robots become more autonomous in executing the task, which is defined and monitored by the physician. The progress of surgical robots is most likely to emerge from the image-guided field, because these systems augment information that is not commonly available. Moreover, unlike humans, robots and imagers are digital devices and may establish a digital platform for image-guided interventions.

Due to the technical challenges involved, image-guided robots are not yet as popular. However, several systems have been developed. Most of these apply to needle interventions, because needle procedures have a large area of utility, are relatively simple, and have the potential to significantly improve upon the traditional manual access. Percutaneous robotic interventions are particularly promising in the field of urology. The kidneys and the prostate are commonly accessed percutaneously for diagnosis and therapy, and improved targeting has the potential to significantly improve the outcomes.

One of the main challenges of image-guided robots is that no imager is perfectly suited. The common ultrasound has relatively reduced imaging quality, and its geometric consistency is not entirely reliable. X-ray fluoroscopy is also real time, but is two dimensional (2D), and its use is limited by the admissible radiation levels. The CT is a "disciplined" geometrically consistent imager, but only a few advanced models deliver real-time 3D images, and this is done at the expense of significant radiation. Finally, MRI-based imagers are slow, notorious for their magnetism related restrictions, and impede direct access to the patient within the scanner for intervention purposes.

As such, the development of image-guided intervention (IGI) robots is a very challenging task. Special systems and methods need to be derived in order to take advantage of the imager's capabilities while accounting for their deficiencies and requirements and still satisfying the combined medical safety, sterility, and precision of the intervention.

A robot's compatibility with a medical imager refers to the ability of the robot to safely operate within the confined space of the imager while performing its clinical function, without interfering with the functionality of the imager.[3] The combination of imager compatibility and clinical requirements has been met with the development of customized systems for specific applications. Several urology examples of these dedicated robots are included in the following table and will be presented subsequently (Table 18.1).

Robotic Percutaneous Access of the Kidney

One of the first robots to be specifically made for urology applications is percutaneous access of the kidney (PAKY),[4] which was developed in our institution. PAKY is a very simple motorized needle driver that enables the active insertion

O. Ukimura and I.S. Gill (eds.), *Contemporary Interventional Ultrasonography in Urology*,
DOI: 10.1007/978-1-84800-217-3_18, © Springer-Verlag London Limited 2009

TABLE 18.1. Several image-guided percutaneous robots for urology.

System	Institution	Status	Imaging modality	Organ
PAKY-RCM	Johns Hopkins, Baltimore, USA	Animal models Human trials	Fluoroscopy and CT	Kidney
AcuBot	Johns Hopkins, Baltimore, USA	Mockup Cadaver studies Animal models Clinical trials	Fluoroscopy and CT	Kidney prostate
B-Rob	ARC, Seibersdorf, Austria	Mockup	Ultrasound and CT	Broad range of percutaneous treatments
InnoMotion	IMB, Karlsruhe, Germany	Animal models Clinical use	MRI and CT	Kidney (ex vivo)
MrBot	Johns Hopkins, Baltimore, USA	Mockup Cadaver studies Animal models	MRI	Prostate
Light puncture robot	TIMC, Grenoble, France	Mockup animal models	MRI and CT	Thoracic and abdominal organs

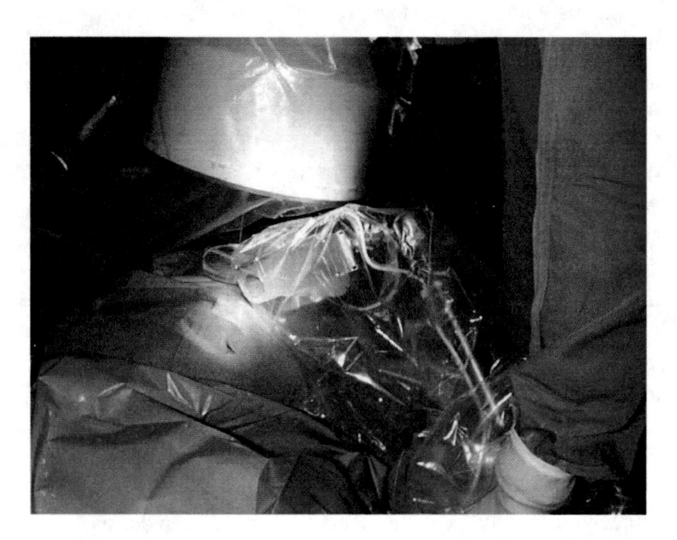

FIG. 18.1. PAKY-RCM in fluoroscopy-guided kidney access

of a needle. This is made of radiolucent materials so that the structure of the driver does not impede the visualization of the kidney. The system helped in accessing the kidney for stone removal interventions and has been used in numerous clinical cases.[5]

In its second version, an automated orientation module was added, the RCM.[6] The entire system comprises three motorized degrees of freedom (DOF): translation allowing insertion of the needle and two rotations allowing orientation of the needle (Fig. 18.1).

Several clinical studies were performed under fluoroscopy guidance and joystick control.[7] Intraoperative access variables (number of access attempts, time to successful access, estimated blood loss and complications) were recorded in a parallel blinded study of 46 patients who underwent either the robotic or standard manual procedure. The robot was successful in obtaining access in 87% (20 of 23) of cases. No statistically significant difference was found between the access variables in the two groups. This was expected because image guidance was not used in controlling the robot, but it showed the feasibility of the robotic procedure and allowed for future image-guided developments. This robot was also successfully tested in telesurgical applications between our institution and several hospitals in Europe[8–11] and Brazil.[12]

The true advantages of robotics are given by their ability to directly use the imaging information. In doing so, however, special algorithms are required in order to coordinate the motion of the robot in the image space. Many groups have contributed to the development of these registration and image-guidance algorithms.[13–15] The photograph in Fig. 18.2 shows a radiofrequency (RF) ablation performed under direct image guidance in the CT scanner.[16]

An IGI robot with full mobility (6DOF) was also made in our laboratory for CT needle interventions, the *AcuBot*.[17] The robot mounts on the mobile table of the CT scanner, has a bridge-like structure over the patient, and its distal part is sufficiently small to fit with the patient in the bore of the scanner. The system was successfully used in several IGI cases for the kidneys and demonstrated outstanding targeting performance and reduced the radiation levels for the patient and medical personnel.[16,18] The robot has also performed the first kidney ablations with CT preplanning of the ablation regions and robotic implementation of the plan (Fig. 18.3).[19]

One of the most advanced IGI robots today is the *Innomotion* robot made by the Innomedic (Herxheim, Germany, http://innomedic.com/). Its most remarkable feature is that it works with MRI scanners, a very challenging engineering development. This started at the Institute for Medical Engineering and Biophysics (IMB), Karlsruhe, Germany.[20,21] Innomedic is the

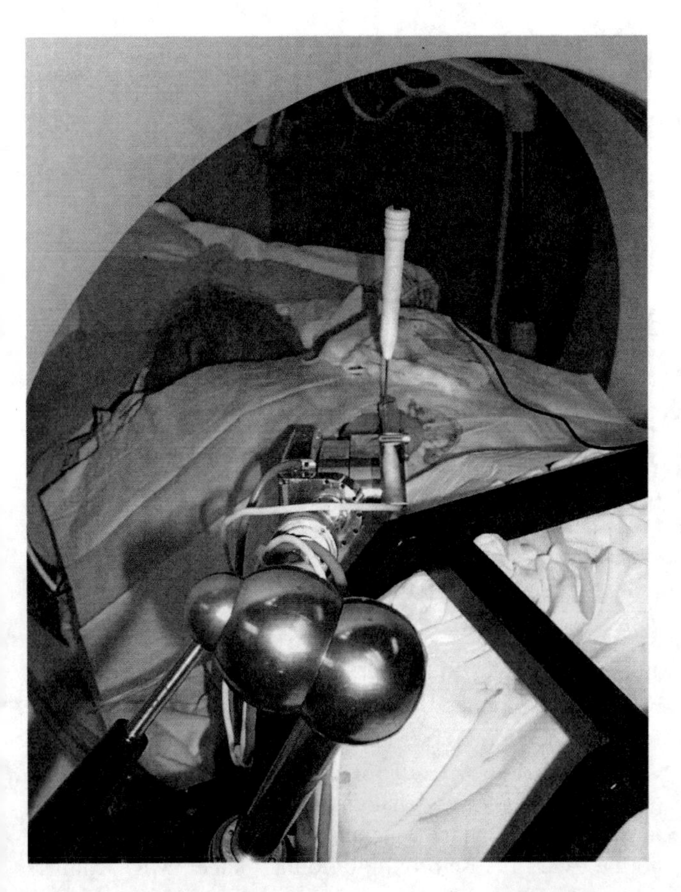

FIG. 18.2. IGI kidney RF ablation with the PAKY-RCM robot in CT scanner

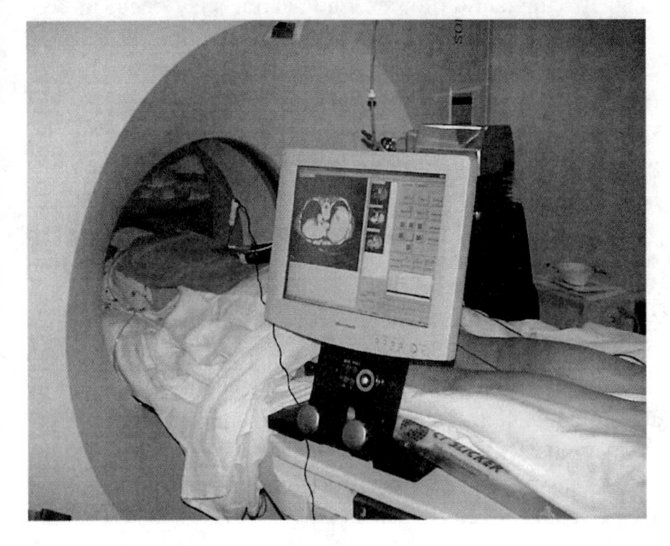

FIG. 18.3. Kidney RF ablation with the AcuBot under CT guidance

first to introduce a commercial MR-IGI system. It includes a five DOF robot to position a needle guide for manual needle insertion and can be used for various abdominal organs including the kidneys. CT-guided procedures can also be performed, because the CT is much less demanding than the MRI.

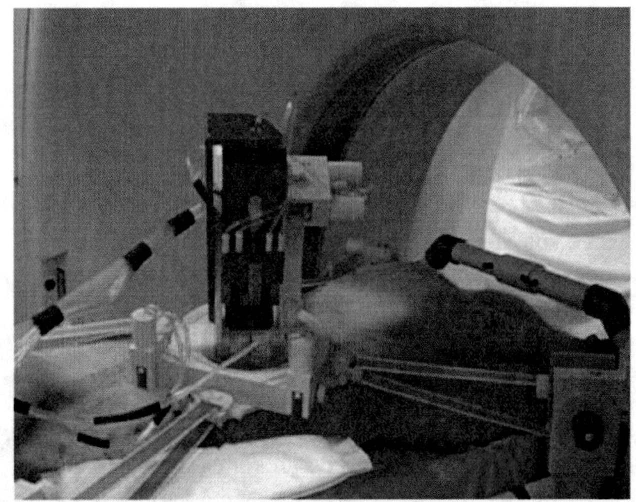

FIG. 18.4. CT-guided animal experiments with the Light Puncture Robot

Another IGI robot for percutaneous interventions is the light puncture robot (LPR),[22] currently under development in the TIMC laboratory (Grenoble, France). This robot is made of plastic (nylon, delrin) for MR compatibility and to reduce artifacts in a CT environment. Like the Innomotion robot, it is designed for multiple application fields. A needle holder is placed on the patient's body supported by four straps (Fig. 18.4). This presents 3DOF (one allowing the inclination of the needle, one for rotation about an axis normal to the patient and a translation for needle insertion) in a compact (15 × 23 cm) light-weight (1 kg) structure. The straps are supported by four pneumatic actuators mounted on a frame placed on the table around the patient. The actuators allow for the translation of the needle holder about the patient's skin (2DOF). The length of the straps can be adjusted according to the patient's size.

The straps allow some flexibility for the needle driver to follow small movements of the skin insertion point (mainly respiratory motion). The driver advances the needle with a relatively fast speed of 9 cm s^{-1}. The setup of the system takes less than 5 min.

All actuators are connected by 7-meter plastic tubes to the robot controller and air compressor, allowing them to be placed outside of the magnetic hazard zone. CT-guided mockup experiments have demonstrated the ability of LPR to reach targets within 1-mm errors. Initial animal experiments on four pigs under general anesthesia with a 17-gauge needle showed errors within 1 cm for liver punctures. These experiments were performed without stopping the respiration, as traditionally performed. Current work is experimenting the use of the robot in the MRI.

Another robot, the B-Rob (Biopsy Robot), was developed by the ARC Seibersdorf Research robotics laboratory in Austria for needle applications guided by X-ray-based imagers. The robot presents two 2DOF arms holding needle guides. The orientation of the needle is changed by positioning the arms. Needle insertion is then manually performed through the needle guide.[23] The first in vitro trials of the system using a penetrable gel phantom showed that B-Rob allows image-guided positioning of a biopsy needle with submillimeter accuracy.[24] Beside biopsy procedures, further clinical applications are under evaluation.

One of the major sources of error for targeting the kidney is the soft tissue deflection and respiratory motion, which is estimated to be about 3 cm in the craniocaudal axis.[25] An active and very challenging research area is now related to respiration tracking algorithms that would allow robots to better target the organs independent of their motion. The main technical difficulty is that current imaging does not completely provide the 3D information required for controlling the robot in real time. Alternatively, the methods most commonly used in robotic interventions are based on respiratory gating and breath stopping, as done in manual interventions.

Robotic Percutaneous Access to the Prostate

Distally from the diaphragm, the movements of the prostate are much more limited, but some motion may be induced by direct interaction of the instruments or transrectal probes.[26] However, immobilization methods may be employed in this case as well.

In view of the high incidence of prostate cancer and the development of minimally invasive techniques for its treatment, many research teams are currently working on robots allowing percutaneous access to the prostate.[27] These systems are usually guided by ultrasound images to perform transperineal biopsies or to implant brachytherapy seeds.

Davies designed a simple robot essentially reproducing the DOF of a brachytherapy template.[28,29] Two DOF are used for needle positioning and one DOF for needle insertion. Rotation around the axis of the needle is added in order to reduce needle deflections. This system is at the stage of a research prototype.

Wei[30] proposed the use of a robot with 6DOF allowing orientation of each needle in all directions. The ultrasound transducer rotates around its axis for reconstruction of a 3D volume. Mockup tests demonstrated a precision on the order of one millimeter.

Our team has also developed a fully automated robot for transperineal prostate access, the MrBot. It is mounted alongside the patient (Fig. 18.4) in the MR imager and can be precisely operated from the control room under image feedback (Fig. 18.5).[31]

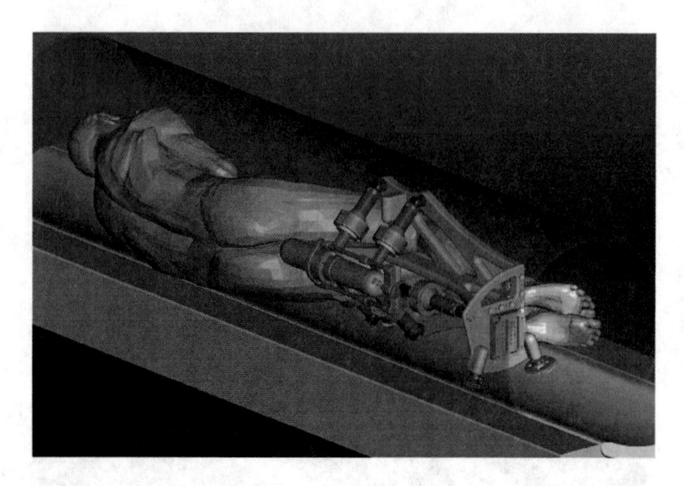

Fig. 18.5. CAD simulation showing the MrBot alongside the man in the left lateral decubitus position in the closed bore of an MRI scanner

In the case of MRI, the design and construction of compatible robots is a very challenging engineering task because most of the components commonly used in robotics may not be used in close proximity to the imager. MRI scanners use very high-density magnetic fields (up to several Tesla), with pulsed magnetic and radiofrequency fields. Within the imager, ferromagnetic materials are exposed to very high magnetic interaction forces, and heating may occur in conductive materials by electromagnetic induction. The use of electricity may cause interference that leads to image artifacts and/or robot signal distortions.

To overcome MRI incompatibilities a new type of motor[32] was designed and used in the new robot. With this the robot is entirely constructed of nonmagnetic and dielectric materials, operates on air, and uses light for the measurements of its sensors. The controller of the robot, containing MRI incompatible materials is distally located outside the imager's room (Fig. 18.6).

The robot has five DOF to place and orient an end effector as desired under MRI guidance. The end effector has an additional DOF to set the depth of needle insertion and 3DOF to manipulate a titanium needle and to deploy brachytherapy seeds automatically.[33] Precision tests in tissue mock-ups yielded a mean seed placement error of 0.72±0.36 mm.[31] With different needle drivers, the MrBot applies to various automated IGI, such as biopsy, therapy injections, and thermal or radiofrequency ablations. The system is presently in preclinical testing with cadaver and animal experiments, but tests show very promising results and clinical trials are expected to commence in the near future.

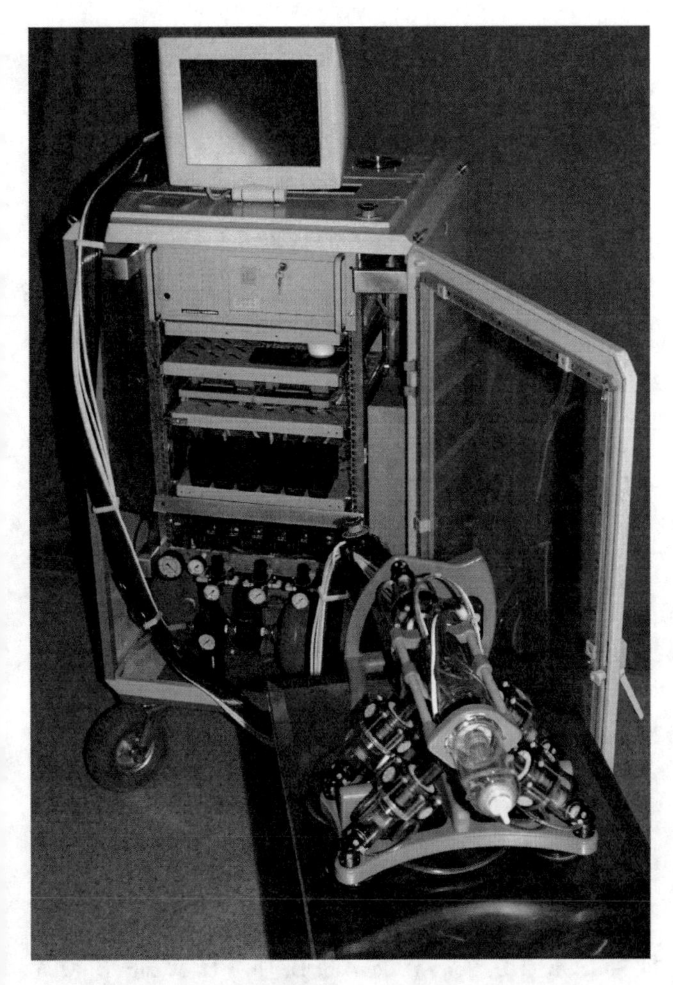

Fig. 18.6. MrBot robot and its control cabinet

Conclusion

Considerable progress has been made in the field of image-guided robots, clinical trials have shown their utility, and a commercial IGI robot is already available for use in Europe. These robots differ considerably from surgeon-driven systems such as the daVinci. In contrast IGI robots bring new dimensions to the typical vision-based surgeries and diagnosis imaging. These also have more autonomous functions, which is not yet of artificial intelligence but base their motions on image feedback. The physician does not directly control the robot, but defines its tasks and monitors its actions based on the image. Clinical performance no longer depends on the physician's 3D cognition and motor skills, and lets him or her free to concentrate on the critical clinical aspects of the intervention. These new characteristics have the potential to improve upon the way that current procedures are done, and also allow for new advanced diagnostic and therapeutic methods to be developed. Image-guided robots are expected to bring a new generation of robots in medicine.

Acknowledgments. The work reported from the author's lab was partially supported by the National Cancer Institute (NCI) of the National Institutes of Health (NIH), the Prostate Cancer Foundation (PCF), and the Patrick C. Walsh Prostate Cancer Foundation (PCW). The contents are solely the responsibility of the authors and do not necessarily represent the official views of NIH-NCI, PCF, or the PCW.

References

1. Davies BL, Hibberd RD, Coptcoat MJ, Wickham JE: A surgeon robot prostatectomy – a laboratory evaluation. *Journal of Medical Engineering and Technology*. 1989; 13(6), 273–277.
2. Taylor RH, Stoianovici D: Medical robotics in computer-integrated surgery. *IEEE Transactions on Robotics and Automation*. 2003; 19(5), 765–781. http://urology.jhu.edu/urobotics/pub/2003-taylor-ieeetra.pdf.
3. Stoianovici D: Multi-imager compatible actuation principles in surgical robotics. *International Journal of Medical Robotics and Computer Assisted Surgery*. 2005; 1(2), 86–100. http://urology.jhu.edu/urobotics/pub/2005-stoianovici-MRCASJ.pdf.
4. Stoianovici D, Cadeddu JA, Demaree RD, Basile SA, Taylor RH, Whitcomb LL, Sharpe WN, Kavoussi LR: An efficient needle injection technique and radiological guidance method for percutaneous procedures. *Lecture Notes in Computer Science*. 1997; 1205, 295–298. http://urology.jhu.edu/urobotics/pub/1997-stoianovici-miccai.pdf.
5. Cadeddu JA, Stoianovici D, Chen RN, Moore RG, Kavoussi LR: Stereotactic mechanical percutaneous renal access. *Journal of Urology*. 1998; 159(5), 56–56.
6. Stoianovici D, Whitcomb LL, Anderson JH, Taylor RH, Kavoussi LR: A modular surgical robotic system for image guided percutaneous procedures. *Lecture Notes in Computer Science*. 1998; 1496, 404–410. http://urology.jhu.edu/urobotics/pub/1998-stoianovici-miccai.pdf.
7. Su LM, Stoianovici D, Jarrett TW, Patriciu A, Roberts WW, Cadeddu JA, Ramakumar S, Solomon SB, Kavoussi LR: Robotic percutaneous access to the kidney: comparison with standard manual access. *Journal of Endourology*. 2002; 16(7), 471–475. http://urology.jhu.edu/urobotics/pub/2002-su-jendourol.pdf.
8. Bove P, Stoianovici D, Micali S, Patriciu A, Grassi N, Jarrett TW, Vespasiani G, Kavoussi LR: Is telesurgery a new reality? Our experience with laparoscopic and percutaneous procedures. *Journal of Endourology*. 2003; 17(3), 137–142. http://urology.jhu.edu/urobotics/pub/2003-bove-jendourol.pdf.
9. Challacombe B, Kavoussi L, Patriciu A, Stoianovici D, Dasgupta P: Technology insight: telementoring and telesurgery in urology. *Nature – Clinical Practice Urology*. 2006; 3(11), 611–617. http://urology.jhu.edu/urobotics/pub/2006-challacombe-nature.pdf
10. Patriciu A, Challacombe B, Dasgupta P, Kavoussi L, Stoianovici D: Robotic telementoring/telesurgical system and randomized evaluation study. *Engineering in Medicine and Biology Society, 2005. Proceedings of the 27th Annual International Conference of the IEEE*. 2005; 2167–2170. http://urology.jhu.edu/urobotics/pub/2005-patriciu-emb.pdf
11. Frimberger D, Kavoussi L, Stoianovici D, Adam C, Zaak D, Corvin S, Hofstetter A, Oberneder R: Telerobotic surgery between Baltimore and Munich [Telerobotische Chirurgie

zwischen Baltimore und München]. *Urologe A.* 2002; 41(5), 489–492.
12. Netto RN, Jr., Mitre AI, Lima SV, Fugita OE, Lima ML, Stoianovici D, Patriciu A, Kavoussi LR: Telementoring between Brazil and the United States: Initial experience. *Journal of Endourology.* 2003; 17(4), 217–220. http://urology.jhu.edu/urobotics/pub/2003-netto-jendourol.pdf.
13. Loser M, Navab, N: A New Robotic System for Visually Controlled Percutaneous Interventions under CT Fluoroscopy *Medical Image Computing and Computer-Assisted Intervention – MICCAI 2000.* Vol 1935/2000 Springer Berlin/Heidelberg, ISBN 978-3-540-41189-5; 2000 pp. 887–896.
14. Patriciu A, Mazilu D, Petrisor D, Kavoussi LR, Stoianovici D: Automatic targeting method and accuracy study in robot assisted needle procedures. *Lecture Notes in Computer Science.* 2003; 1, 124–131. http://urology.jhu.edu/urobotics/pub/2003-patriciu-miccai.pdf.
15. Patriciu A, Stoianovici D, Whitcomb LL, Jarrett T, Mazilu D, Stanimir A, Iordachita I, Anderson J, Taylor R, Kavoussi LR: Motion-based robotic instrument targeting under C-Arm fluoroscopy. *Lecture Notes in Computer Science.* 2000; 1935, 988–998. http://urology.jhu.edu/urobotics/pub/2000-patriciu-miccai.pdf.
16. Solomon SB, Patriciu A, Bohlman ME, Kavoussi LR, Stoianovici D: Robotically driven interventions: A method of using CT fluoroscopy without radiation exposure to the physician. *Radiology.* 2002; 225(1), 277–282. http://urology.jhu.edu/urobotics/pub/2002-solomon-rad.pdf.
17. Stoianovici D, Cleary K, Patriciu A, Mazilu D, Stanimir A, Craciunoiu N, Watson V, Kavoussi LR: AcuBot: A robot for radiological interventions. *IEEE Transactions on Robotics and Automation.* 2003; 19(5), 926–930. http://urology.jhu.edu/urobotics/pub/2003-stoianovici-ieeetra.pdf.
18. Solomon SB, Awad MM, Patriciu A, Stoianovici D, Choti MA: Robotic guided placement of ablation probes for multiple overlapping ablations. *Journal of Vascular and Interventional Radiology.* 2004; 15, S191.
19. Solomon SB, Patriciu A, Stoianovici D: Tumor ablation treatment planning coupled to robotic implementation: a feasibility study. *Journal of Vascular and Interventional Radiology.* 2006; 17(5), 903–907. http://urology.jhu.edu/urobotics/pub/2006-solomon-JVIR.pdf.
20. Felden A, Vagner J, Hinz A, Fischer H, Pfleiderer SO, Reichenbach JR, Kaiser WA: ROBITOM-robot for biopsy and therapy of the mamma. *Biomedical Technology (Berl).* 2002; 47(Suppl 1 Pt 1), 2–5.
21. Kaiser WA, Fischer H, Vagner J, Selig M: Robotic system for biopsy and therapy of breast lesions in a high-field whole-body magnetic resonance tomography unit. *Investigative Radiology.* 2000; 35(8), 513–519.
22. Bricault I, Zemiti N, Jouniaux E, Fouard C, Taillant E, Dorandeu F, Cinquin P. Light puncture robot for CT and MRI interventions: designing a new robotic architecture to perform abdominal and thoracic punctures. IEEE Eng Med Biol Mag. 2008; 27(3):42–50. No abstract available..
23. Kettenbach J, Kronreif G, Figl M, Furst M, Birkfellner W, Hanel R, Ptacek W, Bergmann H: Robot-assisted biopsy using computed tomography-guidance: initial results from in vitro tests. *Invest Radiol.* 2005; 40(4), 219–228.
24. Cleary K, Melzer A, Watson V, Kronreif G, Stoianovici D: Interventional robotic systems: Applications and technology state-of-the-art. *Minimally Invasive Therapy & Allied Technologies.* 2006; 15(2), 101–113. http://urology.jhu.edu/urobotics/pub/2006-cleary-mitat.pdf.
25. Leroy A, Mozer P, Chartier-Kastler E, Richard F, Payan Y, Troccaz J: 3D evaluation of kidney movement during respiration using 2.5D ultrasound. *Engineering and Urology Society – Annual Meeting*, Atlanta; 2006.
26. Keros L, Bernier V, Aletti P, Marchesi V, Wolf D, Noel A: Qualitative estimation of pelvic organ interactions and their consequences on prostate motion: study on a deceased person. *Medical Physics.* 2006; 33(6), 1902–1910.
27. Muntener M, Ursu D, Patriciu A, Petrisor D, Stoianovici D: Robotic prostate surgery. *Expert Review of Medical Devices.* 2006; 3(5), 575–584. http://urology.jhu.edu/urobotics/pub/2006-muntener-ermd.pdf.
28. Davies BL, Harris SJ, Dibble E: Brachytherapy – an example of a urological minimally invasive robotic procedure. *International Journal of Medical Robotics and Computer Assisted Surgery.* 2004; (1), 88–96.
29. Wei Z, Wan G, Gardi L, Mills G, Downey D, Fenster A: Robot-assisted 3D-TRUS guided prostate brachytherapy: system integration and validation. *Medical Physics.* 2004; 31(3), 539–548.
30. Stoianovici D, Song D, Petrisor D, Ursu D, Mazilu D, Muntener M, Schar M, Patriciu A: "MRI Stealth" Robot for Prostate Interventions. Minimally Invasive Therapy & Allied Technologies. 2007; 16(4):241–248. http://urology.jhu.edu/urobotics/pub/2007-stoianovici-mitat.pdf
31. Muntener M, Patriciu A, Petrisor D, Mazilu D, Kavoussi L, Cleary K, Stoianovici D: Magnetic resonance imaging compatible robotic system for fully automated brachytherapy seed placement. *Urology.* 2006; 68(6), 1313–1317. http://urology.jhu.edu/urobotics/pub/2006-muntener-urology.pdf.
32. Stoianovici D, Patriciu A, Mazilu D, Petrisor D, Kavoussi L: A new type of motor: Pneumatic step motor. *IEEE/ASME Transactions on Mechatronics.* 2007; 12(1), 98–106. http://urology.jhu.edu/urobotics/pub/2007-stoianovici-tmech.pdf.
33. Patriciu A, Petrisor D, Muntener M, Mazilu D, Schar M, Stoianovici D: Automatic brachytherapy seed placement under MRI guidance. *IEEE Transactions on Biomedical Engineering.* 2007; 54(8), 1499–1506.

Index

Printed by Publishers' Graphics LLC
SO20120530